Clinical Concepts of Immunology

Clinical Concepts in Medicine Monograph Series

Leighton E. Cluff, M.D.
and
Joseph E. Johnson, III, M.D.
Series Editors

Available Volumes

Cluff & Johnson: *INFECTIOUS DISEASES, 2nd edition*
Toole: *NEUROLOGICAL DISORDERS*

Clinical Concepts of Immunology

ROBERT H. WALDMAN, M.D., Editor

Chairman, Department of Medicine
West Virginia University School of Medicine
Morgantown, West Virginia

The Williams & Wilkins Company • Baltimore

428 E. Preston Street
Baltimore, Md. 21202, U.S.A.

Made in the United States of America

Library of Congress Cataloging in Publication Data

Main entry under title:

Clinical concepts of immunology.

(Clinical concepts in medicine monograph series)
Bibliography: p.
Includes index.
1. Immunologic diseases. 2. Immunology. I. Waldman, Robert H., 1938-
[DNLM: 1. Immunity. 2. Immunology. QW504.3 C641]
RC582.C54 616.07:9 78-3621
ISBN 0-683-08656-1

Composed and printed at the Waverly Press, Inc.
Mt. Royal and Guilford Aves.
Baltimore, Md. 21202, U.S.A.

FOREWORD

In his conceptualization of the body's altered reactivity to foreign substances, Von Pirquet in 1906 relegated "immunity" to a subsidiary role as a subset of "allergy". This broader term was suggested to connote *altered reactivity* while "hypersensitivity" and "immunity" respectively represented *adverse* and *beneficial responses.* During the past century, but particularly in the last three decades since World War II, a veritable explosion of knowledge has expanded *immunology* (now the accepted broader term) into a science in its own right with consequences and implications of importance for most basic biological sciences as well as for the multiple territories of the clinical arena.

Derived from the latin *immunis* (exemption from "charges" or taxes), "immunity" was initially used to describe resistance to attack by infectious diseases. While the concept of resistance to a *second* attack of a disease such as smallpox was recognized in ancient times, the practical application of immunization was clinically established by Jenner and later Pasteur. The theoretical basis of immunology, again initially related to infectious diseases, was laid by pioneers in the last century including Metchnikoff (the theory of cellular immunity), Ehrlich (antibodies) and later by Landsteiner (blood groups) and Bordet (complement). Thus, Von Pirquet and Schick could elaborate the early theoretical framework of the immune system. Our modern conception of the system, particularly as it relates to clinical medicine is the topic of this book.

Clinical Concepts of Immunology is a companion volume in the series *Clinical Concepts in Medicine* which collectively is designed to make available to medical students, house officers, and practitioners a selective survey of clinical problems encountered throughout medical practice. Emphasized in this series are approaches to clinical problems, examples of major disease entities, principles of management—the conceptual framework on which the practice of general medicine is structured. Rather than the exhaustive treatment of the classical comprehensive textbook, this series attempts to present a perspective. By means of selective bibliographies, the reader is directed further to important sources in the literature. Future volumes in the *Clinical Concepts* series, now in preparation, will round out the framework for the remaining areas which collectively comprise the field of general medicine.

LEIGHTON E. CLUFF, M.D.
JOSEPH E. JOHNSON, III, M.D.

PREFACE

Textbooks of immunology tend to fall into two groups, those which emphasize basic immunology (immunoglobulin structure, T cell-B cell interactions, lymphokines, etc.) or those which emphasize "clinical" immunology. The latter usually emphasize the aberrations of the immune system which cause disease. *Clinical Concepts of Immunology* is intended to emphasize the correlation between basic immunology and the clinical situation. In addition to the aberrations, or harmful effects of immune reactions, this book is concerned with the beneficial effects of the immune system. These effects deserve emphasis, we believe, since the immune system apparently evolved as a beneficial mechanism, presumably to protect the host against infectious and malignant diseases, rather than to be a cause of asthma or rheumatoid arthritis. It should also be noted that the study of immune mechanisms in infectious diseases has been, and is likely to continue to be, more successful in improving the health of the population than the other areas of immunology.

In this regard, it is important to remember that immunology historically has been very closely linked to infectious diseases. The first relevant observation was that recovery from many serious infections led to the development of permanent or at least long-lasting protection against a subsequent attack. This fact was first recorded by Thucydides around 430 B.C., with respect to an epidemic of plague in Athens. As a result of this observation, survivors were often given the task of caring for those who had the disease and/or the odious job of disposing of the corpses. The first aim of people interested in this phenomenon, which later came to be known as the scientific discipline of immunology, was to explain it.

Several hundred years ago a second aim of immunology developed: to induce this state of immunity artificially, but without causing severe disease, since it was seen that the immune state was induced not only by severe disease, eg. in survivors of severe smallpox, but also in patients with only mild disease. It is of interest that the second approach, "artificial" immunization, practically, has been much more successful than the first, more basic aim, of understanding the disease induced life-long immunity.

The importance of this overlap of the disciplines of immunology and infectious diseases is obvious, since, along with improved hygiene, public health and nutrition, immunization against infectious diseases has contributed significantly to the more than doubling of life expectancy that has occurred over the past 100 years. As mentioned, it is likely that these contributions of the science of the artificial induction of a state of immunity will continue to play an important role in the continued improvement of human health. One need only consider the potential for development of vaccines against the common malignancies, a vaccine against dental caries, against chickenpox-varicella, the hepatitides and others.

With regard to the organization of this book, it is convenient to arrange the topics relative to the component parts of the immune system: antibody production, cell mediated immunity, and phagocytic function. This division is convenient for teaching purposes, and for presentation of the complex concepts which need to be covered, but the division is quite artificial. The immune system is not a mathematical model, but a biological one, and as is characteristic of biological systems, the whole is greater than the sum of the parts. Dissecting apart the immune system and considering IgG in one compartment, IgA in another, cell-mediated immunity in another, etc., may be likened to trying to appreciate a symphony by listening to each instrument separately.

The book contains three sections, the first on cell mediated immunity, the second on humoral immunity, and a third on non-specific immunity including phagocytosis and some other miscellaneous topics. Each section contains information regarding the function of that arm of the immune system, the results of deficiency states involving the particular area, and the relationship to health and disease.

ROBERT H. WALDMAN, M.D.

CONTRIBUTORS

Abramson, Neil, Clinical Professor of Medicine, University of Florida College of Medicine, Jacksonville, Florida (*Chapter 21*)

Blandford, Gerald, Associate Professor of Medicine, Assistant Professor of Pathology, University of Toronto Faculty of Medicine, Toronto, Ontario, Canada (*Chapter 14*)

Brestel, Eric P., Instructor of Medicine, University of Florida College of Medicine, Gainesville, Florida (*Chapter 24*)

Caldwell, Jacques R., Clinical Assistant Professor of Medicine, University of Florida College of Medicine, Gainesville, Florida (*Chapters 10, 16*)

Cluff, Leighton E., Vice-President, The Robert Wood Johnson Foundation, Princeton, New Jersey, Adjunct Professor of Medicine, University of Pennsylvania School of Medicine, Philadelphia, Pennsylvania (*Chapter 17*)

Delafuente, Jeffrey C., Research Fellow, Department of Medicine, University of Florida College of Medicine, Gainesville, Florida (*Chapter 24*)

Ganguly, Rama, Assistant Professor of Medicine and Microbiology, West Virginia University School of Medicine, Morgantown, West Virginia (*Chapters 1, 2, 5, 7, 13, 22*)

Gifford, George E., Professor of Immunology and Medical Microbiology, and Center for Macromolecular Science, University of Florida College of Medicine, Gainesville, Florida (*Chapter 23*)

Johnson, Joseph E., III, Professor of Medicine, Bowman Gray School of Medicine, Wake Forest University, Winston-Salem, North Carolina (*Chapters, 4, 8*)

Kitchens, Craig S., Assistant Professor of Medicine, University of Florida College of Medicine, and Research Associate, Gainesville Veterans Administration Hospital, Gainesville, Florida (*Chapter 20*)

Klempner, Mark S., Laboratory of Clinical Investigation, National Institute of Allergy and Infectious Diseases, National Institutes of

Health, Bethesda, Maryland (*Chapter 19*)

Lee, J. D., Marshfield Clinic, Marshfield, Wisconsin (*Chapter 7*)

Lee, Martha, Marshfield Clinic, Marshfield, Wisconsin (*Chapter 12*)

Longley, Seldon, III, Assistant Professor of Medicine, University of Florida College of Medicine, and Gainesville Veterans Administration Hospital, Gainesville, Florida (*Chapter 24*)

Panush, Richard S., Associate Professor of Medicine, University of Florida College of Medicine, and Research Associate, Gainesville Veterans Hospital, Gainesville, Florida (*Chapters 15, 24*)

Pfaff, William, Professor of Surgery, University of Florida College of Medicine, Gainesville, Florida (*Chapter 16*)

Quie, Paul G., Professor of Pediatrics, University of Minnesota School of Medicine, Minneapolis, Minnesota (*Chapter 18*)

Schulkind, Martin L., Professor of Pediatrics, University of Florida College of Medicine, Gainesville, Florida (*Chapter 3*)

Shulman, Stanford T, Associate Professor of Pediatrics, University of Florida College of Medicine, Gainesville, Florida (*Chapter 11*)

Waldman, Robert H., Professor of Medicine, West Virginia University School of Medicine, Morgantown, West Virginia (*Chapters, 1, 2, 12, 13*)

Wittig, Heinz J., Professor of Pediatrics, University of Florida College of Medicine, Gainesville, Florida (*Chapter 9*)

Wolff, Sheldon M., Endicott Professor of Medicine, Tufts University School of Medicine, Boston, Massachusetts (*Chapter 19*)

CONTENTS

Section 3.
THE PHAGOCYTIC SYSTEM AND OTHER TOPICS

SECTION
ONE

CELL-MEDIATED IMMUNITY (CMI)

Chapter 1

THE IMMUNE SYSTEM(S)—AN INTRODUCTION

Robert H. Waldman, M.D. and Rama Ganguly, Ph.D.

Immunity refers to the capacity enjoyed by an organism to remain unaffected by harmful agents in its environment and from those arising within itself. The major divisions of resistance mechanisms are: (1) nonspecific or native immunity and (2) specific or acquired immunity. Native immunity refers to the normal animal and its resistance to microorganisms and their toxins. This is an innate endowment to the species with regard to a particular agent. The reverse of this situation refers to specific immunity in which the immunoprotective function of the host is a highly individual property, specifically acquired through the individual's personal experience and exposure to the harmful agent.

Native immunity (see Chapter 22) is the baseline defense in an animal. It is of more importance for our daily welfare than specifically acquired immunity. This is evident when we consider the ubiquity of microbes in an environment and the serious infections seen in patients deficient in some of these natural defense mechanisms. This native immmunity, for the most part, is genetic and the occasional differences in the degree of resistance in individuals of the same species can be accounted for in most instances by differences in environmental and nutritional status. Thus, natural immunity is present in the host as an original grant and, therefore, little attention has been paid to it. In contrast, specific immunity has drawn much scientific attention. Much of our understanding of immunology has emerged from efforts to stimulate acquired immunity.

Acquired immunity results from natural disease processes (called active natural immunity), from artificial exposure to attenuated or inactivated pathogens or their toxins (called active artificial immunity), or may be achieved by receiving antibody, sensitive lymphocytes, or their soluble products from an immune donor (called passive immunity). An example of the latter is the transfer of immunoglobulins in utero from mother to the fetus (passive natural immunity). When such a transfer takes place under artificial conditions it results in passive artificial immunity. An example is the injection of γ-globulin into individuals threatened with hepatitis infection.

Basic Immunologic Concepts

Antigens

Any substance capable of inducing an immune response is an antigen (or immunogen). The most effective antigens are proteins and carbohydrates of high molecular weights. Fatty acids have not been definitely shown to elicit an immune response when administered in a pure state. However, upon conjugation with proteins (called carrier molecules), they may become immunogenic. These substances and many others are, therefore, called "incomplete antigens" and are capable of provoking an immune response only upon conjugation with another high molecular weight substance (usually proteins). They are termed "haptens." Haptens are usually of low molecular weight and are relatively simple in chemical structure. Haptens are capable of reacting specifically with antibodies in vitro or in vivo, but they themselves are incapable of inducing an immune response. Haptens are univalent, i.e., have only one combining site for the antibody.

Antibodies

Antibodies are defined as proteins that are formed by the host in response to an antigen and react specifically with that antigen. The special group of proteins comprising the antibodies are known as "immunoglobulins."

Antigen-Antibody Reaction

It is important to distinguish between the whole antigen molecule and its antigenic determinants. The latter are defined as those restricted portions of the antigen molecule which determine the specificity of the antibody-antigen reaction.

These specific sites are approximately equivalent in volume to only five or six amino acid residues. The most important criterion of immunogenicity of a macromolecule is its "foreignness" to the host, i.e., it should be recognized as nonself to the immunocompetent cells. This recognition acts as a surveillance mechanism against neoplastic cells arising inside the body, as well as against pathogenic invaders. Exceptions to the rule of nonself are formation of autoantibodies to red blood cells (as in autoimmune hemolytic anemia), or proteins of eye lense which anatomically remain sequestered from exposure to immunocompetent cells of the body.

Landsteiner, in a series of elegant studies, explored the chemical specificity of antigen-antibody reactions. He used chemically defined substituents of modified proteins prepared by diazo reactions between aromatic azobenzene and proteins. Antibody to *p*-azobenzene arsonate globulin reacted with this protein and with other proteins containing *p*-azobenzene arsonate substituents, but not with the unsubstituted proteins. On the other hand, *p*-azobenzene arsonate as a hapten was completely capable of inhibiting interactions between antibody and *p*-azobenzene arsonate proteins whereas other aromatic amines usually did not.

Effective immunogenicity is dependent upon various other functions, such as route of administration, physical state of the antigen, and age and sex of the recipient. Steric configuration is also an important determinant of antigenicity of macromolecules. Globular proteins, greater than 40,000 molecular weight, for example IgG (1.5×10^5) and virus particles (40×10^6), are considered to be potent immunogens.

Immunogens that stimulate antibody capable of interacting with antigens from many species are called heterophil antigens (first discovered by Forssman in 1911). All heterophil antibodies (formed in response to heterophil antigens) cross-react with erythrocytes of one species or another, indicating the presence of polysaccharide determinants in the heterophil antigen molecule.

Lipid molecules as haptens are capable of eliciting immune reactions upon conjugation with foreign proteins. A lack of repeated structures (unlike proteins and carbohydrates) may account for the nonimmunogenicity of lipids. Cardiolipin, or Wassermann antigen, an important lipid hapten, is found in a wide variety of plants and in animal tissue. This antigen is used in the serologic test for syphilis. Patients with systemic lupus erythematosis demonstrate the immunogenicity of nucleic acids. Antibodies to single and double stranded DNA are found in the circulation of these patients. Furthermore, when attached to serum albumin, single stranded DNA can become an effective immunogen. Intravenous adminstration of RNA also results in antiribonucleic acid antibody.

The B and T Cell Systems

Gowans and his associates demonstrated that cells of the lymphocyte series are responsible for the immunocompetence of vertebrates. This was followed by the proposal that there were two distinct types of immunocompetent lymphocytes: one which required the thymus gland for development and was responsible for cell-mediated immunity (T lymphocytes); and the other developing independently of the thymus and being responsible for the mediation of the antibody responses (B lymphocytes). In birds and rodents, neonatal thymectomy impairs cell-mediated immunity (CMI), but has much less effect on humoral immunity. In humans, the DiGeorge syndrome (congenital thymic hypoplasia) is

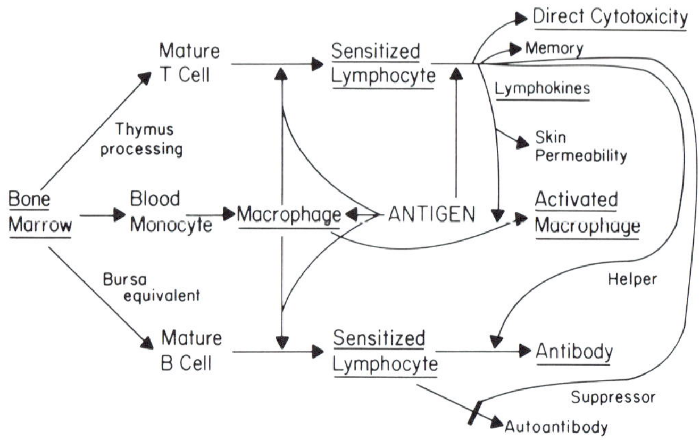

FIG. 1.1. Outlines of the relationships between various cells involved in immunity.

TABLE 1.1 *T and B Cells*

	Location	Characteristics
T cells	Circulating pool: peripheral blood, deep cortical areas of lymph nodes and lymphoid tissues. Non-circulating: thymus	θ antigen positive Ig content of membrane small Forms rosettes in absence of antibody Responsible for cell-mediated immunity Phytohemagglutinin, Concanavalin A, and pokeweed mitogen sensitive
B cells	Medulla of bursa Far cortical areas, germinal centers, and medullary cores of lymph nodes Circulating blood Bone marrow White pulp of spleen Gastrointestinal lamina propria	Secretory lymphocyte or plasma cell Bone marrow dependent Recirculates Cell membranes carry Ig markers Phytohemagglutinin and Concanavalin A insensitive Lipopolysaccharide sensitive Produce rosettes with specific antibodies Short life-span Produce immunoglobulins

associated with deficiency of CMI, although normal humoral responses are present. Conversely, removal of the bursa of Fabricius from birds shortly after hatching impairs the humoral immune response without affecting CMI. In patients with congenital hypo-γ-globulinemia of the Bruton-type, there is a defective humoral immunity with normal CMI.

In protective terms, there seems to be some degree of specialization in T and B cell immunities. Pyogenic infections and those infections involving toxin production are prevented by humoral immunity, whereas CMI is commonly thought to be primarily involved in immune surveillance, in protection against intracellular parasites, and rejection of allograft tissues. In fact, humoral immunity and CMI often act complementarily. Antigenic challenge almost always stimulates both B and T cell responses.

Figure 1.1 outlines the various interactions of the cells involved in immunity. The details will be developed in later chapters. Table 1.1 outlines the location and characteristics of T and B cells.

Chapter 2

CELL-MEDIATED IMMUNITY

Robert H. Waldman, M.D. and Rama Ganguly, Ph.D.

Acquired immunity to some infectious agents does not follow the classical mechanisms of specific antibody interference with infectivity or pathogenicity of microbes by combining with the organism or its toxic products. There is no direct indication that viruses, bacteria, or protozoa, while being protectively accommodated within the cytoplasm of host cells are influenced in any way by antibody. Antibody can rapidly inactivate some intracellular parasites only while in transit from one host cell to the next. Some infectious agents, on the other hand, are quite unaffected by antibody, even during the extracellular phases of their existence. Intracellular organisms with such properties present a special problem of defense and this is met by the body only through measures that drastically change the intracellular environment from one in which the parasite normally prospers to one that will not support its continued survival. Only relatively recently has a mechanism of this type become widely recognized, even though Metchnikoff believed immunity operated in just this manner. This type of immunity operates through the mediation of thymus-derived lymphocytes as opposed to the B cell mediated humoral immunity, which functions through antibody production.

Cell-mediated immunity (CMI) includes those immunologic processes in which thymus-derived sensitized lymphoid cells effect antigen recognition and response. CMI is an important defense mechanism against many microorganisms as well as neoplastic growth arising within the host. It also plays an important role in allograft rejection and the graft versus host reaction. Defective CMI is associated with autoimmune disorders as well as malignant diseases. Delayed hypersensitivity skin reactions are mediated by CMI and have long been used as screening procedures and diagnostic tests for current or past infection.

Antigen Recognition

In CMI, antigen recognition is mediated by macrophages and T lymphocytes. The nature of this specific recognition at the molecular level is not understood, but the cell membrane of the sensitized lymphocytes is believed to play an important role. It has been postulated that the molecule on the surfaces of the sensitized lymphocytes which interacts with the antigenic determinant may be an unknown type of immunoglobulin (IgX), a small number of IgM molecules or its combining sites in the heavy and/or light chains (see later under the B-System), or buried immunoglobulin molecules.

The first requirement for the development of sensitized lymphocytes is the presence of thymus tissue during fetal development. When there is a lack of functional thymus (as in DiGeorge's syndrome) CMI development is defective or absent. The second requirement is previous antigenic exposure. Upon encountering the antigen, sensitized (or committed) lymphocytes undergo synthesis of DNA and replication (blast transformation), resulting in population expansion. Lymphocyte-mediated cytotoxicity and production of soluble mediators, known as "lymphokines," are two other consequences which follow this contact between antigens and the sensitized lymphocytes.

The Thymus

The thymus is a "lymphepithelial" mixture of lymphoid and epithelial cells. In the fetus, at about the sixth week of gestation, it develops from the bronchial pouches of the pharynx as epithelial buds. Subsequently, it dissociates from the point of origin and migrates to the midline of the upper thorax and there it becomes infiltrated with lymphocytes derived from migratory hematopoietic stem cells. These stem cells originate in the yolk sac or liver of the fetus and in the bone marrow of the adult. By radioactive incorporation studies it has been shown that the immigrant cells have a high turnover rate in the thymus. In older animals many of the newly found lymphocytes appear to die in situ. The small proportion of cells that leave the thymus seed the peripheral lymphoid tissues. In younger animals, a much higher proportion provides for the major pool of both long-lived and short-lived T cells. From studies using implanted thymus in Millipore diffusion chambers, it has been demonstrated that some humoral factors elaborated by the thymus influence the outcome of both the function and longevity of T cells.

It is unknown what causes the bone marrow cells to differentiate in the thymus, but there is some suggestive evidence that this may be attributable to some peptide (hormonal?) effect. The thymus acts as the predominant lymphoid organ at a time when the spleen and lymph nodes are barely developed.

Depending upon the patient's age, the thymus varies in size and weight, being at a maximum relative size just before birth. After birth the thymus continues to grow, achieving its maximum size just before puberty (35 g) after which a gradual and continuous involution begins. This age-related decrease in size is characterized by a diminution in the ratio of cortex to medulla and cellular degeneration.

Neonatal thymectomy in mice leads to a deficiency of small to medium lymphocytes at the corticomedullary junctions of lymph nodes and at the pericilliary artery cuffs of the spleen. These areas are known as "thymus dependent" areas of the lymphoid tissues. Thymectomized animals also show a deficit in circulating small lymphocytes. From the functional viewpoint, these animals develop a severe CMI deficiency and a decreased humoral response to some antigens. This is due to a deficit in T cell helper function for antibody production to some antigens (e.g., sheep erythrocytes and bovine albumin). Thymectomy in adult life produces milder defects, probably as a result of the presence of T cells outside the thymus acting as a reservoir.

Thymus-derived lymphocytes do not elaborate antibodies. Subcutaneous injection of immunogens does not result in visible change in the thymus.

The Effector Cell

Mononuclear phagocytic cells are very important for resistance to intracellular pathogens. They participate in all aspects of immune function. They process and present the antigens in a specific manner to the immunocompetent cells, possibly by attaching the antigen to "informational" RNA. In the efferent limb of immunity macrophages phagocytize antigens and bring about the destruction of the foreign particle.

Sensitized lymphocytes, as mentioned above, upon encountering their antigen, undergo blast transformation as well as secreting a variety of lymphokines which have a wide range of activities on the effector macrophages. Macrophages modified by migration inhibitory factor (MIF), for example, become "sticky" (adhering more to glass or to each other). Macrophage activating factor causes an increase in "ruffled borders" of the cell membrane, phagocytic activity, O_2 consumption, hexose monophosphate shunt pathway of metabolism, and H_2O_2 production. This enables macrophages to have an increased killing capacity. Another lymphokine, chemotaxin, induces blood monocytes to emigrate through the walls of vessels and accumulate at the site of antigen. (Table 2.1).

MIF

MIF has been shown to be a relatively heat stable glycoprotein (molecular weight = 35–65,000) synthesized by the lymphocytes within 6–9 hours of exposure to antigen. MIF receptors on macrophages have been

TABLE 2.1. *Some of the Products of Activated Lymphocytes*

1. MIF
2. Macrophage Aggregating Factor
3. Skin Reactive Factor
4. Cloning Inhibitory Factor
5. Lymphotoxin
6. Chemotactic Factor
7. Blastogenic Factor
8. Interferon
9. Lymphnode Permeability Factor
10. TF[a]

[a] Included in the list of lymphokines because it is a soluble factor released from T lymphocytes when they are incubated with antigen.

demonstrated and are sensitive to trypsin and chymotrypsin, but not influenced by neuraminidase. Intradermal injection of a somewhat purified MIF preparation induces a typical delayed hypersensitivity reaction (DHS) in situ, except at a quicker rate.

Two basic approaches are involved in modifying the migration inhibition test for human use: in the indirect techique, MIF is produced by stimulating lymphocytes with antigen and then the lymphokine is assayed with animal indicator cells. The second method is a direct test in which peripheral blood leukocytes (consisting of both lymphocytes and migrating cells) are tested for migration inhibition in the presence of antigen. Both of these in vitro techinques usually correlate with DHS in vivo. The leucocyte migration test differs from the macrophage migration inhibition test in that the migrating cell population represents mainly polymorphonuclear leucocytes rather than macrophages. It remains to be determined if this factor is the same as that responsible for migration inhibition of macrophages.

Chemotaxin

Chemotaxin, another lymphokine, induces emigration of mononuclear cells. Its molecular weight appears to be 80,000 and it migrates with albumin under electrophoretic forces. It has not yet been adequately characterized but it appears to be a distinct entity from MIF and acts synergistically with MIF to attract and accumulate inflammatory cells at the site of activation.

Lymphocyte Proliferation

Sensitized lymphocytes proliferate upon stimulation with antigen. They transform into large metabolically active cells having the morphology of lymphoblasts (blast transformation), increase macromolecular synthesis (of RNA, DNA, and proteins) and undergo enhanced mitotic activity. This proliferation is studied in vitro by incorporation of ^{3}H-thymidine. Nonsensitized lymphocytes can likewise be nonspecifically activated when stimulated by certain plant-derived lectins such as phytohemagglutinin, pokeweed mitogen, and concanavalin A. The biologic effects of these mitogens are similar to those of antigen stimulation of sensitized lymphocytes and also correlate with in vivo DHS reactivities. However, mitogenic stimulation is usually more vigorous and brings about blast formation earlier than that observed with antigens.

Transfer Factor (TF)

Lawrence has shown that extracts of blood leucocytes can transfer the CMI of the leucocyte donor. Recipients become reactive to the antigen within 1–7 days after receiving the extract. This sensitivity usually persists for about 4–12 months, even following injection of extract from only 10^7 cells. It is a dialyzable and stable molecule (molecular weight 10,000), but is inactivated by heat (56°C for 30 min). It is not deactivated by trypsin, RNase, or DNase. Clinically TF has been successfully used for inducing cellular immune capabilitites in patients with deficient CMI (e.g., mucocutaneous candidiasis). TF does not induce antibody formation.

It is thus obvious that only a small number of sensitized lymphocytes accumulated at the site of a CMI response can trigger the entire sequence of the manifestations of DHS. Elaboration of TF probably induces sensitization of "unprimed" T lymphocytes. This could induce, in turn, accumulation of more and more "converted" small lymphocytes to the site of activation. These activated cells further augment the effects by blastogenesis and proliferation as well as by synthesis of lymphokines. This will cause macrophages to emigrate to the site of activation. Thus, the entire sequence of cellular immune response can develop starting from a very small population of thymus-derived sensitized lymphocytes.

Cell Killing by Lymphocytes

If monolayers of target cells are exposed to the action of lymphoid cells from specifically presensitized donors, the lymphocytes cluster around the target cells within a short time. The killer effect of direct cytolysis is characterized by death within 20 hours of a significant number of the target cells. This phenomenon is independent of the presence of antibody and complement, and is highly specific. The destruction of the target cells seems to require intimate contact with the killer lymphocytes, and the destructive phase of this interaction requires synthesis of some (as yet unidentified) agent(s) by the adherent attacking cells.

Subpopulations of Cells Involved in CMI

As indicated above, CMI involves various cellular events, i.e., proliferation of the sensitized lymphocytes, production of lymphokines, and cytotoxicity. The lymphocytes which are involved in the cytotoxic reaction are also commonly called "killer cells". In addition, various functions have been described for T cells. They are involved in some or all of the above cellular events which make up the cellular immune reaction, and in addition there are helper and suppressor T cells. Helper T cells enable or enhance the antibody response to certain antigens. Suppressor T cells depress a variety of immune reactions, including CMI and antibody production and release.

Although CMI and T cell function are most commonly referred to synonymously, this may not be necesarily completely accurate. CMI is a functional concept, i.e., a series of reactions which occur following antigen stimulation, and the T cell is a morphologic entity. Thus, equating CMI and T cell is analogous to equating immunity and the lymphocyte. The reason this is mentioned is that, as will be seen below, there are functions which we ascribe to cell-mediated immunity which may not be a result of T cell function, but this does not detract from their importance in the cellular immune reaction.

The question arises as to whether these various functions are carried out by the same or different cells. This question is made more complicated by the recognition of a third group of lymphocytes, the null cell, in addition to the T and B cell. The null cell is also a morphologic description, being called a null cell because of the absence of the various markers which are used to describe T and B cells morphologically. Soon after its discovery, the null cell was found to have some relationship to antibody-dependent, complement-independent cytotoxicity. This type of cytotoxicity should be differentiated from the type which was first described relative to cell-mediated immunity, i.e., antibody-independent cytotoxicity. As will be seen below, both of these types of cytotoxicity may be a function of the null cell.

An added difficulty is apparent species differences between the types of functions carried out by the different subpopulations of lymphocytes.

The various populations of lymphocytes and their subpopulations have been separated and identified on the basis of suface antigens, rosette formation, various receptors for complement and immunoglobulin, their density, and if they stick to certain substances, such as nylon or glass beads.

A description of the lymphocyte populations and subpopulations, their function and the differences, in the two best studied species, the mouse and human, are shown in Table 2.2.

The data from the mouse model suggest that the same cell at different stages of differentiation is responsible for the various functions. Thus, the multipotential T cells (T_1) differentiates into T_2, which has the suppressor T cell function, and on to the T_3 cell (helper), and finally the T_4 cell (killer). It appears that the stimulus for this differentiation of the T cell is antigenic stimulation.

TABLE 2.2. *Subpopulations of Lymphocytes*

Lymphocyte population	Function	Mouse (surface antigens)	Human
T cell	Multipotential T cell	T1 (TL+, θ+, Ly+, Ly2+, Ly3+)	Present
	Lymphokine production	? all subpopulations (and B cells as well)	Same
	Suppressor	T2 (θ+, Ly1+, Ly2+, Ly3+)	Present
	Helper	T3 (θ+, Ly1+, Ly8+)	Present
	Killer	T4 (θ+, Ly2+, Ly3+, Ly8+)	?
Null cell	Killer	?	Possibly several subpopulations including "natural killer cells" and "autocytotoxic cells"
	Ab dependent killer cell	Yes	Yes
B cell	Ab producer (various classes and subclasses)	Yes	Yes

Human data suggest a different situation. Null cells are negative for surface immunoglobulin and do not form rosettes. A subgroup of null cells, which possesses a receptor for the third component of complement, is cytotoxic for cancer cells. This cell-mediated cytotoxicity is suppressed by a subpopulation of T cells, i.e., suppressor cells. The practical application of these observations for human disease is that, if it is confirmed that the cytotoxic cells are non-T cells, and the inhibitor cells are T cells, it may be possible to enhance tumor protection with suppression of the T cell population, such as by the use of antithymocyte serum.

Summary

CMI is comprised of two principle components: macrophages and lymphocytes. When the pathogen enters the system of a previously sensitized individual, a small number of lymphocytes accumulate and become activated at the point of assault. These activated cells release into the surrounding extracellular fluids several physiologically active effectors. The effectors include migration inhibitory, chemotactic, blastogenic, cytotoxic, and transfer factors and interferon. The ultimate result of these mediators is to attract and retain macrophages and other (nonsensitized) lymphocytes (recruitment) at the site of growth of the foreign agent. Recruited lymphocytes at the site of accumulation become activated, transformed into blast cells and liberate more lymphokines into the area. Thus, through these mediators an amplification of the initial effect is brought about. The initial antigen recognition and binding by the T cell membrane is specific in nature, but this specific reaction results in a sequence of nonspecific effects, e.g., activation of macrophages. The end result is development of delayed hypersensitivity and a heightened resistance to the specific microorganism as well as unrelated organisms. Thus, activation of macrophages by BCG can lead to enhanced resistance both to *Mycobacterium tuberculosis* and *Listeria monocytogenes* or *Bordetella pertussis.* It has also been demonstrated that such activation can also lead to increased resistance to viruses. Macrophages altered by lymphokines have several characteristics: they become "sticky," possess "ruffled borders," enhanced phagocytic capacity, increase in numbers and size of the cytoplasmic organelles, higher O_2 consumption, enhanced activity of hexose monophosphate shunt pathway and H_2O_2 production. Macrophages with these attributes are variously known as "activated," "angry," or "killer" cells. "Killer" functions have also been ascribed to sensitized lymphocytes. In this cytotoxic reaction, the lymphocytes recognize foreign surface antigens on cells and kill by direct contact and cytolysis.

SELECTED REFERENCES

Bloom, B. R., and Bennett, B.: Mechanism of a reaction *in vitro* associated with delayed type hypersensitivity. Science, *153:* 80, 1966.

Boyse, E. A.: A brief account of the use of immunogenetics in studying cell surfaces. In *Membranes and Viruses in Immunopathology*, edited by S. B. Day and R. A. Good. New York: Academic Press, 1972, pp. 105–115.

David, J. R.: Delayed hypersensitivity *in vitro.* Its mediation by cell-free substances formed by lymphoid cell antigen interaction. Proc. Natl. Acad. Sci., *56:* 72, 1966.

David, J. R., and David, R. R.: Cellular hypersensitivity and immunity. Prog. Allergy, *10:* 300, 1972.

Fujimoto, S., Green, M. I., and Sehon, A. H.: Regulation of the immune response to tumor antigens. I. Immunosuppressor cells and tumor bearing hosts. II. The nature of immunosuppressor cells and tumor bearing hosts. J. Immunol., *116:* 791, 1976.

Gershon, R. K.: T cell control of antibody production. Contemp. Top. Immunobiol., *3:* 1, 1974.

Gowans, J. L., and McGregor, D. D.: The immunological activities of lymphocytes. Prog. Allergy, *9:* 1, 1965.

Lawrence, H. S.: Transfer Factor. Adv. Immunol., *11:* 195, 1969.

Ramsey, E . W., Brandes, L. J., Jacob, H. A., and Goldenberg, G. J.: An evaluation of the peripheral leucocyte migration inhibition test as a correlate of delayed cutaneous hypersensitivity. Cell Immunol., *23:* 334, 1976.

Rosenau, W., and Moon, H. D.: Lysis of homologous cells by sensitized lymphocytes in tissue culture. J. Natl. Cancer Inst., *27:* 471, 1961.

Chapter

3

CONGENITAL DEFICIENCY STATES IN CELL-MEDIATED IMMUNITY

Martin L. Schulkind, M.D.

Deficiencies in cell-mediated immunity (CMI) can conveniently be divided into congenital and acquired. This chapter will deal with the congenital deficiencies, which are fortunately relatively rare. They are of great interest, however, because of some recent exciting advances in therapy, and because relationships with other deficiencies, both immunologic and nonimmunologic, and with certain infections and malignancies, have thrown light on the development of the immune system and the role of its various parts in host defenses.

Thymic hypoplasia, also referred to as the DiGeorge or Pharyngeal Pouch syndrome, is a congenital immunodeficiency, clinically characterized by neonatal tetany, unusual facies, and increased susceptibility to infection, in association with the pathologic findings of the absence or hypoplasia of the thymus and parathyroid glands.

The pathogenesis of the syndrome is the abnormal embryogenesis of the third and fourth pharyngeal pouches. The thymus initially develops from the floor of the third and fourth pharyngeal pouches during the sixth to eighth week of embryogenesis and further develops through the twelfth week. At the same time the parathyroid glands, as well as certain aortic arch structures, arise from the same pharyngeal pouches. During the same period of development the nasomedial processes fuse to form the labial philtrum and the external ear is developed. It is probable that events take place at this critical time in development which interfere with pharyngeal development resulting in abnormalities of the thymus, parathyroids, aortic arch, ear, and facial structures.

As a result of thymic hypoplasia the cell-mediated immune system remains undifferentiated. In contrast, the humoral immune system develops normally. The deficiency in CMI is manifested by a lack of cutaneous delayed hypersensitivity responses, failure to be sensitized with substances such as dinitrochlorobenzene, absent or diminished in vitro lymphocyte responses to stimulation by phytohemagglutinin and antigens, an inability to produce lymphokines in vitro and delayed homograft rejection. Interestingly, some infants with this syndrome have been found to have almost normal immunologic responses early in life which subsequently become abnormal.

The patients typically present with hypocalcemic tetany in the first few hours of life as a result of hypoparathyroidism, a characteristic facies with hypertelorism, antimongoloid slant of the eyes, shortened labial philtrum, low set and notched ears, and micrognathia. Those infants who survive the newborn period show an increased susceptibility to infection, manifested by persistent rhinitis, recurrent pneumonitis including infections with *Pneumocystis carinii*, oral candidiasis, and diarrhea. Aortic arch anomalies, such as right-sided aortic arch and tetralogy of Fallot, are common. Associated findings in a few cases are hypothyroidism, bifid uvula, urinary tract infections, and esophageal atresia.

Chest x-ray reveals absence of the thymic shadow; and normal lymphocyte counts, negative skin test responses, and abnormal in vitro lymphocyte responses are found. Serum immunoglobulin levels are usually normal. In addition to these findings the serum calcium is low, the phosphorous is high, and the alkaline phosphatase level is normal.

Early treatment of the patients to control the effects of hypoparathyroidism is lifesaving. After the hypoparathyroidism is controlled and the defect in CMI delineated, transplantation with a fetal (usually 12–20 weeks old) thymus is recommended to correct the immune defect. Immunologic tests should be performed regularly, for after the restoration of CMI, the implanted thymus may be rejected, necessitating the transplantation of another fetal thymus. In addition, the recognition and correction of any cardiovascular anomalies are necessary.

Severe Combined Immunodeficiency

Severe combined immunodeficiency, also referred to as Swiss-type-a-γ-globulinemia, is a congenital deficiency of CMI and humoral immunity. It is characterized clinically by the early onset of severe infections with a rapid unrelenting course and early death. During the 1950's several Swiss investigators described a series of siblings who had diarrhea, candidiasis, lymphopenia, and decreased lymphoid tissue on post mortem examination. Thymic abnormalities as well as a-γ-globulinemia were found.

Combined immunodeficiency occurs with both autosomal recessive and x-linked recessive patterns of inheritance. A deficiency in adenosine deaminase (ADA) has been found in some patients with the recessive form. The role that ADA deficiency plays in the pathogenesis of this immunodeficiency is unclear. However, a recent report describes correction of the in vitro lymphocyte dysfunction by the addition of calf-intestinal ADA to cultures of ADA-deficient patient's lymphocytes. It is the opinion of many investigators that the primary immunologic defect in combined immunodeficiency is in the bone marrow stem cells rather than in the thymus. This concept is supported by the failure of thymus transplants and the success of bone marrow transplants to correct the immunologic deficiency.

The clinical manifestations of this disease are very striking. More than 200 patients with severe combined immunodeficiency have been described with a male to female ratio of 3:1. The major manifestation of combined immunodeficiency is the extreme susceptibility to infections beginning in the first few months of life. Infections are generalized, with skin, respiratory, and gastrointestinal systems involvement and with sepsis being most prominent. Candida infections of the skin and mucous membranes are almost always present and often are the first sign of the disease. Persistent cough and bronchopneumonia is a constant recurrent event and generally the cause of death; with *P. carinii* a prominent cause of fatal pneumonia. Nearly all patients have watery diarrhea starting early in life. Although pathogenic organisms are occasionally cultured, an etiology is not often found. The diarrhea is unresponsive to all forms of therapy except restoration of immune competence. Intermittent episodes of sepsis associated with localized infection such as meningitis occur occasionally and overwhelming infection with varicella, measles, cytomegalovirus, adenovirus, as well as fungi occur frequently. Fatal disseminated BCG infection after intradermal inoculation, as well as progressive vaccinia after inadvertent smallpox vaccination have been described. Characteristically, overwhelming infection due to organisms of relatively low pathogenicity are seen.

Laboratory evaluation shows absence of humoral immunity and CMI. Lymphopenia (total lymphocyte counts $<200/mm^3$) is a common but not invariable finding, and immunoglobulin levels are low. Defective antibody production in response to most antigenic stimulation is present as a manifestation of defective humoral immunity, while absent cutaneous responses to antigens, as well as defective in vitro lymphocyte function, reflect the deficiency in CMI.

Pathologic examination of postmortem tissue reveals a depletion of lymphoid tissue. The thymus is grossly abnormal and is absent in severe cases. The thymus shows histologic findings characteristic of dysplasia, with no corticomedullery differentiation, absent Hassall's corpuscles, and lymphoid cell deficiency. Peripheral lymph nodes are sparse, even at sites of regional infection. The lymph node architecture is markedly abnormal with absence of germinal centers, lymphoid follicles, and plasma cells. Reticulum cells and fibroblasts are the major cells seen.

Variants of Combined Immunodeficiencies

Several variants and partial or incomplete forms of combined immunodeficiency occur, such as combined immunodeficiency with ectodermal dysplasia and short-limbed dwarfism, immunodeficiency with generalized hypoplasia of the hematopoietic system, and the Nezelof syndrome, an autosomal recessive immunodeficiency with lymphopenia and normal and near normal levels of immunoglobulins. The clinical and pathologic findings are similar to those in severe combined immunodeficiency except that the symptoms and course are less fulminant and plasma cells are present in lymphoid tissue.

Chronic Mucocutaneous Candidiasis

There are several forms of this syndrome, with the common theme of persistent Candida infection of the skin, nails, and mucous membranes, often associated with an endocrinopathy. Several immunologic defects have been described, most commonly involving CMI, but no consistent abnormality has been noted.

Immunologic investigation often reveal an absent skin test response to *Candida albicans* extract and occasionally to other skin test antigens. In vitro lymphocyte function studies may reveal a variety of abnormalities, including absent lymphocyte transformation to Candida and/or other antigens and mitogens, and various patterns of abnormal lymphokine production.

The Candida infections most often involve the oral cavity, with finger and toenails being frequently involved. Less commonly involved are the skin of the face and distal parts of the extremities. There is a granulomatous form of the disease with extensive skin involvement. The lesions are keratinized (horny) masses. Only rarely does the infection become systemic. The onset of the Candida infection may be during the first few months of life or may be delayed several years.

Other manifestations of the disease are hypoparathyroidism (most frequent endocrinopathy), hypoadrenalism, hypothyroidism, diabetes mellitus, and pernicious anemia. Most of these patients have autoantibodies to endocrine tissues usually present before the development of clinically evident endocrinopathy.

Antimicrobial treatment is difficult because local application of antifungal agents has not been successful. The most effective therapy has been the use of intravenous amphotericin-B, but its nephrotoxicity prevents prolonged usage. The infection usually recurs after the drug is discontinued. Recently the use of transfer factor as a means of restoring CMI has been effective in clearing the infection in at least a third of the patients and has brought about a striking improvement in the management of patients with this disease.

Wiskott-Aldrich Syndrome (Immunodeficiency with Eczema and Thrombocytopenia)

The Wiskott-Aldrich syndrome is an x-linked recessive immunodeficiency characterized by thrombocytopenia, eczema, and recurrent infection with a characteristic inability to form antibodies to polysaccharide antigens. Abnormal cell-mediated and antibody responses to other antigens have been noted in several patients.

The initial manifestations of the Wiskott-Aldrich syndrome are bleeding episodes secondary to thrombocytopenia, usually followed by a characteristic eczematous rash when the subject is several months of age. Recurrent bacterial and viral infection are common, e.g., otitis media and pneumonia. Later, recurrent herpes simplex infections occur, occasionally resulting in fatal dissemination. Other patients have had severe infections with cytomegalovirus and *P. carinii*. Severe reactions have been noted after immunization with bacterial polysaccharide antigens with an increase in petechiae and eczema and the appearance of purpura. These episodes are similar to exacerbations of the syndrome which are seen after bacterial infections.

The clinical diagnosis of the syndrome can be made shortly after birth in a family with a history of the disease. Characteristic laboratory findings include absent or very low levels of serum isohemagglutinins, normal levels of IgG, increased IgA and IgE, but usually depressed levels of IgM. Patients can usually form antibodies to protein antigens of bacteria but fail in their response to bacterial polysaccharide antigens. Decreased CMI is characterized by impaired cutaneous responsiveness to skin test antigens and in vitro lymphocyte function. The defective CMI becomes more apparent in these patients as they become older. Although many patients with immunodeficiencies have an increased tendency to develop lymphoid malignancy, this propensity seems much greater in patients with Wiskott-Aldrich syndrome. Treatment for this syndrome has been unsuccessful until recently. In an attempt to relieve the thrombocytopenia, splenectomy has often led to a more fulminant course with early death from septicemia. Transfer factor has been found to be effective in many patients, with not only improvement in their CMI and their ability to handle infections but, for some as yet unexplained reason, the bleeding episodes become less frequent and less severe despite the absence of a noticeable change in their platelet counts.

Immunodeficiency with Ataxia-Telangiectasia

Immunodeficiency with ataxia-telangiectasia is an autosomal recessive primary immunodeficiency characterized by telangiectasia, progressive ataxia, and variable immunodeficiency involving the humoral and/or cell-mediated immune system.

In the 1920's Syllaba and Henner described three teen-aged siblings, two males and one female who had progressive ataxia with oculocutaneous telangiectasia, as well as strabismus and athetoses. Several other patients were then described and by the late 1950's a distinct clinical entity was established. Recurrent sinopulmonary tract infections were seen in many of those patients, and in the 1960's several reports appeared describing absent IgA, defective CMI and, most recently, deficiency in IgE. Although most patients with ataxia-telangiectasia have an immunologic deficiency, no consistent pattern has become evident. CMI deficiency has been found in over 60% of the patients, IgA deficiency in 70–80%, and IgE deficiency in 80–90%.

There is no ready explanation for the multisystem involvement in this syndrome although several hypotheses have been proposed. One theory explains the telangiectasia, gonadal abnormalities, and immune deficiency by defective embryogenesis of mesenchyme. This, however, would not explain the central nervous system involvement where the lesions are degenerative and demyelinating and not associated with abnormalities of vascular tissue. Another hypothesis proposes the concept of basic thymic abnormality and relates the multisystem involvement and variable progression of the disease to autoimmunity and/or recurrent infection. An increased incidence of autoantibodies in these patients has been found, some directed against endocrine as well as other affected organs such as liver, gastric parietal cells, and muscle. The variable progression of the disease and involvement of CMI and humoral immunity can also be explained on the basis of immunologic attrition with the immunodeficiency showing a progressive deterioration with time. Several reports have demonstrated normal or near normal levels of immunoglobulins which become deficient with time, as well as an increase in the degree of deficiency in CMI which occurs with the passage of time.

There is considerable variability in the onset of symptoms. The majority of patients develop ataxia during infancy, although in some, ataxia may not be apparent until 4 years of age. In all patients the ataxia progresses slowly to severe disability. The ataxia is cerebellar in type, initially involving posture and gait and later involving movements of intention. Speech is affected and becomes progressively slurred and there are variable choreoathetoid movements. Sensory impairment is rarely seen.

Telangiectasia is seen initially on the bulbar conjunctivae and may be present as early as 1 year of age or as late as 6 years. With time the telangiectasia becomes more prominent.

Several associated abnormal endocrinologic findings have been described, including ovarian dysgenesis, testicular atrophy, abnormalities in growth hormone production, and an unusual form of diabetes mellitus.

Most patients have recurrent sinopulmonary infections leading to bronchiectasis, and symptoms related to this may be the presenting complaint even before the appearance of ataxia or telangiectasia. Death resulting from progressive neurologic deterioration and/or recurrent pulmonary infection is the usual outcome.

The prominent laboratory abnormalities in this disease relate to the deficiencies in CMI and humoral immunity. A variety of abnormalities in immunoglobulin levels has been described including elevated IgA, as well as decreased IgG, IgM, IgA, and IgE. Studies of antibody formation in response to bacterial antigens show variable degrees of deficiency. In addition patients with this syndrome have an increased incidence of autoantibodies to several tissues and also to IgA and and IgG.

Treatment of these patients has been difficult because of the progressive debilitation resulting from the neurologic involvement. Infections can be controlled but not eliminated by judicious antibiotic utilization. γ-Globulin therapy has not been shown to be of benefit. Transfer factor has been used in some patients and leads to correction of specific CMI deficiencies, but with no apparent effect on the course of the disease.

SELECTED REFERENCES

Ammann, A. J., Cain, W. A., Ishizaka, K., Hong, R., and Good, R. A.: Immunoglobulin E deficiency in ataxia-telangiectasia. N. Engl. J. Med., *281:* 469, 1969.

Blaese, R. M., Strober, W., Brown, R. S., and Waldmann, T. A.: The Wiskott-Aldrich syndrome. A disorder with a possible defect in antigen processing or recognition. Lancet, *1:* 2056, 1968.

Boder, E., and Sedgwick, R. P.: Ataxia-telangiectasia: a review of 101 cases. In *Cerebellum, Posture and Cerebral Palsy.* edited by G. Walsh. (Clinics in Developmental Medicine Ser. no. 8), London: The National Spastics Society and Heinemann Medical Books, Ltd., 1962.

Chilgren, R. A., Meuwissen, H. J., Quie, P. G., Good, R. A., and Hong, R.: The cellular immune defect in chronic mucocutaneous candidiasis. Lancet, *1:* 1286, 1969.

Cooper, M. D., Chase, H. P., Lowman, J. T., Krivit, W., and Good, R. A.: Wiskott-Aldrich syndrome: an immunologic deficiency disease involving the afferent limb of immunity. Am. J. Med., *44:* 499, 1968.

DiGeorge, A. M.: Congenital absence of the thymus and its immunologic consequences: concurrence with congenital hypoparathyroidism. In *Birth Defects: Immunologic Deficiency Disease in Man,* edited by D. Bergsma and R. A. Good. Baltimore: Williams & Wilkins Company, *4(1):* 116, 1968.

Gatti, R. A., Meuwissen, H. J., Allen, H. D., Hong, R., and Good, R. A.: Immunological reconstitution of sex-linked lymphopenic immunological deficiency. Lancet, *2:* 1336, 1968.

Gitlin, D., and Craig, J. M.: The thymus and other lymphoid tissues in congenital agammaglobulinemia. I. Thymic alymphoplasia and lymphocytic hypoplasia and their relation to infection. Pediatrics, *32:* 517, 530, 1963.

Kirkpatrick, C. H., Rich, R. R., and Bennett, J. E.: Chronic mucocutaneous candidiasis: model-building in cellular immunity. Ann. Intern. Med., *74:* 955, 1971.

Oppenheim, J. J., Blaese, R. M., and Waldmann, T. A.: Defective lymphocyte transformation and delayed hypersensitivity in Wiskott-Aldrich syndrome. J. Immunol., *104:* 835, 1970.

Peterson, R. D. A., Cooper, M. D., and Good, R. A.: Lymphoid tissue abnormalities associated with ataxia-telangiectasia. Am. J. Med., *41:* 342, 1966.

Pollara, B., Moore, J. J., Pickering, R. J., Gabrielsen, A. E., and Meuwissen, H. J.: Combined immunodeficiency disease. An inborn error of purine metabolism. In *Birth Defects: Immunodeficiency in Man and Animals,* edited by D. Bergsma. Sunderland, Massachusetts: Sinauer Associates, Inc., *11(1):* 120, 1975.

Polmar, S. H., Wetzler, E. M., Stern, R. C., and Hirschhorn, R.: Restoration in *in vitro* lymphocyte responses with exogenous adenosine deaminase in a patient with severe combined immunodeficiency. Lancet, *2:* 743, 1975.

Schulkind, M. L., Adler, W. H., Altemeier, W. A., and Ayoub, E. M.: Transfer factor in the treatment of a case of chronic mucocutaneous candidiasis. Cell. Immunol., *3:* 606, 1972.

Spitler, L. E., Levin, A. S., Stites, D. P., Fudenberg, H. H., Pirofshy, B., August, C. S., Stiehm, E. R., Hitzig, W. H., and Gatti, R. A.: The Wiskott-Aldrich syndrome; results of transfer factor therapy. J. Clin. Invest., *51:* 3216, 1972.

Taitz, L. S., Zarate-Salvador, C., and Schwartz, E.: Congenital absence of the parathyroid and thymus glands in an infant. (III and IV pharynegeal pouch syndrome). Pediatrics, *38:* 412, 1966.

Chapter 4

CELL-MEDIATED IMMUNITY—ACQUIRED DEFICIENCY STATES

Joseph E. Johnson, III, M.D.

Diseases with associated deficiencies in cell-mediated immunity (CMI) which are not congenital in origin are considered to represent "acquired" immunodeficiency disorders (Table 4.1). The circumstances in which acquired deficiency of CMI occurs include a wide variety of neoplastic diseases, infections, and debilitated states and diseases of unknown etiology. In addition, deficiency of CMI may result from treatment with a variety of immunosuppressive agents as well as with radiation. Collectively, these acquired disorders are encountered in clinical medicine much more commonly than the congenital immunodeficiency diseases. In some situations (such as Hodgkin's disease) the deficiency of CMI appears to be a basic or primary condition, in some way inherent to the disease. In other circumstances the deficiency is clearly a consequence of therapy. Except in advanced disease such defects in CMI are more often partial or relative rather than absolute deficiencies. Just as with the congenital immunodeficiencies in which a "pure" cell-mediated (or T lymphocyte) deficiency rarely occurs alone, acquired disorders often show combined deficiencies of both T lymphocyte (cell-mediated) and B lymphocyte (humoral) functions. Thus, although the non-Hodgkin's lymphomas and chronic lymphocytic leukemia appear to represent predominantly B cell disorders, partial deficiencies in T cell function may also occur.

The relatively common finding of combined disorders of both T- and B cell activity (though usually with one form predominating) is perhaps not surprising in view of the complex functional interaction and interdependence of the T and B cell systems now recognized. The complexity is further evident from the delineation of subpopulations of T lympho-

TABLE 4.1. *CMI—Acquired Deficiency States*

Neoplasms
- Hodgkin's disease—basic T cell deficiency
- Non-Hodgkin's lymphomas (lymphosarcoma, reticulum cell sarcoma)—predominant B cell deficiency; partial T cell deficiency.
- Chronic lymphocytic leukemia (especially Sezary syndrome, a rare variety)

Immunosuppressive therapy
- Corticosteroids
- Antilymphocyte sera (antilymphocyte globulins)
- Cytotoxic chemotherapeutic agents
- Antibiotics
- Radiation

Infections
- Leprosy
- Viral Infections
  - Measles
  - Hepatitis
  - Infectious mononucleosis (EB virus)
- Mycobacterial infection (disseminated tuberculosis, others)
- Fungal infections
  - Mucocutaneous candidiasis
  - Coccidioidomycosis
  - Others

Aberrant immune responses
- Sarcoidosis
- "Autoimmune" diseases
  - Lupus erythematosus
  - Rheumatoid arthritis
  - Hashimoto's thyroiditis
- Lymphopenic states
  - Chronic thoracic duct drainage
  - Intestinal lymphangiectasia
- Malnutrition
- Debilitation
  - Metastatic neoplasms
  - Chronic disease states
  - Old age

cytes with essentially opposing functions ("helper" versus "suppressor" activity). Thus the assignment of humoral (antibody) functions to B cells, and cellular immune functions to T cells appears to be an oversimplification. Similarly the distinctions between "congenital" and "acquired" immunodeficiency syndromes may also be somewhat arbitrary. Many patients with immunodeficiency disorders cannot be unequivocally classified, and are grouped under the heading of "common variable immunodeficiency." Certain of the "acquired" immunodeficiency syndromes are quite likely associated with particular immune response genes which influence susceptibility to particular infections, which in turn may lead to particular forms of immunodeficiency.

In this chapter we shall consider the immunodeficiency associated with Hodgkin's disease, the best-studied example of an "acquired" disorder (albeit of still unknown etiology) in which there is a significant, often profound, deficiency of CMI. In addition, the effects of immunosuppressive therapy and radiation will be reviewed. Subsequently, in Chapter 8, disorders in which aberrant immune responses are found (including leprosy and sarcoidosis) will be discussed.

CMI in Hodgkin's Disease and the Lymphoproliferative Disorders

Impairment of immune response in Hodgkin's disease has been recognized since the turn of the century, when, in 1902, Dorothy Reed observed decreased cutaneous reactivity to tuberculin antigen in patients with this disorder. By the mid-1930's, this finding had been confirmed by systematic testing of larger numbers of patients for reactivity to tuberculin. Subsequently, a more general state of cutaneous anergy (loss of skin-test reactivity) was demonstrated by using other allergens including Trichophyton, Candida, and mumps skin-test antigens. More recently other tests of CMI (T cell function) have been used and the characteristics of this significant impairment delineated.

Hodgkin's disease differs from the other "lymphoproliferative" disorders (lymphosarcoma, reticulum cell sarcoma, and lymphocytic leukemia) in several important ways. In Hodgkin's disease there is a pleomorphic, often granulomatous proliferation of lymphoid cells, while in the non-Hodgkin's lymphomas and in lymphocytic leukemia there is typically a much more uniform lymphocytic proliferation. While Hodgkin's disease appears to be associated with a primary defect in T cell function and, therefore, in CMI, the non-Hodgkin's group seem to represent predominantly disorders of the B cell system and therefore, of humoral immunity and immunoglobulins. Nevertheless as indicated, there is often a partial impairment of T cell function in the non-Hodgkin's group as well. An interesting apparent exception is a rare form of chronic lymphocytic leukemia known as the "Sezary syndrome" which is apparently a primary T cell disorder. In this condition, the circulating lymphocytes tend to infiltrate the skin and may be related to the skin disorder, mycosis fungoides. The non-Hodgkin's group in general differ from Hodgkin's not only with respect to the associated immune disorders but also in clinical manifestations, therapy, and prognosis as well.

Characteristics of the Immune Defects in Hodgkin's: Cutaneous Anergy

As indicated, decreased cutaneous reactivity to skin test antigens ("delayed hypersensitivity") was described a number of years ago, and confirmed in numerous studies since (Table 4.2). In general, most studies have pointed to anergy as an early manifestation of the disease process and to correlation of anergy with disease activity. However, one problem with using skin test antigens to test preexisting hypersensitivity is the necessity of relying upon the chance of prior exposure to the particular antigens. This difficulty can be avoided by using direct primary sensitization with an allergen such as dinitrochlorobenzene and subsequent testing for the capacity to become sensitized by this ordinarily "universal" sensitizer. Another potentially confusing variable is the effect of therapy, since both immunosuppressive chemotherapy and radiation may impair immune responses. Recent studies of untreated patients with early disease have indicated little or no anergy in this group. Nevertheless, by using lower concentrations of test antigens and more sensitive techniques, a partial or relative immune deficiency has been demonstrated in such patients. Thus, in untreated stage I disease, patients generally retain the ability to react to strong natural antigens (such as mumps or streptococcal products (SK-SD)) to which they had been previously sensitized (usually in early life) but show relative refractoriness to sensitization with low concentrations of dinitrochlorobenzene. Skin test reactivity at the time of disease onset, however, is not a useful prognostic sign.

In general, skin test reactivity decreases with the progression of the disease, and correlates with the absence of systemic symptoms. Thus, patients with fever, night sweats, pruritus, or weight loss show less reactivity than asymptomatic patients. There is also more correlation with the histologic type of disease, so that patients with mixed or lymphocyte-depleted forms show less reactivity than those with nodular sclerosis and lymphocyte-predominant forms. Although loss of cutaneous skin reactivity may be seen in the advanced stages of many debilitating diseases, including metastatic carcinoma, an important distinction is that anergy is often present in Hodgkin's disease patients who are in good clinical condition.

The occurrence of cutaneous anergy in Hodgkin's disease apparently reflects an underlying associated defect in T lymphocyte function. The exact role of this deficiency in the pathogenesis of the disease—whether cause or effect—cannot yet be clearly defined. However, there can be

TABLE 4.2. *Delayed Hypersensitivity In Hodgkin's Disease*[a]

	Positive skin tests (delayed-type)	
	Hodgkin's	Control
	%	
Mumps	14	90
Candida	19	92
Trichophyton	16	68
Purified protein derivative (tuberculin)	23	71

[a] Adapted from W. W. Schier, et al. Am. J. Med. *20:* 94, 1956.

little doubt that this defect is a regular and integral feature of the basic disease process.

Other Correlates of CMI—Homograft Rejection

The ability to reject skin homografts is thought to be principally a function of CMI. There is evidence, however, that humoral mechanisms may also modify the course of graft rejection. In studies of skin homografts, delayed graft rejection (prolonged graft survival) has been seen in approximately 60% of Hodgkin's patients. Many of the subjects in these studies, however, had previously been treated, so that it is not possible to distinguish clearly effects of the basic disease from those of therapy.

Lymphocyte Numbers and Function

Peripheral lymphocytopenia is a common feature of advanced stages of Hodgkin's in both treated and untreated patients, but most studies have shown low-normal or only minimally depressed lymphocyte counts in early stages. Accompanying the peripheral lymphocytopenia, advanced cases of Hodgkin's often show lymphocyte depletion of lymphoid tissues as well. Normally T lymphocytes comprise approximately 70% of the circulating blood lymphocyte population, and it is not surprising that the quantitative decrease in lymphocytes occurs predominantly in this population. Of particular interest is a recent observation that despite the overall diminution in T lymphocytes in advanced Hodgkin's disease, there is a relative excess of the particular subpopulation of T lymphocytes known as "suppressor" lymphocytes. It is likely that this relative imbalance in T lymphocytes contributes to the immune anomalies in Hodgkin's patients.

Using other in vitro tests of lymphocyte function, including response to phytohemagglutinin (PHA) which normally causes blast transformation of T lymphocytes, Hodgkin's patients show decreased responses. Abnormalities in PHA responsiveness have been found even in early stages of Hodgkin's when testing is carried out with a wide range of PHA concentrations, a more discriminating test than the previously standard single dose. Similar results have been obtained using the mixed-lymphocyte reaction, possibly a more sensitive assay of immunologic competence than PHA stimulation.

Transfer of Delayed Hypersensitivity

As demonstrated by Lawrence, delayed hypersensitivity to an antigen such as tuberculin can be transferred from a tuberculin-sensitive donor to a nonsensitive recipient by injection of donor blood buffy coat cells or a cell-free dialyzable transfer factor derived from the cells. The previously skin-test-negative recipient will then be shown to have positive delayed hypersensitivity skin-test responses to tuberculin. When leukocytes from normal individuals have been used, transfer of delayed hypersensitivity to Hodgkin's patients have usually not been successful. An exception was noted in patients with the nodular sclerosing type of Hodgkin's. The failure to respond to this form of presumed "antigen-information" transfer may simply reflect the underlying diminished capacity to respond to primary immunization in these patients. No studies of transfer experiments from Hodgkin's patients to normals have been reported.

Humoral Immunity in Hodgkin's

A number of studies of antibody response to a variety of antigens in Hodgkin's patients have produced conflicting results. In general, however, it appears that antibody formation in untreated patients and those in relatively early phases is either normal or only minimally depressed. Near the terminal stages of disease, antibody response to immunization becomes markedly impaired. Again, in assessing immunity in advanced stages, it becomes impossible to separate effects of the disease itself from effects of therapy and general debilitation. It may not be surprising that minor defects occur in antibody formation in response to some "weak" antigens in early Hodgkin's, if it is recognized that in some instances, immunoglobulin production is facilitated by an interaction of "helper" subpopulations of T lymphocytes with macrophages and possibly B lymphocytes. Furthermore, it is interesting to speculate that the earlier mentioned relative excess of "suppressor" T lymphocytes in Hodgkin's may actually interfere with humoral immune responses.

Phagocytic Function

Phagocytic function as measured by in vivo clearance of labeled particles from the blood is actually enhanced in advanced Hodgkin's as compared to normals and early, asymptomatic Hodgkin's patients. This may reflect, in part, the reticulum cell hyperplasia of lymphoid tissue in Hodgkin's. In late stages, however, blood granulocyte numbers and function may be impaired, especially in patients receiving cytotoxic therapy.

Susceptibility to Infection in Hodgkin's Disease

Patients with advanced Hodgkin's who have received immunosuppressive therapy represent "compromised hosts" who are particularly susceptible to "opportunistic" infections with a variety of uncommon as well as common pathogens. In one study, 70% of patients with fatal Hodgkin's developed severe infections late in the course of disease. The opportunistic pathogens include viral, fungal, mycobacterial, bacterial, and protozoan agents. Of the viral agents the herpesvirus group is a particular threat, especially the varicella-zoster virus. In fact, herpes zoster is relatively common, even in earlier stages of Hodgkin's disease. It is of interest that the infection more commonly follows the typical dermatome distribution of "shingles," in contrast to disseminated varicella-zoster infections which are more commonly seen in chronic lymphocytic leukemia. This difference suggests that defective CMI may permit the neurotropic dermatome disease but that relatively intact humoral immunity prevents further spread. In contrast the predominant defect in antibody formation in chronic lymphocytic leukemia allows widespread dissemination. Another viral agent of importance in Hodgkin's patients is cytomegalovirus.

Among the fungal agents, Aspergillus, Candida, and Cryptococcus are particular problems. The risk of tuberculosis is especially high in Hodgkin's disease. Septicemia with gram-negative bacilli is a frequent complication especially in the late stages of disease. Protozoan infections with Toxoplasma and Pneumocystis are also seen.

As indicated, the increased susceptibility to infection of patients with advanced Hodgkin's undoubtedly represents the combined immunosuppressive effects of therapy, debilitation, and the disease itself. It is clear, however, that even in untreated patients, the defect in CMI poses the threat of certain types of infections.

Other Immunopathologic Conditions

The consequences of deficient CMI include, not only increased susceptibility to infection, but also potential loss of the surveillance functions of T lymphocytes with resulting decreased ability to limit neoplastic cell proliferation (Table 4.3). Thus in Hodgkin's patients advance of the disease process may be accelerated by the concomitant loss of CMI. In addition, other types of neoplasms may occur simultaneously in this setting. Finally, the imbalance in the immune system may lead to relative over-reactivity of some components of the system (e.g., B lymphocytes) with the consequent appearance of autoallergic disorders such as hemolytic anemia.

Pathogenesis of Hodgkin's Disease—Relationship to the Immunological Defect

The pathogenesis of Hodgkin's disease and of the associated immunodeficiency are not yet clearly understood. Nevertheless, recent detailed observations of the immune system in Hodgkin's disease in particular,

TABLE 4.3. *Potential Consequences of Deficient CMI*

1. Infection—increased susceptibility.
   Opportunistic pathogens.
2. Malignant tumors—increased incidence.
   Loss of "surveillance" function.
3. Autoallergic disorders—deficiency of T cells.
   Leads to overactive B cell responses ?
   (Hemolytic anemia, systemic lupus erythematosus)

and increased knowledge of the functions and relationship of the cellular and humoral immune systems in general permit interesting speculations about possible pathogenetic mechanisms.

An important basic question to be resolved is whether the defect in CMI precedes the disease itself and therefore may be a causal factor or whether it is a consequence of the disease. At present, no evidence exists of an antecedent immune defect in Hodgkin's patients. In untreated patients with early disease, the defect of CMI often appears to be subtle and minimal. As the disease progresses, the immunodeficiency progresses in parallel, suggesting at least an intricate interdependence. One hypothesis suggests that an extrinsic agent, such as a virus, may lead to induction of the malignant disease, probably by direct infection of a subpopulation of T lymphocytes. In the process, a new (tumor associated) surface antigen would be acquired by these cells. Other competent T lymphocytes would then attack the altered cells with a resultant chronic immune reaction. Many of the manifestations of the disease could be explained by this mechanism. Fever, for example, might result from the effect of pyrogenic lymphokines released by the stimulated normal T cells. The hypothesis is further supported by the discovery of specific antigens associated with Hodgkin's disease. Evidence has already been cited indicating the presence of a relative excess of "suppressor" lymphocytes in Hodgkin's patients.

Alternatively, suppression of subpopulations of T lymphocytes might be a consequence of hyperreactivity of B lymphocytes against tumor-specific antigens of neoplastic T cells. Evidence supporting this possibility includes the observation of increased production of IgG by splenic lymphocytes from Hodgkin's patients with specificity for homologous lymphocytes from normal persons.

Either hypothesis would explain the early cutaneous anergy, the progressive loss of T lymphocyte function, and the difficulty of transferring delayed hypersensitivity to Hodgkin's patients. It is, of course, possible that both mechanisms may be operative.

The factors that lead to the initial oncogenic event are even less well understood. If an extrinsic agent such as a virus is a triggering agent, it is quite possible that susceptibility to such infection is related to immune response genes and to the histocompatibility antigens (HL-A system).

Immunosuppressive Therapy

Many chemotherapeutic agents as well as radiation have the potential for interfering with various components of the immunocytologic defense system, including lymphocytes, macrophages, and granulocytes (Table 4.4). The most specific mechanism of suppressing T lymphocyte function (CMI) while leaving B cells (and therefore humoral function) relatively intact is by the use of highly specific antilymphocyte globulins. Usually

TABLE 4.4 *Immunosuppressive Therapy*

	Inhibits induction of delayed hypersensitivities	Suppresses preexisting delayed hypersensitivities
Immunosuppressive agents		
Corticosteroids	+	+
Antilymphocyte sera (antilymphycyte globulins)	+	+
6-MP and azothiaprine	+	−
Cyclophosphamide	+	−
Cytosine arabinoside	+	−
Methotrexate	+	−
5-Flurouracil	±	−
Chlorambucil	±	−
Asparaginase	±	−
Antibiotics		
Chloramphenicol	±	−
Tetracycline	±	−
Rifampin	±	−
Radiation	+	±

some effect on humoral function is also seen. Corticosteroids have profound as well as a potentially wider spectrum of immunosuppressive effects with alterations of granulocyte function as well. Both antilymphocyte sera and corticosteroids affect not only the induction of CMI (i.e., the new acquisition of delayed hypersensitivity) but preexisting delayed hypersensitivity as well. In contrast most of the cytotoxic chemotherapeutic agents predominantly act to inhibit the induction of delayed hypersensitivity rather than preexisting CMI.

Although several common antibiotics such as chloramphenicol and tetracycline can be shown to have immunosuppressive activity, these effects are ordinarily insignificant in usual therapeutic regimens. Finally radiation may have profound effects upon virtually all of the components of the immunocytologic defense system, depending upon the type, dose and duration of therapy.

Conclusion

Acquired deficiency of CMI occurs in a wide variety of neoplastic diseases, infections, debilitated states, and diseases of unknown etiology. Although often less profound than the congenital immunodeficiencies, the acquired disorders are clinically much more common. Hodgkin's disease is a neoplastic disorder in which the associated deficiency of CMI appears to be an intrinsic component of the disease process, may explain certain of the disease manifestations, and is probably involved in its pathogenesis. Immunosuppressive therapy and radiation constitute increasingly important causes of deficient CMI. Infections and other disorders with associated aberrant immune responses will be discussed subsequently (see Chapter 8).

REFERENCES

Aisenberg, A. C.: Immunologic status of Hodgkin's disease. Cancer, *19:* 385, 1966.

Berenbaum, M. D.: The clinical pharmacology of immunosuppressive agents. In *Clinical Aspects of Immunology,* 3rd ed, edited by P. G. H. Gell, R. R. A. Coombs, and P. J. Lachman. Oxford: Blackwell Scientific Publications, 1975, p. 689.

Casazza, A. R., Duvall, C. P., and Carbone, P. P.: Summary of infectious complications occurring in patients with Hodgkin's disease. Cancer Res., *26:* 1290, 1966.

DeVita, V.: Lymphocyte reactivity in Hodgkin's disease: a lymphocyte civil war. N. Engl. J. Med., *289:* 801, 1973.

Eltringham, J. R., and Kaplan, H. S.: Immunodeficiency in Hodgkin's disease. Birth defects. Orig. Art. Series, *11:* 278, 1975.

Faquet, G. B.: Quantitation of immunocompetence in Hodgkin's disease. J. Clin. Invest., *56:* 951, 1975.

Kaur, J., Spurs, A. S., and Galton, D. A.: Increase of T lymphocytes in spleen of Hodgkin's disease. Lancet, *2:* 800, 1974.

Miller, D. G.: Immunological disturbances in lymphoma and leukemia. In *Immunological Diseases,* edited by M. Samter. Boston: Little Brown and Co., 1971, p. 548.

Ng, R. P., Moran, C. J., Alexopoulos, C. G., and Bellingham, A. J.: Transfer Factor in Hodgkin's Disease. Lancet, *2:* 901–903, 1975.

Order, S. E., and Hellman, S.: Pathogenesis of Hodgkin's disease. Lancet, *1:* 571, 1972.

Twomey, J. J., Laughter, A. H., Farrow, S. et al.: Hodgkin's disease. An immunodepleting and immunosuppressive disorder. J. Clin. Inv., *56:* 467–475, 1975.

Young, R. C., et al.: Delayed hypersensitivity in Hodgkin's disease. Am. J. Med., *52:* 63, 1972.

Chapter 5

TUMOR IMMUNOLOGY

Rama Ganguly, Ph.D.

Most malignant growths in experimental animals and humans possess altered somatic antigens. Tumors, induced by chemical carcinogens or oncogenic viruses, as well as those of unknown etiology, elicit immunologic reactions against the tumor. Therefore, the possibility that immunologic reactions may be used for modifying or even controlling malignant diseases is of great interest.

Antigens Associated with Tumors

Tumor-specific antigens (TSA) are dispersed among normal antigens on the cell surface and interact with host cells, including those responsible for immune recognition. These new antigens may be the product of outside information brought to the cell in the form of viral nucleic acid, or through chemical mutation which alters the native information stored in the cellular DNA. These TSA are highly specific for the tumors. Many tumors also possess tumor-associated antigens (TAA), which may be present in several different types of cancer, as well as in some normal tissues. An example of a TAA is carcinoembryonic antigen. The new cellular antigen(s) induce(s) an immune reaction in the host. It is conceivable that effective immunologic surveillance depends on tumor specific antigens being recognized as "nonself" and destroyed by immunocompetent cells of the host. The TSA that behaves like a transplantation antigen is called a tumor-specific transplantation antigen (TSTA). Whether truly nonantigenic tumors exist or whether the available techniques are simply not sensitive enough to detect the antigenicity has not been resolved at present.

There are at least two different ways in which tumor antigens gain access to the circulation: some tumors have cells that spontaneously shed (or even secrete) large amounts of their membrane structures into the circulation; and some tumors do not shed antigens spontaneously but do so when they come under immunologic attack by the host.

In vitro studies also indicate that tumor cells, when maintained in tissue culture, spontaneously liberate soluble TSTA into the medium. This antigen can be detected in sera from animals with tumors. There is also suggestive evidence that the propensity to shed surface antigen may be an important determining factor in the malignancy of a tumor, in that it constitutes an escape mechanism from the host's restraint. In the primary tumor, shedded TSTA in large quantities could combine with and neutralize both specific effector cells and humoral antibody. This local neutralization of immune functions may then be followed by overwhelming antigenic load in regional lymph nodes, and finally systemic escape may occur.

Bodily Defense and Malignancy

The first line of defense in preventing neoplastic growth is "immunologic surveillance" which recognizes as foreign small numbers of malignant cells and destroys them. Interference with this surveillance system may occur when the immune system is compromised, as in congenitally immunologically-deficient patients, in kidney allograft recipients undergoing prolonged immunosuppressive therapy, and in other situations such as in viral infections, during which transient immunosuppression may occur. The latter is also referred to as the "sneak in" mechanism by which a tumor gains a foothold due to a temporary immunologic lapse and then overwhelms the host's immune functions simply by its rapid growth. It has been observed that the incidence of cancer in immunodeficiency states and in recipients of renal allografts is far greater than normal. However, other factors, apart from defective immune surveillance, may also be responsible for the malignancies. These include changes in immunogenicity of tumor cells and modulation of TSTA of tumor cells in such a way that the host's immune system cannot recognize or respond to TSTA. Other mechanisms include production of "blocking antibody" that paradoxically interferes with the killer effects of immune lymphocytes (vide infra). In experimental animals, incubation of a very small number of tumor cells that should be handled by the host's immune system, with blocking antibody, often results in establishment of growth, even in the presence of well-documented host immunity. Another postulated mechanism is through inhibitor T cells.

Host Immune Response to Malignancy

Once the neoplastic growth has been established, the new cellular antigens elicit a response in the host that clearly indicates recognition of the abnormal or "nonself" cells. This immune response to an antigenic tumor, like that to a kidney allograft, may be expressed by the host in terms of both cellular and humoral reactivities. Very little is known about the nature of the cells effective in tumor immunity. In in vitro cytotoxicity tests for tumor immunity, for example, both T and B cells have been implicated under different conditions. The host immune response is also evidenced from histologic studies indicating inflammatory reactions, for example, in breast cancer, with a hyperplastic appearance of regional lymphoid tissue, especially in T cell-dependent areas. There is suggestive evidence that a higher degree of this inflammatory reaction is related to a better prognosis. Another indication of the host's immune response to the tumor is borne out by the fact that the tumor-bearing animal shows endogenous resistance to reimplantation of tumor cells administered subcutaneously.

In Vitro Tests for Cell-Mediated Immunity

Evidence for lymphocyte-mediated immunity to tumors in vitro was first published by Yoshida and Southam in 1963. They demonstrated that spleen cells from mice had cytotoxic effects on cultured sarcoma cells, when the donors were previously sensitized to the same (chemically-induced) sarcoma. Hellström et al. developed a quantitative technique for measuring such cytotoxicity of lymphocytes toward tumor cells. Subsequently, in various experimental animals, cell-mediated cytotoxicity has been demonstrated using various types of tumors.

A variety of tests have been developed to measure the cellular immune response against tumors. The colony inhibition test is done by plating target cells in Petri dishes, the cells forming colonies which are counted 4 days later. If the target cells are injured, it is reflected in a decreased number of colonies. This method was first used for measuring the effects of antibodies in the presence of complement. The colony inhibition test has been modified for target cells which do not attach to plates (leukemia cells) by plating in agar. These tests have been used as micro assays requiring less materials. Using a radioactive label of target cells with various isotopes, it is also possible to determine the degree of damage by measuring released radioactivity in the media.

Macrophage migration assay is another test system used for measuring the cellular immune response to TAA. The blastogenic response of lymphocytes of patients in the presence of their tumor cells has been studied in vitro using radioactive thymidine incorporation as a measure of DNA synthesis.

Another cell of importance in tumor destruction is the macrophage, which operates through collaboration with T cells. Being activated by a variety of lymphokines liberated from activated lymphocytes (chemotactic factor, migration inhibitory factor, and macrophage activating factor) macrophages kill malignant cells with which they come in contact.

Humoral Immunity

The second major component of the immune response to tumor antigens is antibody synthesis. In the presence of complement, IgM and IgG antibodies are cytotoxic for tumor cells. Antibodies also can mediate killing of neoplastic cells in collaboration with lymphoid cells. Thus, the host's response to neoplastic growth may be mediated at both cellular and humoral levels involving various cell types almost in an orchestral fashion.

Sera obtained from animals or patients with tumors can specifically abrogate lymphocyte mediated killing of tumor cells. These "blocking factors" can act by modulating the tumor cells after combining with surface antigens, so that the neoplastic cells are not recognized by effector lymphocytes. Blocking factors may also act by direct action on lymphocytes, although the mechanism is not well understood. These blocking factors may be complexes formed between antigens shed from the tumors and antibodies formed by the host. A blocking effect, as evident in the microcytotoxicity assay, can also be demonstrated by the macrophage migration assay. In the presence of serum from tumor-bearing animals, macrophage migration, which would be inhibited without the serum being present, occurs. Thus, there is inhibition of migration inhibitory factor release. Furthermore, sera from cancer patients contain soluble inhibitors or nonspecific blocking factors for cell-mediated immunity, which can, for example, reduce the lymphocyte blastogenic response to phytohemagglutinin.

Sera from mice with spontaneously regressed (Moloney virus-induced) sarcoma have been found to contain a specific factor which can neutralize the blocking activity of sera from mice with growing Molony sarcomas. The nature of such factors has not been delineated fully, but they are probably antibodies with specificity directed against tumor antigens rather than against the combining sites of the blocking immunoglobulins. Possibly they act by neutralizing antigenic sites of the blocking antigen-antibody complex, so that the effector immune lymphocytes can no longer be blocked.

Thus it would appear from the above that, in response to tumor antigens, the host reacts by forming multiple clones of reactive cells: the potential killer cells, and plasma cells producing various types of antibodies directed toward TSA. Some of these antibodies integrate with antigen products of tumors, forming blocking antibodies, which in turn can materially affect functions of the effector immune lymphocytes. They can also interfere with antibody-armed macrophage functions as well as antibody-mediated lympholysis. So, there are various ways in which the tumor-specific defense mechanisms might be abrogated. One salient feature is that the immune response (even under optimal experimental conditions) is incapable of handling a large amount of tumor cells, indicating that the tumor burden of the host should be removed or reduced to as small as possible by surgical procedure and/or other conventional therapy.

Immunotherapy

It has been observed that nonspecific augmentation of immunity may be useful in destruction of tumor cells. As a result, clinical trials have been initiated attempting to nonspecifically stimulate immunity by inoculation with BCG. Complete tumor remission has been seen following BCG administration into subcutaneous metastases in a few melanoma patients. Encouraging results also have been obtained in leukemia patients in whom the tumor load has been significantly reduced using chemotherapy. On the other hand, studies in animals with solid tumors indicate that tumor enhancement occurs after BCG administration and that an increase in blocking antibodies may also result following such therapy. Other nonspecific immunostimulants besides BCG have also been studied, e.g., dinitrochlorobenzene in treating skin carcinoma, *Corynebacterium parvum* or levamisole in lung cancer. The mode of action of nonspecific stimulants is not well understood, but has been postulated to be mediated through nonspecific enhancement of specific lymphocyte-tumor cell interaction or nonspecific tumor cell destruction resulting from interaction with the sensitizing antigen (nonspecific stimulant) in close proximity to the malignant cells.

Attempts have been made to use specific immunotherapy against neoplastic disease, using modified tumor cells as "vaccines." Examples are killed tumor cells from the same patient or from another patient bearing antigenically similar tumor, in vitro altered autologous tumor cells with enhanced immunogenicity and antigenic extracts from tumor cells. Various techniques have been applied to increase immunogenicity of tumor cells. One of the methods is to treat the tumor cells with the enzyme neuraminidase, which removes a coating of sialic acid from the cell surface. Such antigens, when introduced into the patient, hopefully augment cell-mediated antitumor immunity in terms of direct cytotoxicity of lymphocytes as well as the levels of unblocking and cytotoxic antibodies. It is desirable at the same time that this would not stimulate the development of tumor-enhancing antibodies. Unfortunately, such vaccines have still to be developed and caution is necessary to application since many aspects of host-neoplasm interactions are only poorly understood.

Transfer of tumor immunity has also been attempted more recently using immune RNA or transfer factor. Both these entities have been shown to stimulate lymphoid cells in vitro and are nonimmunogenic to the host. Transfer factor transfers memory of cellular immunity without

TABLE 5.1. *Some Recent Adjuvant Immunotherapy Trials in Humans*[a]

Disease	Adjuvant therapy	Number of patients studied	Comments
Acute leukemia	BCG intradermal during remission period	14 patients in 2 different studies	5 showed remission over 90 days. Improved results when combined with active immunotherapy.
	Bordetella pertussis by intramuscular injection	8	Relapse period lengthened but not greater than 455 days.
Malignant melanoma	BCG injected into local lesion	22 patients in 4 different studies	13 showed regression of lesions. One deteriorated and developed blocking factor in serum.
	Vaccinia virus inoculated into skin lesions	Total 48 patients treated in 4 different studies	13 patients showed improvement from disappearance of tumors to regression of skin nodules.
Skin carcinoma and other skin tumors (including squamous and basal cell carcinoma, mycosis fungoides, breast carcinoma metastatic to skin)	Topical chemical sensitizer (e.g., dinitrochlorobenzene) applied repeatedly to skin tumor sites	Total 77 patients studied in 3 different studies	Complete or partial regression for several months occurred in some but follow-up is not clear.
	BCG vaccination in combination with methotrexate and isoniazid	16	13 reached clinical remission for longer periods compared to retrospective controls.
Other widespread tumors	BCG vaccination	43	Survival at 2 years superior to that of a control group.
Bronchogenic carcinoma	BCG vaccination	71	Survival at 2 years superior to that of a control group.

[a] Modified from Baker M.A., and R.N. Taub: *Progress in Allergy,* New York, S. Karger, vol. 17, 1973, pp. 227–299.

TABLE 5.2. *Some Recent Trials of Active Immunotherapy in Cancer Patients*[a]

Disease	Active immunotherapy	Number of patients studied	Comments
Advanced solid tumors (including colon, stomach, cervix, uterus, ovary, lung, and breast)	Living tumor cells or DNA extracts of cells mixed with Freund's adjuvant	253 in 2 different studies	No clinical improvement noticed in most patients.
	Microsomal and mitochondrial fractions of autologous tumor cells mixed with adjuvant.	20	7 showed temporary regression of masses and 10 converted to positive delayed skin reactivity status.
	Tumor cells mixed with Freund's adjuvant and hyaluronidase	25	An unspecific number had temporary regression of lesions; 22 had rise in antibody titer.
	Whole tumor cell vaccine	14	12 had rise in serum protein fractions that produced tumor necrosis upon injection into lesions.
	Tumor homogenate mixed with Freund's adjuvant	12	Tumor shrinkage with histological changes of delayed hypersensitivity
	Crude tumor homogenate	181	23% showed shrinkage of measurable lesions and improvement in cellular and humoral responses to tumor antigens.
	Autologous tumor cell preparations	32	Studied only in breast cancer patients. Had better survival than controls.
	Tumor cells coupled to rabbit γ-globulin ± Freund's adjuvant	75 in 4 different studies	15 showed improvement in terms of either clinical remission, regression or prolonged survival.

[a] Modified from Baker M.A., and R.N. Taub: *Progress in Allergy,* New York, S. Karger, vol 17, 1973, pp. 227–299.

TABLE 5.2—*continued*

Disease	Active immunotherapy	Number of patients studied	Comments
Malignant melanoma	Irradiated autochthonous cultured cells	19	Clinical remission of 2–3 years in 2 with antibodies to melanoma cells.
	Neuraminidase treated cells in combination with BCG and autologous stimulated lymphocytes	22	6 patients achieved complete regression of disease.
Choriocarcinoma	Paternal leukocytes plus rabbit antisera to seminal fluid.	1	Clinical remission in metastastic disease
	BCG + paternal skin grafts	21	8 clinical remissions but only 1 clearly due to immunotherapy
Acute Leukemia	Pooled irradiated leukemic cells ± BCG	20	12 showed remission from 3–6 years
	Pooled irradiated leukemia cells ± BCG	15	11 patients still alive after 2 years (well controlled study)
	Autologous irradiated tumor cell vaccine ± chemotherapy	12	Remission in 1 and 6 of 9 converted to skin reactivity to leukemic cells.
	Vaccination with leukemic cells and infusion of remission plasma and leukocytes	12	3 complete remission up to 6 months and 5 partial remissions.
Chronic myelogenous leukemia	Cultured human leukemia cells combined with BCG	6	Regression of splenomegaly seen and survival better than 11 controls
Burkitt's lymphoma	Autochthonous irradiated tumor cells + adjuvant + chemotherapy	11	6 patients achieved long-term remission, probably better than chemotherapy alone.

TABLE 5.3. *Some Recent Trials of Adoptive Immunotherapy in Humans*[a]

Disease	Adoptive therapy used	Number of patients	Comments
Acute leukemia	Bone marrow transplantation: (a) identical twins: conditioned with irradiation	7	No clinical benefits
	also vaccinated with stored leukemic cells and leukocyte infusion	4	2 showed remissions of 8–13 months
	(b) nonmatched allografts	81 in two different studies	Frequent GVH reaction, 4 patients with established graft died of recurrent leukemia in 9–20 months
	(c) HL-A matched allografts: Methotrexate given to suppress graft versus host	7	1 achieved remission of 200 days
	Cyclophosphamide given prior to irradiation to augment immunosuppression	12	5 remission, longest > 600 days
	Cyclophosphamide and irradiation before transplantation	9	Median survival of all patients = 90 days. Two patients in remission at 8 and 11 months
	Cyclophosphamide before infusion of compatible bone marrow	12	Graft Versus host reaction frequent.
	Infusion of unstimulated peripheral leukocytes	24	2 remissions at 75 and 200 day
	Infusion of autologous remission leukocytes	18	Increase in duration of remission in treated group as compared to control
Malignant melanoma	Peripheral leukocytes from remission patients	1	Remission in skin lesion for 5 years
	Cross-implantation of tumors and cross-transfusion of white cells in patient pairs	143 in 3 different studies	7 clinical remissions from 8 months to 4 years: clinical response in 24 patients
	Transfer factor	1	Regression of skin nodule

[a] Modified from Baker M.A., and R.N. Taub: *Progress in Allergy*, New York, S. Karger, vol. 17, 1973, pp. 227–299.

TABLE 5.3—*continued*

Disease	Adoptive therapy used	Number of patients	Comments
Various advanced malignancies (involving gastrointestinal tract, lung, kidneys, breast, cervix, ovary, testicle, and sarcoma)	Thoracic duct lymphocytes infused	6	1 clinical remission for 6 months
	Cross implantation of tumors and cross-transfusion of white cells	74 in 3 different studies	In 12 clinical response was noted. Favorable responses were frequent in patients with small amount of tumor.
	Transfer factor	40	Regression of tumors in 7 patients and clinical improvement for up to 17 months.
Leukemia	Heteroantisera: antisera raised in horse, sheep, guinea pig, made against pooled leukemic cells, normal human cells, human lymphocytes.	26 in 3 different studies	2 patients achieved remission for 2 years with horse antisera to pooled leukemic cells; transient decrease in counts in patients with chronic lymphocytic leukemia.
	Alloantisera: Plasma from volunteers injected with acute or chronic leukemic cells or normal lymphocytes	13 in 2 different studies	No benefits excepting transient leukopenia
Clear cell carcinoma	Plasma from patient in remission	1	Clinical remission at least for 15 months

changing humoral functions, which is considered an important attribute. There is no good animal model, so experiments have to be done directly upon humans, severely limiting the extent of studies. Another limitation to this approach is the lack of availability of the source of such factors. It has been suggested that search for reactive normal donors should be made, e.g., mothers of neuroblastoma children. Alternatively, patients whose own tumors have regressed spontaneously or been cured may serve as donors. Various applications of immunotherapy in the treatment of cancer in recent human trials have been summarized in Tables 5. 1–5.3.

In conclusion, intensive investigation is presently being carried out to understand the mechanism of action of the host-neoplasm interaction. Such studies have shed light in delineating the biology and etiology of a variety of tumors. Attempts are being made to diagnose early and use immunotherapy. However, the present status of knowledge does not yet permit replacement of conventional treatment procedures by immunotherapeutic approaches.

SELECTED REFERENCES

Baldwin, R. W.: Immunological aspects of chemical carcinogenesis. Adv. Cancer. Res., *18:* 1, 1973.

Davey, G. C., Currie, G. A., and Alexander, P.: Spontaneous shedding and antibody induced modulation of histocompatibility antigens on murine lymphomata: correlation with metastatic capacity. Br. J. Cancer, *33:* 9, 1976.

Ganguly, R., Cusumano, C. L., and Waldman, R. H.: Suppression of cell-mediated immunity after infection with attenuated rubella virus. Infect. Immun., *13:* 464, 1976.

Hellstrom, K. E., and Hellstrom, I.: Immunological enhancement as studied by cell culture techniques. Ann. Rev. Microbiol., *24:* 373, 1970.

Hellstrom, K. E., and Hellstrom, I.: Lymphocyte-mediated cytotoxicity and blocking serum activity to tumor antigens. Adv. Immunol., *18:* 209, 1973.

Kersey, J. H., Specter, B. D., and Good, R. A.: Immunodeficiency and cancer. Adv. Cancer Res., *18:* 211, 1973.

Levy, J. P.: Antigens associated with C type RNA virus induced tumors. In *Progress in Immunology.* Edited by L. Brent, and J. Holborow. Amsterdam: North-Holland, 1974, pp. 3249–3259.

Oettgen, H. F.: Immunotherapy of Cancer. N. Engl. J. Med., *297:* 484, 1977.

Old, L. J. A., Boyse, E. A., Clarke, D. A., and Carsswell, E. A.: Antigenic properties of chemically induced tumors. Ann. N. Y. Acad. Sci., *101:* 80, 1962.

Simmons, R. L., Rios, A., Lundgren, G., Ray, P. K., McKhann, C. F., and Haywood, G. R.: Immunospecific regression of methylcholanthrene fibrosarcoma with the use of neuraminidase. Surgery, *70:* 38, 1971.

Chapter 6

TRANSPLANTATION IMMUNOLOGY

William Pfaff, M.D.

The laws governing the immune response to intraspecies transplantation were established in the 1940's and 1950's by the Nobel Laureate, Sir Peter Medewar. He recognized the arousal of immune defenses against genetically dissimilar rodent skin grafts and described the histologic and immunogenetic features of the response that has been termed "graft rejection." He also discovered a means of circumventing rejection in the experimental animal, notably the establishment of neonatal tolerance, a genetically specific state of nonreactivity induced by transplantation of tissue from a putative donor to a neonatal or embryonal recipient.

About 25 years ago, human investigation was begun. In the absence of effective immunosuppression, organ grafting was followed by short-lived function which was soon lost when rejection supervened. There was a measure of success using near-lethal total body radiation. Survivors of radiation sickness were found to be immunodeficient and a graft was placed shortly after recovery from the acute symptoms. A few years later it was shown that 6-mercaptopurine ablated immune reactivity to soluble foreign antigens. This led to the development of a related compound, azathioprine, as the premier cytotoxic agent to blunt the immune response to a graft. When combined with adrenocorticosteroids, fairly predictable success was noted, and these agents remain the principle means of immunosuppression today.

Large scale development of clinical renal transplant programs occurred throughout the 1960's. Surgical techniques were standardized, experience was gained with immunosuppressive drugs, septic complications were encountered, and their management was deciphered. The sum of this era was that organ transplantation evolved from a clinical experiment to become a rational alternative for the practical management of end-stage renal disease.

The potential for replacing a vital organ applies equally to kidney, heart, liver, or other critical structures. However, prolonged replacement of organ function by artificial means while awaiting a donor, during malfunction induced by the operative procedure, or during periods of decreased function imposed by graft rejection is restricted to the kidney. Hemodialysis, and to some extent peritoneal dialysis, can substitute for absent excretory function. Nonetheless, the ability to replace the diseased heart and liver has been convincingly shown. Because of the greater level of experience, this discussion will in the main, be limited to the kidney.

Selection of a Donor Combination

Current options are limited to a living related donor or an unrelated cadaver donor. In the past, a number of transplants were performed from unrelated living donors, but were largely discontinued after it became clear that there was no advantage over the use of a cadaveric graft.

The ideal living related donor is an identical twin, for no genetic barriers are breached. Immunosuppression might be avoided with the exception that chemotherapy could be of potential advantage in averting recrudence of autoimmune disease if such had provoked the initial renal failure.

Barring the availability of a monozygotic twin, the most favorable source of a graft is a sibling with identical cell surface antigens, discovered by means of serologic white blood cell typing (tissue typing). The next most favorable group would be living related donors who share some though not all of these same membrane antigens: parents, siblings, and in some instances more distant relatives.

Cadaver donors are generally the victims of central nervous system disease or trauma. As with all kidney donors, it must be certain that the donor is free of pathologic processes that might compromise graft survival such as preexisting hypertension, significant systemic vascular disease, disseminated infection, or malignancy. In the United States, the death of the donor is generally made on neurologic grounds, thus permitting normal renal perfusion until the time of nephrectomy. This avoids the ischemic injury that necessarily accompanies cardiac death. As will be seen, the benefits of tissue typing are not as apparent in heightening graft success as is the case with living related donors.

Tissue Typing and the Histocompatibility Complex

Human leukocyte antigens (HLA) permit serologic discrimination of individuals. There are two subgroups, termed HLA-A and HLA-B. Approximately 20 antigens have been recognized in each subgroup. These subseries are mutually exclusive. The antigens are paired, a linkage embracing an antigen from each subgroup. This pairing, called a haplotype, persists in genetic transmission, so that a given haplotype will be found in generation after generation.

The HLA system has thus been useful in recognizing immunologically ideal donors within a family. The relationship of parent to child is consistent. Except in instances of chance shared antigens between mates, each parent contributes two HLA antigens, a haplotype to a child, and thus differs from a child in not sharing the two remaining antigens. In current slang, the child-parent relationship is termed a half-match. Simple Mendelian distribution determines the relationship between siblings. Chance dictates that a potential kidney recipient would have a 1:4 probability of sharing all four antigens with a sibling, a 2:4 probability of sharing two antigens, and a 1:4 probability of sharing no antigens.

The HLA system is identified by and mediated through antibodies. However, it is genetically linked to a cell-mediated immune system, and therein lies the particular advantage of intrafamilial grafting. The cell-mediated immune response between individuals can be predicted by an in vitro reaction termed the mixed leukocyte culture (MLC). Lymphocytes from one individual, when mixed with those of another, recognize foreign antigens and proliferate in preparation for immune attack. This proliferative phase can be quantitated by adding radioactive thymidine to the culture medium and measuring its incorporation in the reacting subpopulation. By this means it is possible to confirm maximum shared genetic information and predict minimum antigenic barriers to transplantation. If there is no reaction, there is predictably a high graft success rate. Recently developed laboratory techniques recognize some of the individual antigens responsible for this cell-mediated immunity reaction and foretell specific identification of this system in the future.

There is good correlation of tissue typing with graft success and is most notable with living related donors. HLA and MLC identical donor-recipient combinations are likely to result in 90% functional graft survival 1 year after transplantation. Sharing of one-half of the available measured genetic information in the histocompatibility complex yields a 1 year graft survival of 70%. When there is an absence of shared genetic information, living donor renal graft survival statistics are virtually the same as cadaver donor grafts.

The positive role of tissue typing is less clear in an unrelated donor-recipient relationship. Within a family, antibody and cell-mediated determinents are linked, and except in unusual circumstances of cross-over of chromosomes, a maternal or paternal package is delivered intact. In the general population, chance sharing of antibody-mediated antigens is unlikely to be accompanied by shared cell-mediated antigens. At best, four shared A and B locus antigens (HLA identical cadaver donor) confers a 1 year grafting success rate of 70%. The relative advantage of lesser degrees of sharing is a moot point, seemingly of value in countries of inbred population, and less important in countries with an outbred populace. There appears to be some advantage from the data in the United States.

Perhaps the main profit of tissue typing is in avoiding selection of a graft for a presensitized recipient, an individual who, as a result of prior antigen exposure through blood transfusion, an earlier transplant, or pregnancy, has developed complement fixing antibodies directed against HLA-A and B antigens. The existence of such antibodies is discerned by screening potential recipients against a panel of lymphocytes that includes all of the known HLA antigens. While data are not uniform to this point, most series show an advantage in transplanting a well-matched graft. Certainly knowledge of past and current specific antibodies (e.g., anti-HLA-A2) permits avoidance of this antigen in selecting a donor-recipient combination.

Immunosuppression

The mainstays of immunosuppression are cytotoxic drugs, principally azathioprine (Imuran) and corticosteroids (generally prednisone and its analogues). These are sometimes supplemented by biologic agents to produce lymphocytopenia, such as horse, rabbit and goat anti-human lymphocyte serum, anti-thymocyte serum, or their derivative globulin fractions. Local graft radiation has also been used.

Cytotoxic Agents

Immune reactivity to a new antigen was shown to be blocked by simultaneous administration of 6-mercaptopurine. This drug was modified by adding an imidazole ring to allow oral administration and is known as azathioprine (Imuran). By itself, it is a moderately effective immunosuppressant for organ transplantation, but will rarely provide long-term success when used as a sole agent. The limiting side-effect of azathioprine is bone marrow suppression, which is generally dose dependent. In a smaller number of patients, apparent hepatic toxicity or febrile drug reactions may prohibit continuation of the drug.

The only other cytotoxic drug that has been used with relative effectiveness has been cyclophosphamide (cytoxan). While clearly effective, it has been reported to be inferior to azathioprine in direct experimental comparison.

Adrenocorticosteroids

Prednisone is a necessary evil in immunosuppression, although it is not particularly effective as a sole agent. It alters virtually every phase of the immune mechanism—macrophage function, lymphocyte population, blastogenesis, and lymphocyte expression. Unfortunately many of these effects will also be reflected in secondary immune suppression, the ability to respond to an antigen or organism with which the recipient has had prior experience. This is in contradistinction to azathioprine, which will not greatly retard an anamnestic response. Of equal import, adrenocorticosteroids have remarkably diverse effect on innumerable metabolic processes that are, in the main, deleterious when the drug is used in unphysiologic dosage.

Biologic Agents

Antilymphocyte serum was meant to supplant a somewhat more cumbersome technique of mechanical depletion of lymphocytes that used chronic thoracic duct fistula. Both modes seek to abolish the defender of our antigenic integrity, the lymphocyte. The mechanical means involves cannulation of the thoracic duct, collection of many liters of lymph each day, centrifugation to remove the cellular components, and systematic return of the fluid component, all without breaking aseptic technique. This requires a hospital environment with supporting personnel, a good deal of expense, and a foreseeable termination, that is, relatively early transplant—for the procedure seems most effective when it precedes rather than follows a transplant. Because it is so cumbersome and so expensive, few programs have pursued research with this technique. The efficacy is real, though, and recent data from Vanderbilt University report noteworthy increased survival in cadaveric organ grafts. Unfortunately the procedure cannot be applied to a large number of patients and its refinement is hampered by the same disadvantage that condemns pharmalogic immunosuppression, namely that it is general rather than selective, inviting infectious complications.

Antilymphocyte serum was recognized as a potential immunosuppressant in the early 1960's. This agent is made by introducing lymphocytes of the recipient species into another species to induce antibody formation. The resultant serum or its component immunoglobulin is injected into the graft recipient before and after grafting with the purpose of reducing the recipient lymphocyte population. It has been an extraordinarily effective tool in experimental transplantation, particularly in rodents. It has not been nearly as effective in humans. While success has been described in both uncontrolled and controlled clinical experiments, there have been repeated reported and unreported failures to confirm these results. The species used and the modes of preparation of the agent have varied, as have route and dosage of administration. There has been sufficient success in both experimental and clinical circumstances to warrant continued trials.

Constraints

The principle reason for isolated failure of a renal graft is immune rejection. Despite the immunosuppressive agents, the defense mechanisms may remain sufficiently intact to result in graft destruction. There are predisposing factors, other than the antigenic differences that have been described:

(1) Although the information is scattered and incomplete, there is a degree of correlation of graft rejection with pretransplant evidence of immune reactivity. Of particular note is the fate of second grafts. Individuals who were able to maintain a first graft for prolonged periods of time are likely to accept a second graft. When a first transplant is lost to abrupt and early rejection, the second graft is usually subject to a similar fate. In more controlled circumstances, qualitative and quantitative response to a new antigen, such as dinitrochlorobenzene may predict a patient's reactivity to an organ graft.

(2) There is a growing body of evidence that patients who have never received a blood transfusion paradoxically have a lower rate of graft survival than individuals who have had prior exposure to whole blood. The explanation of this phenomenon has thus far been elusive. The human data suggest that blood transfusion induces antibody formation by immunoreactive prospective recipients, makes positive cross-matches likely, and thus practically eliminates these individuals from the recipient pool. Conversely, the patient who has received multiple transfusions without the production of antibody may well be an immunologic weakling, and in a similar fashion fail to respond to his graft.

(3) Opelz and Terasaki have recently reported significant and major differences in graft survival in various racial combinations. Cadaver organ grafting from Caucasian to Caucasian resulted in a 1 year graft survival of 49%. Black recipients receiving cadaver kidneys from black donors had a 1 year success rate of 33%. Caucasian recipient graft survival was intermediate when the kidney was from a black donor. Interchange of Caucasian and Oriental combinations occurred with less frequency, but the small number of Oriental kidneys in Caucasian recipients was the least successful subgroup, with a graft survival of only 18%. Racial differences in immune responsivity and antigenic strength are potential explanations.

(4) All nonspecific immunosuppression presents an opportunity for proliferation and invasion of microorganisms with which the host has not had previous contact. Despite immunologic memory, adrenocorticosteroids impede the response to organisms that *are* familiar. The list of offenders is thus lengthy, but sepsis, the most common cause of death after organ transplantation, is often the result of infectious organisms that are not commonly encountered in general medical care. *Pneumocystis carinii, Cryptococcus neoformans,* nocardia, and cytomegalovirus are fairly typical infections in graft recipients. Sometimes effectively restrained by specific antimicrobial therapy, it is often necessary to discontinue or curtail graft-sustaining immunosuppressive drugs to limit invasive infection.

(5) Patients who have developed renal failure as a result of immune or metabolic processes are at some risk for recrudesence after grafting. For example, the patient with oxalosis is almost surely going to deposit calcium oxalate in the graft, for the transplant, though helpful in reducing the concentration, does not modify the overproduction that is responsible for insidious precipitation in the vasculature as well as the kidney parenchyma. Glomerulonephritis is an encompassing diagnosis that would appear to embrace a variety of disease entities. Specific subtypes, such as electron-dense membrano-proliferative glomerulonephritis, recur with high frequency. The recurrence of systemic immune disease seems likely, though limited experience with renal transplants in patients with lupus erythematosus has not as yet been associated with high frequency of recurrence. The combination of azathioprine and prednisone is doubly

effective, staving off rejection and in all likelihood maintaining a remission of the systemic disease in a highly selected group of stable patients. The same drug combination is frequently ineffective in controlling classic chronic nonspecific glomerulonephritis.

Too little time has passed to judge the recurrence rate of diabetic glomerulopathy, but the lengthy induction period after the onset of juvenile diabetes, 10–20 years, would lead one to guess that the other vascular manifestations will limit survival before recurrence appears.

Prospects for the Future

Renal transplantation has served as the first clinical model for replacement of failed vital organs. The immunologic laws are identical for other structures and success, particularly with trained cardiac and liver transplant teams, is hindered largely by technical barriers and the lack of an analogue of renal dialysis to temporarily support the recipient when rejection interrupts function.

Patient survival statistics after cadaveric renal transplantation are improving, but graft survival may actually be lessening. The remarkable success of many patients supports the feasibility of application to larger numbers only if we can discriminate potential failures before grafting. Recognition of an immune responder, now a preliminary area of investigation, may allow avoidance of a graft combination which will result in unquenchable rejection.

Modification of the host response to donor antigen and to this antigen alone is the most desirable means of achieving graft success. The induction of nonreactivity, akin to Medawar's neonatal tolerance, has seemed a promising route but has not been achieved. Another manipulation has centered on inducing graft protective immune mechanisms before or at the time of grafting.

Suggested supplementary reading.

1. Advisory Committee to the Renal Transplant Registry. The 13th Report of Human Renal Transplant Registry. Transplant. Proc. *9:* 26, 1977.
2. Mills, S. A., Siegler, H. F., and Wolfe, W. G.: Incidence and management of pulmonary mycosis in renal allograft patients. Ann. Surg. *182:* 617, 1975.
3. Opelz, G., and Terasaki, P. I.: Prolongation effect of blood transfusion on kidney graft survival. Transplantation, *22:* 380, 1976.
4. Rider, A. K., Copeland, J. G., Hunt, S. A., Mason, J., Spector, N. J., Winkle, R. A., Bieber, C. P., Billingham, M. E., Dong, E., Griepp, R. B., Schroeder, H. S., Stinson, E. B., Harrison, D. C., and Shumway, N. E.: Status of cardiac transplantation. Circulation, *52:* 531, 1975.
5. Stazl, T. E., Porter, K. A., Schroter, G. P., Halqrimson, C. G., Weil, R., Hoelscher, M., and Reid, H. A.: Orthotopic liver transplantation in 93 patients. Surg. Gynecol. Obstet., *142:* 487, 1976.
6. Thomas, F., Mendez-Picon, G., Thomas, J., Peace, K., Flora, R., and Lee, H. M.: Effect of antilymphocyte-globulin potency on survival of cadaver renal transplants. Lancet, *2:* 671, 1977.

Chapter 7

PASSIVE ENHANCEMENT OF CELL-MEDIATED IMMUNE RESPONSE

Rama Ganguly, Ph.D. and J. D. Lee, M.D.

Although specific immunity to infection was recognized over 2000 years ago in China and Greece, progress was slow until the late 19th century when the unravelling of the mechanisms of immunity was begun. At that time, the demonstration that the serum of diphtheria-immune animals neutralized diphtheria toxin and prevented illness led to concentrated efforts towards understanding antibody-mediated immunity. That antibody-mediated immunity did not explain all observable phenomena was largely ignored until the 1940's when it was demonstrated that delayed type hypersensitivity (DHS) could be transferred from one animal to another by leukocyte transfusion but not by serum. This fundamental observation not only provided an immunological tool for analysis of the mechanisms of DHS but also clearly differentiated the latter from those responses mediated by serum immunoglobulins. From this, it was clear that an antibody-independent cell-mediated immune response existed. This type of response was subsequently shown to also mediate contact hypersensitivity, graft rejection, as well as immunity to some pathogens e.g., brucella, salmonella, and listeria. These pathogens are intracellular parasites and are, therefore, largely inaccessible to the action of serum antibodies.

Like the humoral response, the cell-mediated mechanism is specific for the immunizing agent, and an anamnestic response is elicited when the host has previous exposure to the pathogen/antigen. That this specificity resides in the T lymphocytes is further proved by the fact that treatment with anti-T-serum obliterates this response.

Unlike the humoral system, however, exposure of an immune animal to an intracellular pathogen results in a transient state of increased resistance to other unrelated intracellular pathogens. Therefore, even though the initiation of the cell-mediated response is specific, requiring the interaction of sensitized lymphocytes with the specific antigen, the resulting protection is relatively nonspecific. The state of increased nonspecific resistance is associated with and dependent upon macrophage activation i.e., increase in macrophage number, phagocytic ability, and bactericidal activity. That lymphocytes are capable of inducing macrophage activation is demonstrable in vitro after exposure of sensitized lymphocytes to antigen. This does not occur with nonsensitized lymphocytes and can be shown to be related to elaboration by the lymphocytes of lymphokines. The activity of these may also be demonstrated in vivo.

Thus, the results and benefits of the cell-mediated immune (CMI) response are brought about, at least to a major extent, by activated macrophages, and are to some extent independent of the cause of activation. The CMI response may be enhanced by (1) creation of a lymphocyte population which can react with the required antigen; or (2) activation of macrophages by other means, e.g., drug, alternate antigen, mitogens, etc.

Immunization is the oldest method of enhancement, dating back in the Middle Ages when the Turks used intranasal administration of crusts from smallpox lesions as vaccine. The discovery of attenuated organisms by Jenner in 1796 made immunization a much safer procedure and since that time immunization has been one of the most important steps in disease control, second only to public health measures. A large number of vaccines has been developed and some of them mediate protection by inducing a CMI response. In individuals in whom immunity cannot be actively induced because of an acquired or congenital defect in the immune system or in those who do not have time for active immunization, immunity can be passively produced by transfusion of lymphocytes from an immune individual. Such a transfusion, however, will also transfer cellular antigens and this will lead in 5–15 days to the destruction of transfused lymphocytes arising from the recognition of "nonself" antigens by the host lymphocytes or it may lead to death of the host due to graft versus host reaction as is found in immunologically incompetent animals.

In 1949, Lawrence demonstrated that, in man, intact lymphocytic cells are not required for transference of cell-mediated activity, but the same effect can be produced by infusion of disrupted leukocytes. In addition, the duration of the transferred immune responses was measured in months instead of days. This transfer factor (TF) is defined by its ability to convert a population of unsensitized lymphocytes to a sensitized population capable of responding to those antigens to which the donor was capable of responding. This appears then to transfer the immunologic memory of the donor to the recipient. TF has been difficult to characterize since it can be assayed only in humans. It is inactivated by heat at 56°C for 30 min, but not by trypsin, RNase, or DNase. It is dialyzable, retains its activity upon long-term storage, and has a molecular weight of less than 10,000. Recipients become reactive to antigen 1–7 days after receiving the extract and after receiving extract from as few as 10^7 total lymphocytes. TF is very weakly antigenic or nonantigenic, it is also unaffected by the action of anti-immunoglobulin serum and is too small to be an informational molecule. Lymphocytes sensitized by exposure to TF appear capable of synthesizing new TF.

TF has been used in the following clinical situations: (1) congenital immunodeficiency diseases, e.g., Wiskott-Aldrich syndrome, (2) infectious diseases in which acquired defects in CMI are associated with chronicity and progression of disease in face of standard therapy, and (3) cancer (see Chapter 5).

Since CMI is important in intracellular infections, TF would be expected to be of value only in viral, fungal, and mycobacterial infections. Unfortunately, most chronic diseases of this sort have spontaneous remissions and exacerbations, so that placebo-treated controls are necessary in order to clearly evaluate responses to therapy.

Successful therapeutic application of TF has been reported by Kempe in a child with disseminated vaccinia, who showed progression of lesions after treatment with serum with high titer antibody. Development of cutaneous reactivity after treatment with TF was also noted simultaneously. Similar successful therapeutic application of TF in adults has been reported by O'Connell and coworkers. These workers observed that clinical recovery from the infection was associated with acquisition of DHS to vaccinia virus after transfer of viable leukocytes bearing TF obtained from vaccinia-sensitive donors. This patient also developed concomitant local DHS to vaccinia virus in pock sites widely spread on the skin. A relapse was observed in this patient after this temporary relief and a second course of viable sensitized cells were promptly reinfused. This time, the patient was cured without further relapse.

Successful therapeutic use of TF has been achieved in a child with disseminated candidiasis persisting for several years. This patient was refractory to treatment with amphotericin and repeated administration of immunoglobulin. David achieved successful treatment of patients with chronic disseminated candidiasis with TF from a candida-sensitive donor and this recovery was accompanied by appearance of positive skin reactivity as well as production of migration inhibitory factor by the patient's leukocytes when exposed to antigen in vitro. There are other reports of successful application of TF in the treatment of disseminated coccidioidomycosis. Graybill and coworkers prepared TF from either leukocyte extract or from supernatants of sensitive leukocytes incubated with coccidiodin which was then dialyzed out of the cell-free supernatant solution. Both this antigen-liberated TF and extract TF were found to be effective in two of three patients suffering from disseminated coccidioidomycosis, resisting chemotherapy with amphotericin for several years. These two patients showed clinical remission for a long period of time. All three patients showed migration inhibitory factor production, whereas positive DHS and lymphocyte transformation were observed in two and one of them, respectively.

TF was successfully used for treating patients with anergic leprosy. Four patients received TF and five others received whole lymphocytes in this study. The latter group (five patients) rejected the lymphocytes they received as a homograft forming TF. Erythematous changes within leprous skin lesions, erythema nodosum, and arthralgia were manifested in various degrees in patients of both groups. Positive DHS to *Mycobacterium leprae* antigens was noted in seven of these nine patients, indicating a conversion rate of more than 77% in contrast to only 15% DHS conversion in patients treated with chemotherapy alone. Long-term follow-up of these patients, however, was not reported.

TF has been used for the treatment of Wiskott-Aldrich syndrome, with prompt conversion to positive delayed hypersensitivity and eradication of the severe infections. Two of three patients with Swiss-type a-γ-globulinemia responded to TF with positive delayed skin reactivity.

Of other viral infections, subacute sclerosing panencephalitis, a chronic progressive encephalitis thought to be attributable to measles virus and accompanied by anergy to measles antigen, has been studied. Approximately half of the patients were able to respond to measles antigen after TF treatment but this did not appear to affect the clinical course. Application of TF in patients with malignancy has been made with various degrees of success. These are discussed in detail in Chapter 5. Various clinical applications of TF are shown in Tables 7.1 and 7.2.

As discussed above, the benefits of a specifically-induced CMI response may be obtained to some degree by macrophage activation from any cause. This can be achieved through exposure of the patient to an antigen to which he is sensitive such as BCG or dinitrochlorobenzene and using the activated macrophages for a purpose unrelated to the initial stimulus. BCG has been used to enhance CMI in the treatment of warts, recurrent herpes simplex and herpes progenitalis. Dinitrochlorobenzene application to warts has been used, as has repeated small pox immunization for recurrent herpes simplex infection. However, no controlled trials have been performed. There is no evidence that any of these are more effective than other means and complications of therapy are not uncommon.

Enhancement by drugs has received some attention since the demonstration that levamisole can enhance some immune responses. Levamisole is an antihelminthic used widely against intestinal parasites in animals and humans. In vitro levamisole increases the responsiveness of lymphocytes to antigens and mitogens. Effects on phagocytic function and

TABLE 7.1. *TF Immunotherapy in Infectious Diseases: Summary of Various Reported Studies*[a]

Disease	TF[b] source	Immune reactivity			Clinical improvement
		DHS	MIF[c]	LT[d]	Number improved/number tested
Viral					
Measles	Rubeola positive		+	0	2/2
Subacute sclerosing panencephalitis	Rubeola positive		+	0	3/7
Congenital herpes	Herpes positive				1/1
Mycobacterial					
Leprosy	Lepromin positive	+		0	6/9 reversal[e]
Tuberculosis	Tuberculin positive	+	+	+	1/1
Fungal					
Coccidioidomycosis	Coccidiodin positive	+	+	+	2/3
Candidiasis	Candida positive	+	+		0/2
	Candida positive	+	+		1/1
	Candida positive	+		+	1/1
	Candida positive	+	+	+	2/5
	Candida positive	+	+		1/7
	Candida positive	+	+	+	1/1
	Candida positive	+	+	0	5/5
	Candida positive	+		+	1/1
	Candida positive	+			2/2

[a] Modified from: Lawrence, H. S.: Selective immunotherapy with transfer factor. In *Clinical Immunobiology*, edited by F. H. Bach and R. A. Good. New York, Academic Press, vol. 2, 1974, p. 115.

[b] Highly purified dialysate preparation.

[c] Migration inhibitory factor.

[d] Lymphocyte transformation developed.

[e] Coincident with the acquisition of lepromin sensitivity, the patients proceeded to initiate delayed hypersensitivity inflammatory reactions in multiple local skin depots of previously tolerated lepra bacilli which was considered a good prognostic sign.

chemotaxis have been also reported. In animals, enhanced reticuloendothelial function, as measured by carbon clearance, has been shown. Decreased mortality from staphylococcal and herpes infections in mice and rats, and increased resistance to induction and growth of tumors in animals have been demonstrated. In humans, skin test reactivity, as a manifestation of CMI, may be increased.

Clinically, the drug has been used with good results in the treatment of warts, but good controls are lacking. Recurrent herpes simplex infection appeared to respond to levamisole, but again, no definite conclusion can be drawn, since adequate controlled studies have not been done. Lev-

TABLE 7.2. *Immunotherapy with TF in Various Diseases in Humans*[a]

Congenital	Acquired immuno-deficiency	Cancer	Infectious disease
Wiskott Aldrich	Sarcoid	Melanoma	Vaccinia
		Sarcoma	Herpes
Swiss-type a-γ-globulinemia	Kwashiorkor marasmus	Nasopharyngeal carcinoma	Measles
			SSPE
			Candidiasis
Ataxia-telangiectasia			Coccidioidomycosis
Combined deficiency			Leprosy
			Tuberculosis
Dys-γ-globulinemia			

[a] Modified from: Lawrence, H. S.: Immunotherapy with transfer factor. In *Clinical Immunobiology,* edited by F. H. Bach and R. A. Good. New York Academic Press, vol 2, 1974, p. 115.

amisole requires extensive testing, with well-controlled studies, as well as research into its mechanism of action, before its clinical application as an immunostimulant can be recommended.

Agents that have been tested recently for systemic viral infections include iododeoxyuridine and cytosine arabinoside. Both of these agents have been shown to have significant side effects resulting in suppression of most immune functions. This severely limits their use in viral infections where CMI and interferon production are thought to play key roles in the host-defense mechanisms. Therefore, a considerable research interest has been generated in studying clinical potentials of agents that augment cellular immune responses and induce interferon formation. These include, apart from TF and levamisole, polynucleotides, and bacterial adjuvants such as BCG, tilerones, and statalon. Most of these reports relate to laboratory and animal studies. Pending their encouraging results from such investigations, large scale clinical studies will be required before they are accepted for clinical use.

The *p*-acetamidobenzoic acid salt of inosine dimethylamino-isopropanol (1:3 molar ratio) has been reported to have antiviral effects. In various clinical studies, this agent has been shown to enhance antibody synthesis in patients with viral infections. This agent also was shown to protect mice and hamsters from influenza and herpes virus infection, respectively, and this effect was interfered with by antilymphocyte globulin or cortisone acetate. This indicates the mechanism of action of isoprinosine may be mediated also through cellular immune response. Another recent report by Hadden and coworkers suggests that this agent significantly augments mitogen-induced lymphocyte proliferation, which is not dependent upon a direct action of this agent on cyclic nucleotide regulatory pathways. Further clinical evaluation of this agent is required to assess its immunopotentiating properties.

Recent studies indicate that mycobacterial cell wall fractions have adjuvant properties and have the ability to induce DHS as well as enhanced antibody response to immunogenic stimulation. It has been delineated that the peptidoglycan moiety is the adjuvant active unit in the chemical structure of the cell walls of mycobacteria. Such active fractions are also found in other organisms, like nocardia and corynebacteria. Recent data suggest that Streptococcus, Staphylococcus, Bacillus, Escherichia, Neisseria, Moraxella, Proteus, and anaerobic coryneforms also possess cell wall properties which are active as adjuvants for the induction of DHS and enhanced antibody synthesis. These data certainly suggest that an important area for future research is the development of immunoenhancing agents of significant clinical application. Chedid and coworkers have described the biologic properties of a nontoxic water soluble adjuvant (Neo-WSA) obtained by lysozyme digestion of delipidated mycobacterial cells. Neo-WSA is capable of inducing nonspecific resistance to infection in mice challenged 10 min later with *Candida albicans.* No protection was noted if Neo-WSA was administered 6 days before challenge. These studies clearly separate Neo-WSA from bacterial endotoxins, which are classical inducers of nonspecific resistance to infection.

SELECTED REFERENCES

Buckley, R. H., Lucas, Z. J., and Hattler, B. G.: Defective cellular immunity associated with chronic mucocutaneous moniliasis and current staphylococcal botryomycosis. Clin. Exp. Immunol., *3:* 153, 1968.

David, J. R.: Mediators of Cellular Immunity. Proceedings of an International Conference held at Brook Lodge, Augusta, Michigan, April 20–30, 1969; edited by H. S. Lawrence and M. Landy. New York: Academic Press, 1969.

Editorial: Levamisole. Lancet, *1:* 151, 1975.

Elin, R. J., Wolf, S. M., and Chedid, L.: Non-specific resistance to infection induced in mice by a water-soluble adjuvant derived from *Mycobacterium smegmatis.* J. Infect. Dis., *133:* 300, 1976.

Hadden, J. W., Hadden, E. M., and Coffey, R. G.: Isoprinosine augmentation of phytohemagglutinin induced lymphocyte proliferation. Infect. Immunol., *13:* 382, 1976.

Kempe, C. H.: Studies on smallpox and complications of smallpox vaccination. Pediatrics, *26:* 176, 1960.

Lawrence, H. S.: Transfer factor. Adv. Immunol., *11:* 195, 1969.

Lawrence, H. S.: Transfer factor and cellular immune deficiency disease. N. Engl. J. Med., *283:* 211, 1971.

Levin, A. S., Stites, D. P., and Spitler, L. E.: Induction of delayed hypersensitivity in a Wiscott-Aldrich patient by transfer factor. Clin. Res., *18:* 428, 1970.

O'Connel, C. J., Karzon, D. T., and Barrow, A. L.: Progressive vaccinia with normal antibodies; a case possibly due to deficient cellular immunity. Ann. Intern. Med., *60:* 282, 1964.

Van Eygen, M., Znamensky, P. Y., Heck, E., and Raymaekers, I.: Levamisole in prevention of recurrent upper respiratory-tract infections in children. Lancet, *1:* 382, 1976.

Waldman, R. H., and Ganguly, R.: Therapeutic efficacy of inosiplex (isoprinosine) in rhinovirus infection. Ann. N.Y. Acad. Sci., *284:* 153, 1977.

Chapter

8

DISEASES OF ABERRANCY OF CELL-MEDIATED IMMUNITY

Joseph E. Johnson, III, M.D.

Alterations or abnormalities in cell-mediated immunity (CMI) occur in a broad spectrum of diseases and in widely varying gradations of severity. The most pronounced disorders include the congenital syndromes of thymic hypoplasia and severe combined immunodeficiency (discussed in Chapter 3). Acquired disorders include neoplasms such as Hodgkin's disease in which deficiency of CMI appears integrally related to the basic disease process and parallels the clinical course (see Chapter 4). Acquired immunodeficiency may also result from immunosuppressive therapy, in which the suppression of CMI may vary from profound to trivial (see Chapter 4). In addition, aberrations or deviations from normal responses occur in certain infections, such as leprosy, mycobacterial and viral diseases as well as sarcoidosis and the "autoimmune" diseases. The aberrancies of immunity in these disorders may also vary in severity from relatively incidental and insignificant changes, as in some of the common viral infections, to intricate involvement in the pathogenesis and clinical expression of the disease (as in leprosy and sarcoidosis). These conditions will be discussed in greater detail in this chapter as examples of diseases of aberrancy of CMI.

Leprosy

Infection with *Mycobacterium leprae* produces a wide spectrum of disease ranging from the tuberculoid form, in which the disease is relatively limited, host cell-mediated immune response relatively intact and effective and prognosis good, to the lepromatous form in which widespread dissemination of mycobacteria occurs, cell-mediated responses are impaired and prognosis poor. In between ranges a continuum of mixed or intermediate forms. The contrasts between the two polar extremes of leprosy present useful insights into the role of the immune response in both protection from and pathogenesis of disease. Contrasting characteristics are listed in Table 8.1. In the tuberculoid form, the more limited and demarcated clinical lesions histologically show infiltrations of lymphocytes and macrophages into infected areas with the production of granulomatous foci. The relative effectiveness of this defensive host response is indicated by the paucity of mycobacteria found in the lesions and the limitation of their spread. The lesions appear to represent cell-mediated immune responses, and there is additional evidence of preservation of delayed hypersensitivity responses both to antigens of the leprosy mycobacteria as well as to other antigens. Thus, injection of *M. leprae* antigens (lepromin) intradermally evokes a slowly evolving but strong delayed-type hypersensitivity reaction. Humoral antibody responses in this form of the disease are minimal in contrast to the predominant cell-mediated immune responses.

In lepromatous leprosy, on the other hand, extensive diffuse involvement of skin occurs with massive numbers of extracellular bacteria and relatively few lymphocytes or macrophages. There is widespread involvement of lymph nodes with predominant destruction of paracortical ("thymic-dependent") areas. In this form of the disease, cell-mediated immune responses are defective as evidenced by the typically weak or negative lepromin skin test as well as moderate depression of delayed-type hypersensitivity responses to other antigens (cutaneous anergy). Antibodies to *M. leprae* antigens are formed in larger quantities and may give rise to immune complex or Arthus-type reactions ("lepra reactions") in these patients. The host defense is clearly less effective in this form of the disease, and is typically associated with a massive total body load of bacilli (up to 1×10^{12}). Prognosis is accordingly relatively poor in this less common and more serious form of disease.

Between the polar extremes, mixed or intermediate varieties occur and present a spectrum in which delayed type hypersensitivity responses correlate inversely with hyperglobulinemia and antibodies to *M. leprae*.

TABLE 8.1. *Leprosy—Polar Forms*

	Tuberculoid (Mixed)	Lepromatous
Clinical		
Nerves	Predominant involvement	±
Skin	Limited, demarcated	Extensive, diffuse
Histopathology	Granulomatous foci	Diffuse infiltrate
Bacteria in lesions	Rare	Massive
Lymph nodes		Paracortical destruction
Lepromin skin test	Positive	Negative
CMI defect	Mild	Profound
Antibodies to *M. leprae*	±	+
Prognosis	Good	Poor

Furthermore, patients may show changes in the form of the disease which reflect alterations in the immune status. Such changes may occur spontaneously or under the influence of therapy. The "reversal reaction" in lepromatous patients, for example, represents a shift toward more pronounced delayed hypersensitivity, and improving prognosis.

The heterogeneity of the clinical manifestations in leprosy apparently reflects the variable immune response of the patient and seems to depend upon the relative balance between cell-mediated responses and antibody responses. A similar range of manifestations can be produced experimentally in mice by carrying out thymectomy, irradiation, and then partial restoration with either T or B cells. Undoubtedly the immunosuppressive effects of the infection itself, especially in the lepromatous form, contribute further to the generalized defect of CMI and progression of disease.

The observed defects in CMI in lepromatous disease are listed in Table 8.2, and although "specific" anergy (to *M. leprae* antigens) is more pronounced, there is a broad depression of CMI response to nonmycobacterial antigens as well. With successful antibiotic therapy, reversal of the impaired reactivity to nonmycobacterial antigens occurs, while specific impairment of response to *M. leprae* antigens tends to persist, probably reflecting the very slow reduction in body load of *M. leprae* over many years.

The pronounced impairment of CMI in lepromatous disease has been attributed to the widespread destruction of paracortical areas of lymph nodes (a major locus of T lymphocyte "traffic"). A similar effect has been produced in murine (rat) leprosy in which a marked alteration of T lymphocyte circulation occurs, apparently as a consequence of widespread "trapping" of these cells in the lymphoid organs and spleen, paralleling the granulomatous destruction of the "lymphocyte-trafficking" areas.

If the host response is the principal determinant of the form of disease produced by infection with *M. leprae,* the factors which direct the host response are obviously of great interest. While there is no clear evidence of a genetic basis for the variations in host responses in leprosy, it is of interest that in heavily infected populations, the lepromatous form occurs

TABLE 8.2. *Lepromatous Leprosy*

Defects in CMI	
Delayed hypersensitivity (skin test)	Depressed (anergy)
Skin allograft rejection	Prolonged
Lymphocyte transformation (mitogen stimulation in vitro)	Decreased
Migration inhibitory factor production (lymphocytes in vitro)	Decreased
Circulating T lymphocytes	Decreased
Lymph nodes—"thymus-dependent (paracortical) areas"	Decreased lymphocytes

in only a limited proportion (about 1%). It has been suggested that the heterogenity of host response results in a variable balance of antibody and cell-mediated responses, accentuated by the immunosuppressive effects of the infection. Mitigating against a genetic explanation is the occurrence of reversal reactions resulting in shifts along the spectrum of disease.

The importance of CMI in defense against certain types of infections (generally "intracellular") is well demonstrated in leprosy in which CMI responses are predominantly protective while humoral (antibody) responses are not only ineffective in protection but mediate pathogenic (immune-complex) reactions.

Attempts at "reconstitution" of CMI responses using either living allogenic cells from lepromin-positive donors or transfer factor prepared from such cells has been encouraging, producing possible "reversal reactions" in some patients. This technique may prove to be a useful adjunct to antibiotic therapy.

Other Infections

A variety of other infections is also associated with depression of cell-mediated immune responses (Table 4.1). Prominant among these are viral infections, including measles and hepatitis, disseminated tuberculosis and coccidioidomycosis, and cutaneous leishmaniasis. The mechanisms by which depression of CMI occurs in these disorders appear to be quite varied. Viruses may directly infect particular subpopulations of T lymphocytes for example. On the other hand, some evidence suggests that in the case of measles, the primary effect is on the function of macrophages rather than directly upon T lymphocytes, since macrophages are necessary effector cells for many cell-mediated immune responses. Alternatively certain viruses (e.g., Newcastle disease virus) appear to attach to surface receptors on T cells and result in temporary but severe disruption of lymphocyte circulation from blood to lymph. Other viruses appear to have cytopathic effects on thymus-dependent areas of the spleen and lymph nodes. Other possible mechanisms include the elaboration of inhibitor substances (negative mediators or chalones) by infected T lymphocytes.

The specific cutaneous anergy to tuberculin seen in 35–50% of adult patients with disseminated (miliary) tuberculosis may result from a specific "desensitization" by the sudden hematogenous antigen load. Conversely in some patients loss of CMI due to other causes may itself result in inadequate defense leading to reactivation of latent infection and consequent dissemination. An additional factor which may play a part in both disseminated tuberculosis and coccidioidomycosis is the granulomatous involvement of the "thymic-dependent" areas (white pulp of the spleen and paracortical areas of lymph nodes).

Sarcoidosis

Sarcoidosis was first described as a skin disease but subsequently was recognized to be a systemic disease characterized by widespread noncaseating epithelioid and giant-cell granulomatosis. Clinical presentation may be in many forms varying from acute onset with fever, arthritis, and erythema nodosum to insidious development of pulmonary hilar lymphadenopathy. In addition to lymph nodes, many other organs may be involved including lungs, liver, spleen, skin, eyes, bones, and parotid glands. The hallmark of sarcoidosis—the noncaseating granuloma—is similar to the granuloma seen in mycobacterial, fungal, and other diseases such as berylliosis. In fact, the granuloma appears to represent a host defense response involving the cell-mediated immune system—a defensive effort to localize and destroy an invading organism or foreign body. In the case of sarcoidosis, however, the invader or pathogenetic agent has not been identified. A variety of etiologic candidates has been proposed, including mycobacteria, pine pollen, and other particulate antigens, but causal relationships have not been established.

Of particular interest in sarcoidosis have been the associated immunologic aberrations—a combination of deviations from normal unique to this disorder. One intriguing consideration is that sarcoidosis might represent an abnormal host immune response, possibly genetically determined, to a common extrinsic agent (or agents). Detailed family studies to date, however, have failed to confirm a correlation between sarcoidosis and genetic markers such as histocompatibility antigens. In any event, it seems likely that understanding of the immunologic abnormalities may represent the key to the enigma of the etiology and pathogenesis of sarcoidosis.

Immunologic Aberrations in Sarcoidosis

The most striking immunologic abnormalities in sarcoidosis consist of the depression of delayed hypersensitivity, the evidence of increased or hyperactive humoral (B cell and circulating antibody) responses and the Kveim-Siltzbach skin test phenomenon.

Impairment of CMI is indicated by the finding of cutaneous anergy to a variety of skin test antigens including tuberculin, mumps, trichophytin, and candida and refractoriness to sensitization by dinitroclorobenzene. In addition, there are decreased numbers of circulating T lymphocytes, and impaired lymphoblast transformation after mitogen stimulation (Table 8.3). Paradoxically, there is evidence of increased activation of T lymphocytes, as suggested by the finding of spontaneous morphologic transformation of T lymphocytes in long-term cultures of peripheral blood lymphocytes from sarcoid patients. Spontaneous release of migration inhibitory factor by these lymphocytes has also been demonstrated.

TABLE 8.3. *Immunologic Findings in sarcoidosis*[a]

Immunologic enhancement	Immunologic impairment
In vitro	
Spontaneous morphologic lymphoblastic transformation	Diminished lymphoblastic transformation in response to phytohemagglutinin stimulation
Spontaneous migration inhibitory factor release	Serum factor(s) inhibiting lymphoblastic transformation
Activated circulating monocytes	
In vivo	
Diffuse granulomata	Cutaneous anergy
Increased numbers of circulating B lymphocytes	Decreased numbers of circulating T lymphocytes
Hyper-γ-globulinemia	
Circulating antigen antibody complexes	

[a] Adapted from: Kateria, et al.: Am. Rev. Resp. Dis. *113:* 315, 1976.

These findings suggest the possibility that lymphocytes (and probably monocytes) in sarcoidosis may be circulating in an already activated or hyperreactive state.

With respect to humoral immune responses, immunoglobulin levels are increased as are the numbers of activated B lymphocytes. Furthermore, increased antibody levels to Epstein-Barr, herpes simplex, rubella, measles, and parainfluenza viruses are found in groups of sarcoid patients. Sarcoid patients also show enhanced antibody responses to mismatched blood as well as occasional "biologic false-positive" tests for syphillis. Circulating antigen-antibody complexes have been found in some patients with sarcoidosis.

The Kveim-Siltzbach test is an intradermal skin test using a fine saline suspension of sarcoidal tissue from spleen or lymph nodes. In sarcoid patients after 4–6 weeks, a small papule forms at the test site, which on biopsy is shown to be a noncaseating granulamatous reaction. Of patients with sarcoidosis, 60–80% have a positive test, especially in the earlier phases of the disease and in patients who present with erythema nodosum or lymphadenopathy. A reported incidence of false-positive tests in a variety of other diseases, including leprosy, regional ileitis, ulcerative colitis, and lymphadenopathies of varying etiologies has been attributed to the use of two particular lots of "defective" skin test materials. Using validated preparations, the false-positive reaction rate has been reported to be only 2%. Despite its use in diagnosis, the exact nature of the reaction remains puzzling. If it represents a hypersensitivity reaction to some component of a specific causal agent present in the suspension, it is intriguing that the reaction may diminish and disappear as the disease wanes, in contrast to the specific tuberculin and similar fungal antigen reactions in other infections. Alternatively, the reaction may be "nonspecific" with respect to a particular agent, but rather reflect some basic immunologic abberation associated with active disease. Neither possibility can be excluded at present.

Comparison with Hodgkin's Disease

Because of similarities in the granulomatous tissue reactions in Hodgkin's disease and sarcoidosis as well as the evidence of similar immunologic abnormalities, it is of interest to compare CMI in the two disorders. In both conditions, cutaneous anergy tends to parallel disease activity. Despite the similarities there are important differences (Table 8.4). In general, cell-mediated immune function is more severely depressed in Hodgkin's disease (see Chapter 4). This is reflected in greater refractoriness of Hodgkin's patients to dinitrochlorobenzene sensitization and to transfer of delayed hypersensitivity. Hodgkin's patients also show delayed homograft rejection in contrast to sarcoid patients. The addition of cortisone to tuberculin used in the intradermal skin test produces reversion to a positive test in only a small percentage of Hodgkin's patients compared to about half of sarcoid patients. Finally, unlike Hodgkin's patients, sarcoid patients do not show significant evidence of increased susceptibility to opportunistic infection. This again may represent the relatively greater suppression of CMI in Hodgkin's, or may reflect differing underlying immunologic aberrations.

Pathogenesis of Sarcoidosis

Several pathogenetic mechanisms have been postulated in sarcoidosis centering about unusual etiologic agents or aberrant host immune responses, possibly to common or multiple agents, or some combination of these possibilities. Detailed studies of the specific immunologic aberrations in sarcoidosis as summarized above have led to hypotheses which attempt to explain and integrate these observations in light of current understanding of the immunologic system. Such an hypothesis, recently advanced by Kateria and associates, is outlined in Figure 8.1. It is assumed that the initiating etiologic event is an "insult"—an infectious agent or foreign antigen which leads to sensitization of the host and in addition to alteration of lymphoid cells. A chronic immune reaction might

TABLE 8.4. *Sarcoidosis and Hodgkin's Disease*

CMI	Hodgkin's	Sarcoid
Dinitrochlorobenzene sensitization	−	±
Transfer of tuberculosis sensitivity (cells or transfer factor)	−	±
Homograft rejection	Delayed	Normal
Cortisone-tuberculin test	−	+ (50%)
Increased susceptibility to infection	+	−

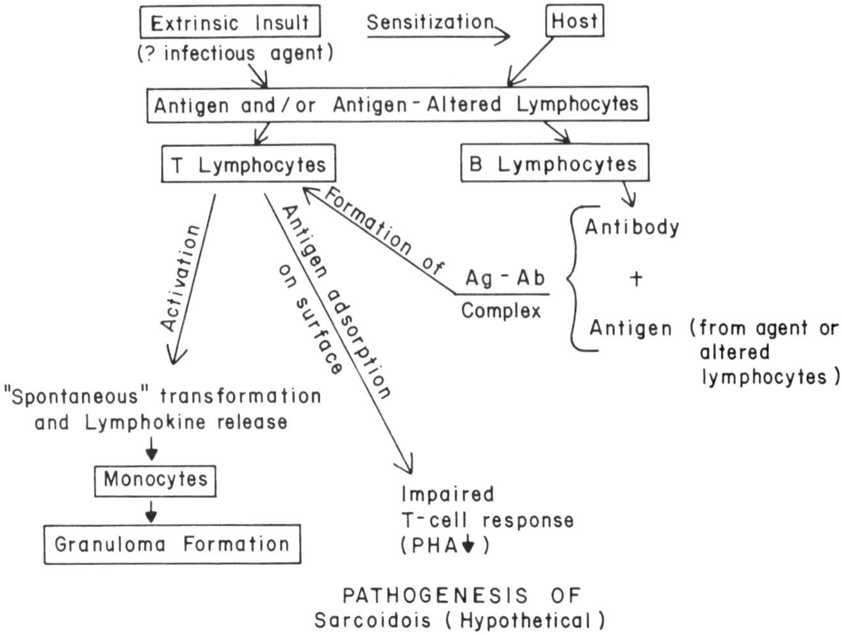

FIG. 8.1.

then be initiated with either the original agent or altered lymphocytes serving as a continuing antigen source. Hyperreactivity of both T and B lymphocytes is postulated. Antibodies synthesized by B cells could produce antigen-antibody complexes which if absorbed on the surface of T lymphocytes might impair T lymphocyte function (? by masking surface receptors). Antigen-antibody complexes might also serve as a continuing stimulus for activation of T lymphocytes (which would result in the observed enhanced spontaneous lymphoblast transformation and lymphokine release). T cell activation in turn might lead to monocyte-macrophage activation and formation of granulomata. Collectively, this sequence and interaction could explain the principal immunologic aberrations outlined in Table 8.3. Qualitative and quantitative changes in T lymphocytes would result in depression of cell-mediated immune functions including cutaneous anergy, decreased numbers of circulating T cells and decreased in vitro responses to phytohemagglutinin.

Still unanswered are the nature and specificity of the initiating agent(s) and the determinants (genetic or otherwise) directing the host responses.

Other Conditions with Aberrant Immune Responses

As indicated in Table 4.1, aberrant immune responses may be seen in a variety of "autoimmune" diseases including lupus erythematosus (see

Chapter 14). In these diseases, CMI deficiency may occur in association with other disordered immune responses but usually is not predominant.

Lymphopenic states such as chronic thoracic duct drainage, directly deplete the predominantly T cell population of the thoracic lymph and sometimes lead to profound depression of CMI. Malnutrition and other debilitated states may also lead to deficiencies in both CMI and humoral immunity.

SELECTED REFERENCES

Bode, F. R., Pare, P., and Fraser, R.G.: Pulmonary Diseases in the Compromised Host. Medicine, *53:* 255, 1974.

Bullock, W. E.: Anergy and infection. Adv. Intern. Med., *21:* 149, 1976.

Edelman, R., Suskind, R., Olson, R. E. and Sirisinha, S.: Mechanism of defective delayed hypersensitivity in children with protein-caloric malnutrition. Lancet, *1:* 506, 1973.

James, D. G., Neville, E., and Walker, A.: Immunology of sarcoidosis. Am. J. Med. *59:* 388, 1975.

Kantor, F. S.: Infection, anergy, and cell-mediated immunity. N Engl. J. Med., *292:* 629, 1975.

Kataria, Y. P., Sagone, A. L., LoBuglio, A. F., and Bromberg, P. A.: In vitro observations on sarcoid lymphocytes and their correlation with cutaneous anergy and clinical severity of disease. Am. Rev. Resp. Dis. *108:* 767, 1973.

Lim, S., Kiszkiss, D. F., Choi, Y. S., Gajl-Peczalska, K., and Good, R. A.: Immunodeficiency in leprosy. Birth Defects, *11:* 244, 1975.

Niklasson, P. M., and Williams, R. C.: Studies of peripheral blood T and B lymphocytes in acute infections. Infect. Immun., *9:* 1, 1974.

Remington, J. S.: The compromised host. Hosp. Pract. April 1972, p. 59.

Siltzbach, L. E.: The course and prognosis of sarcoidosis around the world. Am. J. Med., *57:* 847, 1974.

SECTION TWO

HUMORAL IMMUNITY

Chapter 9

FUNCTION OF THE HUMORAL IMMUNE SYSTEM

Heinz J. Wittig, M.D.

Structure of Immunoglobulins, (Fig. 9.1)

The association of antibodies with the γ-globulin fraction of animal sera was first demonstrated by Tiselius and Kabat 1939. Porter suggested the basic four-chain structure of immunoglobulins with two light and two heavy chains cross-linked by disulfide bonds. Light chains (molecular weight 22,000) have 213 (λ) or 214 (κ) amino acid residues of which 108 constitute a "variable", the remainder a "constant" region. Intrachain disulfide bonds render these chains capable of loop-formation which form the basis of an intricate tertiary structure. In the variable portion this tertiary structure exposes certain portions (the "hypervariable" portions) to the surface for antigen-binding sites. Heavy chains are about twice the length of light chains. One fourth of the length of heavy chains constitute the variable portion, and the remainder the constant portion, which is characteristic in its amino acid sequence for IgG (γ chain), IgA (α chain), IgM (μ chain), IgD (δ chain), and IgE (ϵ chain). Variable lengths of the heavy chains and their carbohydrate content account for different molecular weights of the five immunoglobulins.

The constant portion of heavy chains can be subdivided into three parts of approximately equal size, the amino acid sequence of each showing some homology. There is also some homology among different species and for the constant portion of the light chains. These homologous portions have a molecular weight of about 11,000 to 12,000 and are similar in their amino acid sequence to β-2 microglobulins. β-2 Microglobulins are a component of histocompatibility antigens and may constitute the phylogenetic precursors of humoral immunity. They are membrane-associated and occur in small quantities in the serum and urine of normal animals.

Classification, (Table 9.1)

Monomeric Immunoglobulins

IgG. Molecular weight: 150,000. There are four subclasses, IgG-1, IgG-2, IgG-3, and IgG-4 which are contained in human sera in amounts of 70, 19, 8, and 3%, respectively, of total IgG content. The subclasses differ in their ability to bind complement, with IgG-1 and IgG-3 binding complement well, IgG-2 poorly, and IgG-4 not at all. Normal IgG levels in adult sera are between 8 and 16 mg/ml of serum.

IgD. Molecular weight 150,000. Function of IgD is unknown, although it is present in human sera in quantities of 0.003 –0.4 mg/ml of serum.

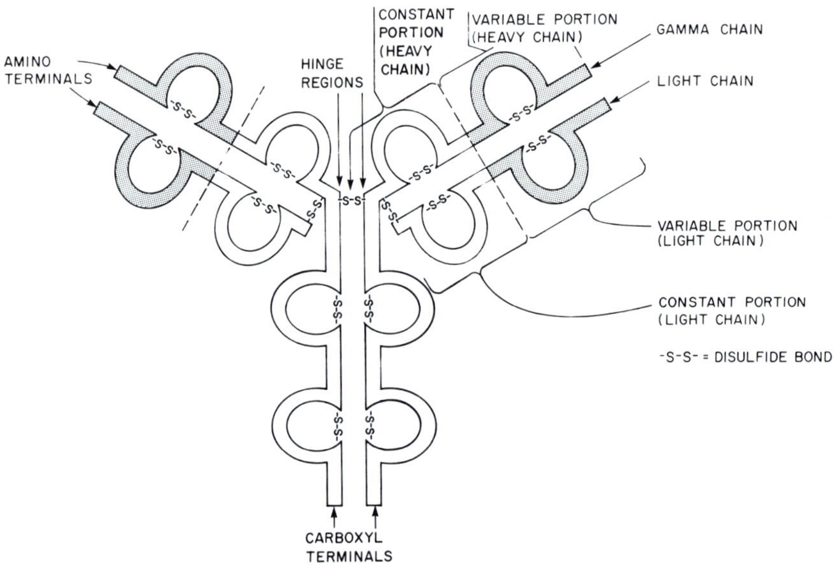

FIG. 9.1. Model of IgG molecule with important "landmarks" noted.

TABLE 9.1. *Properties of Human Immunoglobulins*

Properties	IgG	IgA	IgM	IgD	IgE
Serum concentration	800–1800 mg/100 ml	140–420 mg/100 ml	50–190 mg/100 ml	0.3–40 mg/100 ml	10–600 ng/ml
Complement fixation	+	0[a]	++	0	0
Placental passage	+	0	0	0	0
Secretory	0	+	0	0	+
Skin sensitizing (> 24 hr)	0	0	0	0	+
Size ($S_{20,w}$)	6.5–7.0	7, 11	18–20	6.2–6.8	8.0
Light chain types	κ, λ	κ, λ	κ, λ	κ, λ	κ, λ
Heavy chain types	γ	α	μ	δ	ϵ

[a] Not by classical pathway (see Chapter 10).

IgD does not appear to bind complement. It appears on the surface of B cells early in the course of events that lead to antibody formation.

IgE. Molecular weight 200,000 (ϵ chains are about 100 amino acids longer than γ chains). IgE contains skin-sensitizing antibody of atopy. Normal levels: 10–600 ng/ml of serum. Elevations up to several thousand nanograms are found in atopic patients and in patients with helminthic infestations.

Serum IgA. Molecular weight 180,000 due to higher carbohydrate content than IgG. There are sublcasses (IgA-1 and IgA-2). IgA does not fix complement by the classical pathway (see Chapter 10). Normal serum levels are 1.4–4.2 mg/ml of serum.

Polymeric Immunoglobulins

IgA. This occurs as dimers, trimers, and higher polymers which are connected to each other via disulfide bonds at the "hinge region" of the heavy chains. This linkage is further strengthened by the "J-chain." Polymeric IgA is only produced by plasma cells of mucosal association while IgA produced elsewhere (lymph nodes etc.) is monomeric. IgA dimers and trimers pass through mucosal surfaces into secretions, and, during this passage, become associated with "secretory component" which is produced in epithelial cells. Secretory component has a molecular weight of about 60,000. Its function is not completely known, but is thought to (1) aid IgA-precursor lymphocytes to "home" to mucosal sites, (2) aid in transport of IgA from the submucosal plasma cells through the epithelial cells onto the luminal surface, and (3) protect the molecule against proteolysis.

IgM. The vast majority of IgM occurs in the serum as a pentamer and has a molecular weight of 900,000 due to the added weight of about 100 amino acids per μ chain as compared with γ chains. The five monomers of pentameric IgM are linked at the hinge region of the heavy chains with one J-chain reinforcing this linkage (Fig. 9.2).

Phylogeny

Plants

Plants have no actual antibodies. Two lectins (pokeweed mitogen and concanavalin A) have hemagglutinating properties but no structural resemblance to immunoglobulins.

Invertebrates

Moth larvae have a bactericidin, suggesting some humoral protective mechanisms. This substance is of low molecular weight and is probably not protein.

Spiny lobsters possess a bactericidin which appears to be of protein nature and resembles antibody.

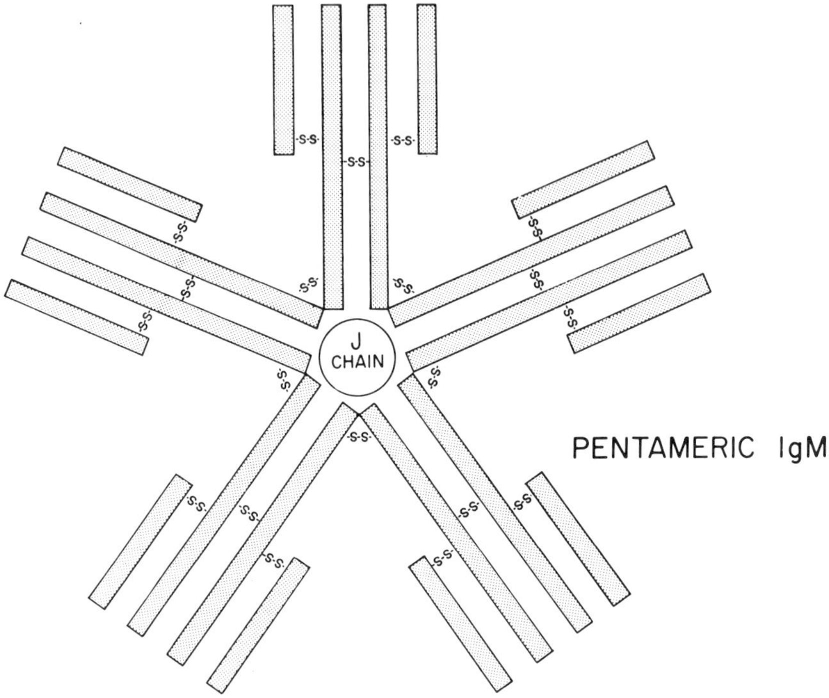

FIG. 9.2. Model of IgM.

Oysters and horseshoe crabs both are capable of producing a hemagglutinin with polypeptide chains of molecular weight 22,500 which are reminiscent of light chains in their structure.

Cyclostomes

Good and Papermaster found hagfish to have a serum globulin which resembles immunoglobulins chemically but could not induce antibody formation in that animal. Hagfish also have white cells which resemble lymphocytes but do not respond with delayed hypersensitivity to antigenic challenges or attempts of transplantation. Thoenes and Hildemann used repeated antigenic stimulation with keyhole limpet hemocyanin, and were able to show good antibody formation of a 28S size which they suspected to be a dimer of 19S IgM.

Lampreys are cyclostomes which abound in the Great Lakes of North America and were found by Marchalonis and Edelman to produce 6S and 14S antibodies to bacteriophage f_2. Both types of antibodies appeared to be antigenically identical and possessed heavy and light chains which were, in contrast to immunoglobulins of higher animals, not covalently linked. Otherwise they resemble IgM chemically.

Higher Fish

All higher fish are able to produce monomeric and polymeric antibody of IgM characteristics.

Amphibians and Reptiles

Amphibians retain the fish's ability to make IgM antibody, but in addition produce the more efficient IgG type antibody which has significant immunologic memory. These characteristics hold true for the reptile family.

Birds

Birds can produce very efficient IgG (also called IgY by some investigators) and IgM antibodies. Birds have a characteristic lymphoid organ attached to the cloaca which is associated with the genesis of humoral immunity: the bursa of Fabricius (anatomist in Padua, late 16th century). Glick and his associates found that removal of this organ inhibits the development of humoral immunity. Birds also possess a well-defined thymus.

Ontogeny

The development of fetal and neonatal humoral immunity is, in part, described in Chapter 11. Important aspects of this subject are tolerance and the development of the complement system.

Tolerance during Neonatal Development

The neonate is equipped with adult levels of IgG which is obtained from the maternal pool. Selective transfer for IgG across the placenta excludes IgM, IgA, IgD, and IgE antibodies of maternal origin.

This maternally transferred IgG conveys a considerable degree of immunity to the fetus and neonate for certain bacterial and viral infections.

If the fetus becomes infected with rubella virus from the mother during the first trimester of pregnancy, this precedes the fetal ability of recognizing rubella as nonself and the fetus makes no antibody to the virus. If infection occurs after the first trimester, a high antibody titer to rubella virus results, but there still may be inadequate defense against the viral infection because of the survival of virus in an intracellular environment which may elude humoral antibody function.

Passively transferred maternal antibodies may either suppress or enhance the baby's own immunologic response. Perkins et al. observed that there is diminished immunity from polio vaccination in the presence of maternal antibody. A similar effect was described by Smith on the immune response to Salmonella immunization. However, Levi et al.

showed that at a certain antigen/maternal antibody ratio the infant's responses to pertussis, diphtheria, and tetanus antigens is enhanced, as compared to the response to antigen alone.

Development of the Complement System

C3 and C4 have been detected in the serum of human fetuses older than 15 weeks, C3 levels being about half of adult levels by the 24th week of gestation.

Function

IgG

Like other immunoglobulin classes, the multivalency of IgG enables it to form a lattice and, thereby, precipitate with antigenic material. The larger precipitate particles are easily phagocytized and eliminated. The defense against bacterial infection is primarily mediated by the complement system, through chemotactic activity and opsonization of bacterial cells which will be described in greater detail in Chapter 10.

Aside from its precipitating and complement-fixing properties, IgG acts as neutralizing antibody for toxins and viruses, and as the "blocking antibody" which is measurable in the wake of hyposensitizing therapy in allergic disease. The impact of deficiencies of IgG antibody is discussed in Chapter 11).

IgM

IgM, due its large molecular size, is primarily present in the intravascular space. It has a strong complement-binding capacity and contains most of the antibodies against somatic 0-antigens of gram-negative bacilli, cold agglutinins, isohemagglutinins, the Wasserman antibody, heterophile antibody, and rheumatoid factor. In patients with absent IgA there have been IgM antibodies found in secretions.

IgM is a more primitive antibody than IgG and appears to precede IgG during an immune response. IgM production, unlike IgG, does not increase on repeated stimulation with the same antigen.

IgA, (Fig. 9.3)

The vast majority of IgA in the serum is monomeric, while secretory IgA exists predominantly as dimers (see "Structure of Immunoglobulins"). Of great interest is the control of production and secretion of mucosal IgA. Pertaining to this is a recent patient reported by Strober et al. who described a 15-year-old boy with chronic intestinal candidiasis who had abundant monomeric serum IgA but complete absence of IgA in salivary and jejunal secretions. Biopsy of the jejunum showed absent secretory component production. Treatment with bovine colostrum induced clinical improvement.

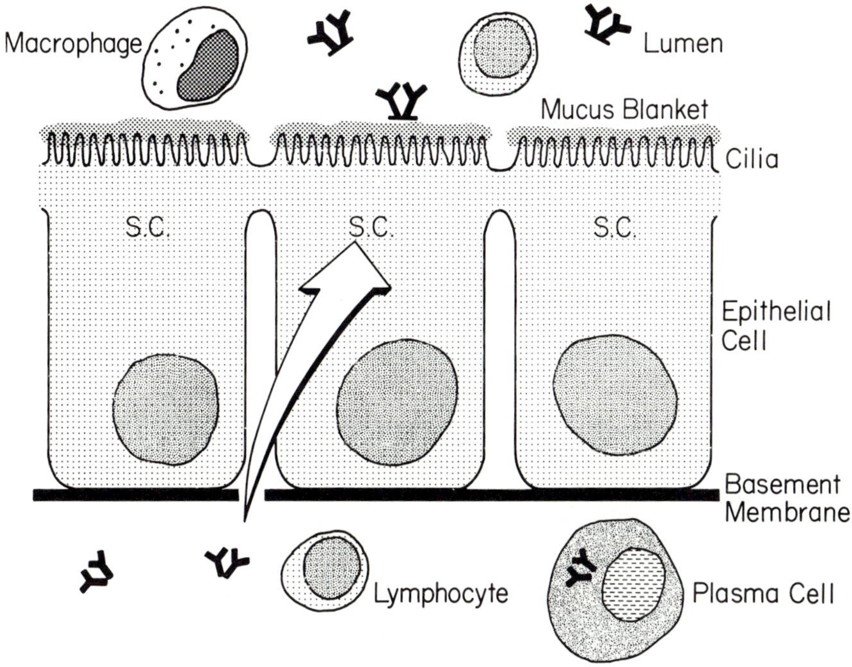

FIG. 9.3. Mucosal surface, such as respiratory epithelium, showing various host defense mechanisms, including production and transport of secretory IgA. S.C. = secretory component. "Double Y's" represent IgA dimer. "Double Y's" with bar underneath represent IgA with S.C., i.e., secretory IgA.

The authors raised the question of whether (1) secretory IgA producing B cells home to the intestinal lamina propria only if secretory component is produced by the adjacent epithelial cells in such tissues, or (2) secretory component is only produced in epithelial cells if dimeric IgA is produced by the B-cell population of the respective lamina propria.

Secretory IgA constitutes the first line of defense against infection and/or ingress of foreign protein at the mucosal level. Because of its poor ability to fix complement, IgA can neutralize viral and other foreign antigens at the mucosal level without danger of secondary tissue damage. The significance of the role of secretory IgA is exemplified by the pathogenesis of infantile bronchiolitis due to respiratory syncytial virus infection. Since IgA is practically absent from the young infant's mucosal coverings the virus combines with maternally transferred IgG antibody with resulting complement fixation, chemotaxis of leukocytes, and tissue damage by leukocytic proteolytic enzymes. The older child handles the infection of syncytial virus simply by its neutralization by secretory IgA with inconsequential morbidity. Low secretory IgA in the gut has been thought to be associated with food allergy, particularly to cow's milk proteins. Aside from the gastrointestinal and respiratory tracts, the urinary tract, salivary glands, the genital mucosae, and the conjunctivae all bear a protective coating of secretory IgA.

IgD

The function of IgD is unknown. Patients who are allergic to penicillin sometimes contain high titers of penicillin-specific IgD in their sera. In one series of atopic children, serum IgD levels were found to be lower than those of a normal control group. IgD antibody to insulin has been observed in some diabetic patients.

IgE

This most recently discovered and most sparsely represented serum immunoglobulin has been the subject of extensive study during the last decade, primarily because of its detrimental role. Most normal humans have some IgE. How much of this is normal and how much indicative of some pathology is still a matter of discussion. IgE levels are not, like those of other immunoglobulins, measured in terms of milligrams or even micrograms per unit of serum, but rather in nanograms per milliliters or International Units (IU), with one IU being approximately 2 ng. Most tabulations of IgE measurements in normal populations indicate a non-Gaussian distribution with the mode lying in a low level and scattered high levels forming a tail of the curve towards high levels in an asymmetric fashion. Most tabulations, therefore, use a geometric mean and geometric standard deviations which make the data more Gaussian in appearance (Fig. 9.4). Recently revised IgE norms, based on measure-

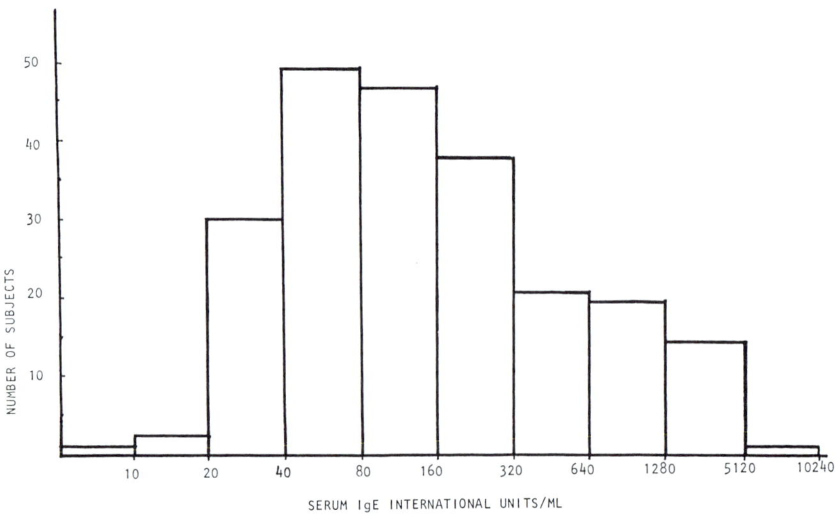

FIG. 9.4. Serum IgE levels in individuals without allergic disease.

ments in a Swedish population, were geometric means for 2 year olds of 10 IU, for 10 year olds of 39 IU, and for adults of 26 IU, indicating a rise of IgE levels in early childhood and a fall in adulthood.

In atopic patients and in patients with helminthic infestations, levels are up to 50,000 IU. Figure 9.5 represents the IgE measurements of 277 patients with bronchial asthma expressed as geometric means for age groups. The data suggest that asthma of younger patients is more strongly associated with high IgE levels than that of older adults. The genes for high IgE levels appear to be present in about 13% of the Caucasian population. However, individuals lacking the genes can be induced to produce large quantities of IgE upon intense contact with the antigens from nematodes. Genetic studies appear to indicate that the control of serum IgE levels is multifactorial, with contributions both from the X-chromosome and from chromosome 6 which carries the HLA loci.

The function of the IgE molecule is associated with its ability to attach itself to the membrane of mast cells. If two IgE molecules are situated on a mast cell surface in close proximity and are bridged by an antigen, a series of poorly understood events is initiated resulting in the extrusion of mast cell granules and liberation of mediators which, in turn, cause the allergic tissue reaction. Histamine, the most important of these mediators, effects capillary leakage (edema), smooth muscle contraction (asthma, diarrhea), and stimulation of afferent neural elements (pruritus, vagal reflexes).

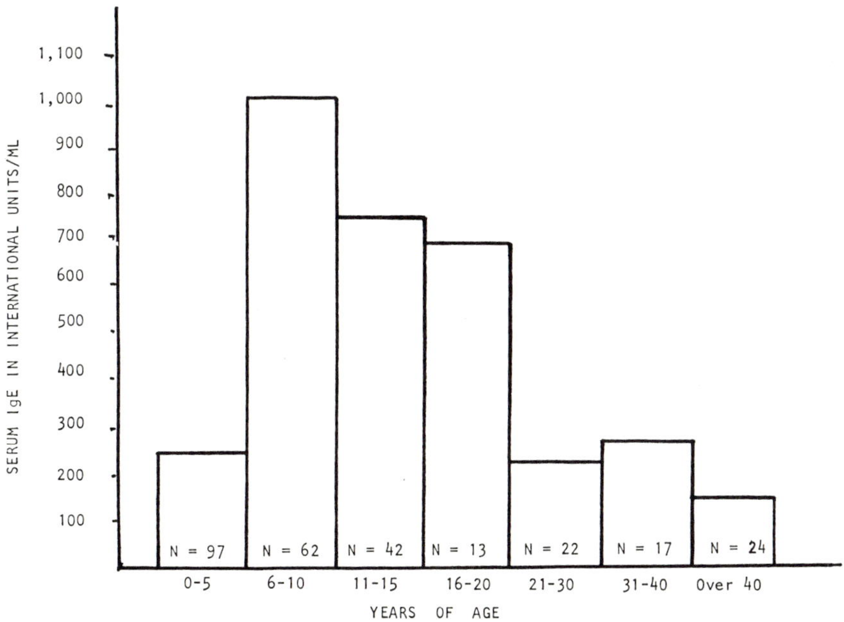

FIG. 9.5. Mean geometric serum IgE levels by age groups—patients with asthma.

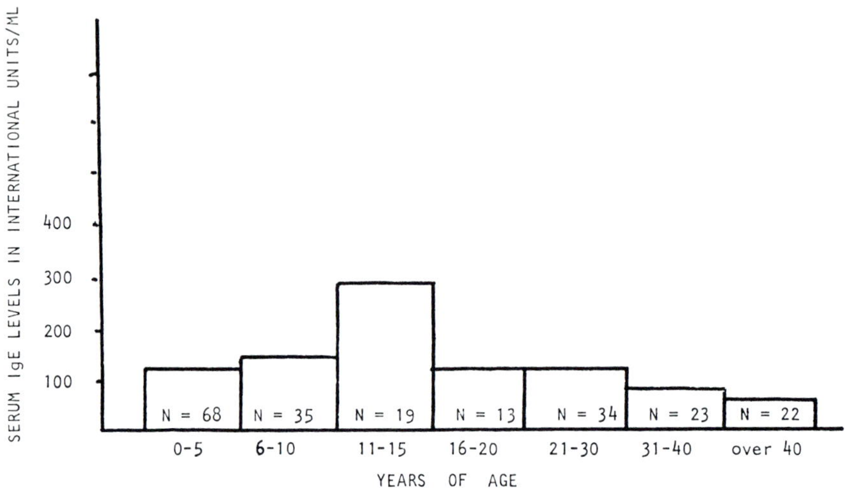

FIG. 9.6. Mean geometric serum IgE levels by age groups—patients with hayfever, hives, etc. but without asthma.

IgE-producing B cells are largely concentrated in the lamina propria of skin and of mucosal surfaces (similar to IgA) and the concentration of such B cells in certain organs of atopic patients may determine the specific organ involvement of their allergic manifestations. Consequently, if such increased B cell aggregations occur in areas of large surfaces (e.g., skin in atopic dermatitis or lung in bronchial asthma), many B cells will be stimulated by antigens to secrete large amounts of IgE which is reflected in a high serum level. If the anatomical involvement is small (e.g., nose, eye) the atopic reaction may be severe in that respective organ and yet not involve enough B cells to result in a significantly elevated serum IgE level (Fig. 9.6). This limits the value of serum IgE measurements in labeling a person as atopic or nonatopic. Measurements of secretory IgE may solve the dilemma in such situations.

SELECTED REFERENCES

Clem, L. W., and Small, P. A.: Phylogeny of immunoglobulin structure and function. I. Immunoglobulins of the lemon shark. J. Exp. Med., *125:* 893, 1967.

Devey, M., Carter, D., Sanderson, C. J., and Coombs, R. R. A.: IgD antibody to insulin. Lancet, *2:* 1280, 1970.

Gerrard, J. W., Horne, S., Vickers, P., MacKenzie, J. W. A., Goluboff, N., Garson, J. Z., and Maninga, C. A.: Serum IgE levels in parents and children. J. Pediat. *85:* 660, 1974.

Gleich, G. J., Bieger, R. C., and Stankievic, R.: Antigen combining activity associated with immunoglobulin D. Science, *165:* 606, 1969.

Glick, B., Chang, T. S., and Jaap, R. G.: The bursa of Fabricius and antibody production. Poult. Sci., *35:* 224, 1956.

Good, P. A., and Papermaster, B. W.: Ontogeny and phylogeny of adaptive immunity. Adv. Immunol., *4:* 1, 1964.

Huggins, K. G., and Brostoff, J.: Local production of specific IgE antibodies in allergic rhinitis patients with negative skin tests. Lancet, *2:* 148, 1975.

Kjellman, N-I. M., Johansson, S. G. O., and Roth, A.: Serum IgE levels in healthy children quantified by a sandwich technique (PRIST). Clin. Allergy, *6:* 57, 1976.

Levi, M. I., Kravtov, F. E., Levova, T. M., and Fomenko, F. A.: The ability of maternal antibody to increase the immune response in infants. Immunology, *16:* 145, 1969.

Marchalonis, J., and Edelman, G. M.: Phylogenetic origins of antibody structure. III. Antibodies in the primary immune response of the sea lamprey, Petromyzon marinus. J. Exp. Med., *127:* 891, 1968.

Porter, R.: The structure of gammaglobulins and antibodies. In *Symposium on Basic Problems in Neoplastic Disease,* edited by A. Gelhorn and E. Hirschberg. New York. Columbia University Press, 1962, p. 177.

Smith, R. T., Eitzman, D. V., Catlin, M. E., Wirtz, E. O., and Miller, B. E.: The development of the immune response. Characterization of the response of the human infant and adult to immunization with Salmonella vaccines. Pediatrics, *33:* 163, 1964.

Strober, W., Krakauer, R., Klaeveman, H. L., Reynolds, H. Y., and Nelson, D. L.: Secretory component deficiency. A disorder of the IgA immune system. N. Engl. J. Med., *294:* 351, 1976.

Tiselius, A., and Kabat, E. A.: An electrophoretic study of immune sera and purified antibody preparations. J. Exp. Med. *69:* 119, 1939.

Chapter 10

THE COMPLEMENT SYSTEM

Jacques Caldwell, M.D.

The complement system is comprised of a group of proteins normally present in plasma and other extracellular fluids in a precursor state. Appropriate stimuli alter these proteins so that they interact in a sequential fashion, reminiscent of the clotting cascade. The end result of these enzymatic interactions is the generation of a variety of biologically active substances which promote an inflammatory response. These biologically active substances are very important in promoting host defense against infection, in modulating lymphocyte responses, and perhaps even in rejection of certain tumors.

Generation of the biologically active principles of complement can be accomplished in at least two ways: (1) activation of the classic complement pathway by antibody-antigen interaction and (2) by activation of the alternative or properdin pathway which is probably less efficient than the classical complement pathway and which is antibody independent (Fig. 10.1). Activation of either pathway produces enzymes which cleave the third component of complement. Fragments from C3 have chemotactic and anaphylatoxic properties and sustain further propagation of the complement enzymatic chain.

Activation of the classical complement pathway is affected by interaction of IgG subclasses 1, 2, and 3 or IgM with antigen. Such antigen-antibody reactions result in conformational changes in the Fc portion of the antibody molecule allowing binding to a portion of first complement component, C1q—a highly positively charged subunit which is responsible for binding to antibodies and to other negatively charged substances. Binding results in alterations in the other two subunits of C1—C1r and C1s and the conversion of C1s from a precursor to an active serine esterase enzyme. The antigen-antibody-C1 complex subsequently cleaves the next two interacting molecules of the complement sequence, C4 and

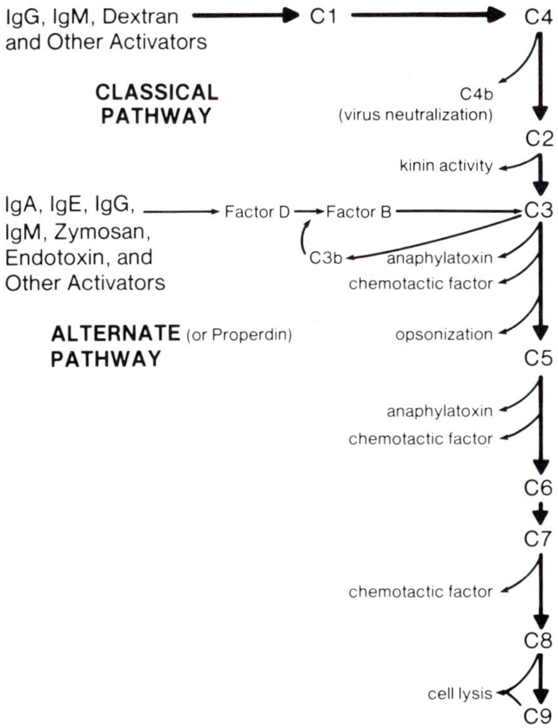

FIG. 10.1. Simplified representation of complement system, showing both the classical and alternate pathways.

C2, which are the natural substrates of C1s. The attachment of C4 to an immune complex containing a virus antigen produces the first biologically important effect of complement, enhancement of virus neutralization. Thus the attachment of antibody, C1, and C4 to certain viruses impairs the ability of the virus to infect the cells and to propagate.

After splitting and fixation of a large piece of C4 to the antigen-antibody complex, C2 is split. A large fragment of C2 affixes to the antigen-antibody complex and generates a second enzyme—C3 convertase—which is capable of cleaving the C3 molecule. The smaller split products of C4 and C2, which do not attach to the immune complex, may combine independently of the immune complex to form a highly vasoactive substance which is capable of enhancing protein leakage from the intravascular space.

Splitting of C3 results in the production of two fragments; a small fragment, C3a, with a molecular weight of about 9000. It has two important biologic activities. It is an anaphylatoxin, i.e., it is capable of releasing histamine and other mediators from mast cells and it is a potent chemotactic factor for polymorphonuclear leucocytes and eosinophiles. A larger fragment of C3, C3b, has several functions. Attachment of C3b to the immune complex renders the complex "biologically sticky" i.e., it is capable of attaching to specific receptor sites on polymorphonuclear leucocytes and macrophages. Cells or bacteria with C3b attached to their surface adhere to the C3b receptors on phagocytic cells, thereby increasing the efficiency with which the phagocytic cells can ingest the substances. Attachment of C3b to B lymphocytes stimulates the production and release of lymphokines.

The next reacting complement component is C5. Cleavage of C5 produces two major fragments: C5a, a low molecular weight fragment which has anaphylactoid and chemotactic functions similar to C3a, and is chemotactic for both polymorphonuclear leucocytes and monocytes; and the large molecular weight fragment, C5b, which is capable of attaching to the immune complex; it may play a role in opsonization and phagocytosis of yeast.

C5b, C6, and C7 interact to form a trimolecular complex, C567, which also has chemotactic activity for polymorphonuclear leucocytes. The interaction of C5 with C6, C7, C8, and C9 forms a molecular complex which attacks and disrupts the osmotic integrity of certain cell membranes and allows osmotic lysis to ensue. It is important to recognize that not all cell membranes are susceptible to lysis by complement. The most susceptible types of cells seem to be those belonging to the hematopoietic system.

In the last several years, a second means of generating the biologic products from C3-9 has been described in some detail. This is the properdin or alternative pathway of complement activation. This pathway can be activated by certain polysaccharides, by lipopolysaccharide such as endotoxin, by certain bacterial products, and complexes containing IgA.

The first protein initiating factor, is poorly defined but is activated by a variety of substances such as endotoxin, inulin, polymerized flagellin, pneumococcal polysaccharide, pokeweed mitogen, and yeast cell walls. Activation results in loose association of a split product of native C3, C3b with a third protein, factor B of the alternative pathway system. The C3b-B complex is then acted upon by factor D which, in the presence of magnesium ion, results in the production of a C3 cleaving enzyme which splits C3 into its subunits, C3a and C3b. The C3b-factor B complex can attach to cell membranes and in the presence of the stabilizing influence of the protein properdin can lead to the self-assembly of the membrane attack complex composed of C5-9, with resultant lysis of the cell.

Measurement of Complement Proteins

Clinical measurement of complement proteins has proved useful for the diagnosis and follow-up of the clinical course of certain illnesses. In general, measurement of only three of these proteins, C4, C3, and C1 inhibitor, has been clinically relevant. The easiest method of measuring these proteins is by radial immunodiffusion in gel (Mancini technique). For most purposes, this technique is perfectly adequate for quantitating complement; however, it fails to distinguish between native and inactivated complement proteins. This distinction is sometimes important in clinical disease. Measurement of enzymatically active (native) complement components can be performed by making use of their ability to participate in the lysis of sensitized sheep erythrocytes. A standard concentration of sensitized sheep erythrocytes is incubated with an excess amount of all complement components except the one being measured. Dilutions of the biologic fluid which are being assayed are added, and, after incubation, the lysis of the red cells can be measured spectrophotometrically. The degree of lysis can be related to the amount of the complement enzymatic activity.

Measurement of complement components is helpful to the clinician in relatively few clinical settings. Measurement of the C1 inhibitor (C1 Inh) is useful for establishing the diagnosis of hereditary angioedema. In this disease the C1 Inh is congenitally absent or, in about 10% of patients, the C1 Inh protein is produced but is biologically inactive. C4 levels are also low in hereditary angioedema as a result of the unimpeded action of activated C1 on C4. In the normal individual C4 destruction by C1 is limited by the C1 Inh. Occasionally, low levels of C1 Inh occur in patients with acquired angioedema who have 7S IgM in their serum.

Measurement of C4 in serum can be very helpful in following the course of patients with certain immune complex diseases such as systemic lupus erythematosus. The activity of these diseases is characterized by the presence of circulating antigen-antibody complexes which activate C1 and lead to C4 consumption. In patients with lupus, active disease is signaled, in over 75% of cases, by the finding of a low C4 as measured by the Mancini technique. If measurements of C4 activity are conducted by the hemolytic assay, low levels of C4 are found in nearly 90% of individuals with active disease.

In years past, the concentration of C3 was used to determine the activity of lupus erythematosus, particularly of lupus nephritis. Most investigators find that low levels of C3 are found in only about a third of patients with recognizable nephritis. In patients with lupus nephritis whose disease has been brought under control by the administration of long-term steroid therapy, a spuriously low level of C3 may be found; this does not necessarily reflect active tissue destruction by circulating immune complexes but reflects decreased synthesis of the C3 protein.

Complement in Human Disease

Several excellent reviews of the role of complement in human disease have appeared in recent years. This summary, then, will not be exhaustive but will give the general principles underlying the relevance of the complement system to human illness.

Congenital absence or abnormalities in the structure of complement components have received much attention recently. The first such disease to be recognized was hereditary angioedema which is due to a lack of, or defect in, the structure of the inhibitor of the first complement component, C1 Inh. The C1 Inh deficiency is inherited as an autosomal dominant, and the disease is characterized by periodic episodes of angioedema which may involve the face, oral cavity, extremities, gastrointestinal tract, or larynx. Involvement of the gastrointestinal tract produces vomiting, cramps, and frequently mimics intestinal obstruction. Involvement of the larynx may lead to asphyxiation and death. Attacks of angioedema are frequently triggered by trauma (see Chapter 16).

Several kindreds of individuals with deficiency of the second complement with component, C2, have been reported. Members of these families experience an increase in the incidence of collagen diseases—particularly systemic lupus erythematosus. However, many persons with a deficiency of C2 remain clinically normal.

Congenital deficiencies of the subunits of the first complement component have been described. C1q deficiency has been associated with hypo-γ-globulinemia. Deficiencies of C1r and C1s have been seen in patients with systemic lupus erythematosus and nephritis. A patient with C4 deficiency had lupus erythematosus.

C3 deficiency has been reported in at least three individuals. These patients had defects in the generation of chemotactic factors and in opsonization, as one would suspect, and were subject to repeated pyogenic infections such as pneumonia, otitis media, meningitis, and septicemia.

A deficiency of the inhibitor of the third complement component has been described in one individual. This inhibitor slows the breakdown of C3 by the alternative pathway. This patient has low levels of C3 and has evidence for continual cleavage of C3. He has a positive Coombs' test, due to C3b on his erythrocytes. The patient suffers repeated bacterial infections with gram positive organisms and experiences episodes of urticaria when showering. This latter phenomenon probably results from the release of large amounts of anaphylatoxin from the uninhibited activation of C3 with consequent release of histamine from mast cells. Urine histamine is elevated in this patient.

Deficiency of C5 has been found in a patient with systemic lupus erythematosus. Infants with Leiner's syndrome have a dysfunctional C5 protein and experience diarrhea, seborrheic dermatitis, and frequent episodes of infection. Fresh plasma transfusion corrects this defect. Two cases of C6 deficiency have been reported. These individuals were healthy—although one girl suffered from Neisseria arthritis. A girl with C7 deficiency, acrosclerosis, Raynaud's phenomenon, and telangiectasia has been described. The relationship between the C7 defect and the collagen disease is unknown. C8 deficiency was associated with gonococcemia.

Acquired Diseases in which Complement is Involved

Immune Complex Disease

Antibodies of the IgG subclasses 1, 2, and 3 and of the IgM classes can complex with antigen and activate complement. Such immune complexes can be entrapped in the interstices of adjacent endothelial cells of small blood vessels, within the joint space, or on serosal surfaces. A complement-induced inflammatory response may ensue at the site of entrapment. The anaphylatoxins generated from C3 and C5 act directly on blood vessels to promote increased vascular permeability and allow intravascular materials to transude into the tissue spaces. Anaphylatoxins also promote increased vascular permeability and vasodilatation by releasing histamine from mast cells. Local tissue edema and erythema result. Chemotactic factors derived from C3, C5, and C567 attract polymorphonuclear leukocytes to the site of the immune complex entrapment. The polymorphonuclear cells attempt to phagocytize the immune complexes and in the process release lysosomal enzymes. Several of these enzymes can directly destroy many constituents of the connective tissue. Tissue injury ensues and organ function is compromised.

Many examples of immune complex diseases exist and are discussed in detail in Chapter 14.

In systemic lupus erythematosus anti-DNA antibody is thought to interact with circulating DNA. Tissue destruction, exposure to excessive amounts of sunlight and other factors, incompletely understood, enhance release of DNA from cells, which can then interact with specific antibody. One of the most sensitive ways of predicting tissue destruction and of following the disease response to therapy in patients with systemic lupus erythematosus is by following the C4 levels at monthly intervals. Serum C4 levels frequently remain depressed after the patient has clinically recovered and may fall days to weeks before clinical evidence of reactivation of disease appears.

In rheumatoid arthritis the major immunologic reaction appears in the joint space. In the patient with a nonimmunologic effusion of the joint space (such as occurs in trauma, gout, or degenerative arthritis) the joint fluid C4 is approximately 65–75% of the C4 concentration in the serum. Ratios of joint fluid to serum C4 levels below 60% are found in the fluids of patients with adult or juvenile rheumatoid arthritis. Measurement of this ratio of joint fluid to serum C4 can be helpful in the diagnosis of cases of mono- or polyarticular arthritis.

In most cases of rheumatoid arthritis the serum C4 is normal or elevated. There is a subgroup of rheumatoid patients with low normal or low C4 levels. The prognosis of the disease in these patients is worse than in other patients; generally these patients are not as responsive to therapy as normocomplementemic rheumatoids and have a far higher incidence of the systemic complications of rheumatoid arthritis—such as cutaneous or systemic vasculitis, nodules, or involvement of the central nervous system, gastrointestinal tract, lung, etc.

Patients with subacute bacterial endocarditis frequently have evidence of peripheral embolization (e.g., Roth spots, Osler nodes, focal glomerulonephritis) which are thought to be complexes of bacterial antigen, antibody, and complement.

Serum C4 has been found to be low during the period of schizont rupture in malaria and immune complexes containing antibody and complement have been found in the kidneys of patients with the nephrotic syndrome secondary to malaria.

The prodromal phase of hepatitis is occasionally associated with a polyarticular arthritis, urticarial rash, and low serum C4. This suggests antigen-antibody immune complex disease. This syndrome usually clears at the time of the appearance of jaundice. In hemorrhagic fever and shock associated with dengue multiple complement components are found to be low; the turnover rate of C3 and C1q is markedly elevated indicating complement consumption in this illness, probably by circulating immune complexes.

Membrane-Associated Diseases

Several hematologic diseases result from the interaction of antibody, cell membrane, and complement. The attachment of C3b to the membrane of red blood cells or platelets enables fixed macrophages of the reticuloendothelial system to remove these cells from the circulation. Macrophage membranes contain receptors specific for C3b which greatly enhance entrapment and phagocytosis of particulate antigens to which C3b is attached (discussed in more detail in Chapter 18).

In blood transfusion reactions, in cold agglutinin disease, autoimmune hemolytic anemia, paroxysmal cold hemoglobinuria, and idiopathic thrombocytopenic purpura antibodies attach to antigenic determinants on the cell membrane. Complement components are activated and affix to the membrane. If sufficiently large amounts of antibody and complement are deposited upon the cells intravascular hemolysis may occur; usually however, the extravascular removal of cells from the circulation by macrophages of the spleen and liver occurs. In drug-induced hemolytic anemia the drug may stimulate the formation of antibody to a constituent of the red cell membrane (as in methyldopa-induced hemolytic anemia) or to the drug itself (as in penicillin-induced hemolytic anemia). In the situation in which antibody to the cell membrane is stimulated, activation of complement by the antibody-cell membrane complex affixes complement to the membrane with the resultant destruction of the cell. In the penicillin model, in which antibody is formed to the drug, the red cell membrane serves as an innocent bystander. Penicillin readily adsorbs onto red blood cells and complexes of antibody with penicillin can similarly be adsorbed to the red blood cell. Complement subsequently is affixed to the cell membrane and lysis of red cell ensues.

Complement components have been found in the diseased kidneys of patients with multiple types of renal disease. Components of the classical and alternative pathways have been found in kidneys of patients with systemic lupus erythematosus and acute poststreptococcal glomerulonephritis. In patients with membranoglomerulonephritis deposits of C3 and factor B of the alternative pathway have been found on renal biopsy material. Most of these patients have normal levels of C1, C4, and C2 but reduced levels of factor B and properdin—thus indicating alternative pathway activation. Many patients with this disease have in their serum a substance, C3 nephritic factor, that activates the alternative complement pathway.

In Goodpasture's disease antibody and complement can be found both on the basement membrane of the glomeruli and also the basement membrane of the lungs.

Complement has been implicated in several dermatologic diseases. Complement components have been found deposited at the site of the disease process. In pemphigus vulgaris, C3 can be found in the region of the intercellular cement. In bullous pemphigoid, discoid lupus, and systemic lupus erythematosus complement component deposits have been found in the region of the dermal-epidermal junction. Serum complement levels in patients with these diseases (except for systemic lupus erythematosus) are usually normal.

Graft rejection of transplanted organs involves cellular and humoral events. Complement consumption can be demonstrated most dramatically in the hyperacute rejection phenomenon but a closer scrutiny has demonstrated that complement is also consumed from the serum of patients undergoing gradual rejection of transplants suggesting that complement probably is involved in the transplant destruction process.

SELECTED REFERENCES

Frank, M. M., and Atkinson, J. P.: Complement in clinical medicine. Dis. Month, Jan., 1975.

Ruddy, S., Gigli, I., and Austen, K. F.: The complement system of man. N. Engl. J. Med., *287:* 489, 545, 592, 642, 1972.

Ruddy, S., and Colten, H. R.: Rheumatoid arthritis. Biosynthesis of complement proteins by synovial tissues. N. Engl. J. Med., *290:* 1284, 1974.

Ruddy, S., and Austen, K. F.: Activation of the complement system in rheumatoid synovitis. Fed. Proc., *32:* 134, 1973.

Schur, P. H. Complement in lupus. Clin Rheum. Dis. *1:* 519, 1975.

Agnello, V. Complement deficiency states. Medicine, *57:* 1, 1978.

Chapter 11

HUMORAL DEFICIENCY STATES

Stanford T. Shulman, M.D.

This discussion will be limited to disorders characterized by immunoglobulin deficiencies and will not touch upon those diseases in which there may be deficiency of other humoral immune factors, such as complement components. The categories of disorders to be considered include: (1) a physiologic state; (2) an exaggeration of a physiologic condition; (3) two kinds of "primary" immunodeficiencies; and (4) those humoral immunodeficiency disorders which are secondary to other disease processes.

Fetal and Neonatal Humoral System ("Physiologic Deficiency")

Over the past 10 years it has become apparent that, in contrast to earlier dogma, the fetus and neonate are capable of antibody production. B lymphocytes, which mature into the cells responsible for antibody production, and which are identified by the presence of surface immunoglobulin, have been identified in the fetus long before birth. IgM- and IgG-bearing lymphocytes are detectable in human fetal liver as early as 9 weeks gestation, while IgA-bearing cells are detectable by the 11th week. By the 14th week of gestation, the percentage of B lymphocytes in blood and in spleen which bear surface IgM, IgG, and IgA, are well within the normal adult range. The ability of these fetal B lymphocytes to synthesize and secrete immunoglobulin was established by experiments which showed that spleen cells from 20-week fetuses in cell culture produced immunoglobulin. It thus seems likely that the very low levels of circulating immunoglobulin of fetal origin for the most part reflect lack of antigenic stimulation rather than lack of ability to produce antibody. Evidence that the human fetus is capable of antibody synthesis is available from the experience with infants born after intrauterine infection, for elevated levels of total IgM and of IgM antibody specific for the infecting agent are present. Because IgM is not transplacentally passed, its presence reflects fetal synthesis.

However, some experimental data suggest that fetal and neonatal animals may be deficient in macrophages responsible for antigen recognition or processing, and that this fact may lead to some degree of impairment of antibody production. Studies in several species including fetal sheep and neonatal opposums (which are extremely immature at birth) have demonstrated that the ability to respond to various antigens develops sequentially in a stereotyped manner. Whether this phenomenon reflects maturation of a particular cell population has not yet been conclusively demonstrated. At the time of birth, neonatal (cord) blood contains small amounts of IgM and IgA and approximately 105 to 140% of the maternal level of IgG. In addition, a small amount of IgG synthesized by the fetus is present.

The ability of the human newborn to synthesize specific antibody upon antigenic stimulation has been assessed in a number of studies. These data show that transplacentally acquired maternal antibody is immunosuppressive and that this effect is antigen specific. A number of studies showed (1) that passively acquired anti-Salmonella H antibodies would inhibit the neonatal H agglutinin response; (2) that infants older than 13 days frequently produced H agglutinin titers comparable to those found in adults; and (3) that the ability to produce Salmonella O agglutinins did not appear until 3 to 9 months of age, confirming the sequential acquisition of the ability to respond to different antigens. In addition, it was found that the quality of the infant's anti-H response differed from that of adults by consisting exclusively of IgM antibody for 20 to 30 days after immunization, which contrasts with the response of adults who switch from IgM to IgG antibody synthesis within 5 to 15 days. These studies confirmed that, although certain differences exist in the infant's antibody response as compared to that of adults, the newborn certainly is capable of responding to antigenic stimulation by producing antibody.

Transient Hypo-γ-globulinemia of Infancy

Transient hypo-γ-globulinemia of infancy is the first nonphysiologic humoral deficiency state to consider. This self-limited deficiency is characterized by an exaggeration of the normal lag in onset of the production of significant quantities of immunoglobulins, resulting in a lower and longer depression of serum immunoglobulin levels, as compared to normal. This is particularly common in premature infants and is followed by complete recovery without evidence of a permanent immune deficiency. By 9 to 15 months of age, complete recovery generally has occurred. The great majority of these infants escape without significant infection although an occasional infant with transient hypo-γ-globulinemia will develop a serious bacterial infection. The etiology of transient hypo-γ-globulinemia is unknown, although it has been speculated that it may result from maternal isoimmunization by an IgG allotype possessed by the infant but not by the mother; however, there is little substantiating evidence to support this.

The diagnosis of transient hypo-γ-globulinemia should be considered when the sum of the serum concentrations of the three major classes of immunoglobulin is less than 400 mg/100 ml. Patients who are identified as suffering from this problem may benefit from several monthly injections of γ-globulin, with reevaluation of serum immunoglobulin levels 1 month or more after the last injection to determine whether the patient has recovered.

Congenital Humoral Immunodeficiency

A variety of disorders exist which represent congenital defects in the development of the humoral immune system. These constitute the most common forms of primary immunodeficiency, accounting for 50–75% of the total. The age at which the diagnosis of antibody deficiency is made varies; in a large British study, 17% of the diagnoses were made in infants under 1 year of age, 41% in children ages 1–15, and the remaining 42% in adults. It is clear that there is a male predominance of approximately 2 to 1 and that this is most pronounced in childhood. For example, in the first year of life, 82% of cases of humoral immunodeficiency are diagnosed in males. In this group of disorders, cell-mediated immunity is intact, as evidenced by skin test responses and by in vitro studies.

The classification of primary humoral immune disorders remains unclear despite attempts to organize these disorders. The organization used here ignores etiologic considerations and is used for convenience.

X-Linked A-γ-globulinemia

The condition characterized by congenital absence of immunoglobulins is known as Bruton's a-γ-globulinemia. This disorder was first described by Colonel Ogden Bruton in 1952, and within several years it was apparent that these patients lacked the serum proteins we now call immunoglobulins and that most but not all cases appeared in male infants and children. The reason that this first of the immunodeficiencies became apparent at that time in history clearly related to the advent of antibiotics. In the preantibiotic era, patients with immune deficiency disorders apparently did not survive their early episodes of serious infection so that they could manifest the repeated infections which would lead one to suspect a deficiency in host defenses.

The infections to which such patients are unduly susceptible include those produced by encapsulated bacteria, especially the pneumococcus and *Haemophilus influenzae*. Viral and fungal infections are handled appropriately. Septic arthritis, meningitis, septicemia, pneumonitis, sinusitis, and mastoiditis are particularly common among untreated patients with a-γ-globulinemia. These infections generally begin after the first 9–12 months of life but occasionally some years later. The protective effect of transplacental IgG is thus apparent for most of the first year of life. Clinical examination of a-γ-globulinemic children frequently reveals sparse lymphoid tissue, including lymph nodes, tonsils, and adenoids. The lateral neck x-ray of such patients characteristically shows deficient adenoidal tissue. A-γ-globulinemic patients lack plasma cells in lymph nodes, marrow, and gastrointestinal tract, and the lymph nodes lack the germinal centers characteristic of normal lymph nodes. The thymus is normal, and cell-mediated immunity is intact by all parameters.

The treatment of a-γ-globulinemic patients with intramuscular injections of γ-globulin in a dosage of 0.6–0.8 ml/kg every 4 weeks is generally sufficient to maintain an IgG level more than 200 mg/100 ml and to protect against systemic infection. However, most a-γ-globulinemic patients nevertheless develop slowly progressive chronic sinusitis and chronic pulmonary disease with bronchiectasis. For this reason, adherence to a rigorous program of postural drainage and pulmonary therapy is essential to slow the progression of the latter complication. Several additional complications of a-γ-globulinemia include predisposition to *Giardia lamblia* infestation with malabsorption, which generally responds to treatment with metronidazole, an increased incidence of *Pneumocystis carinii* pneumonitis, and an increased incidence of neoplasia, although not as strikingly as in other immune deficiency states.

As immunology has developed increasing sophistication, it has become apparent that the group of patients with sex-linked a-γ-globulinemia is heterogeneous and probably represents more than a single immune defect. The majority of these patients lack both circulating immunoglobulins and circulating B lymphocytes, i.e., lymphocytes which bear surface immunoglobulin, although they have been shown to have normal numbers of "pre-B" cells (contain cytoplasmic immunoglobulin). In addition, two smaller groups of patients with sex-linked a-γ-globulinemia have been identified: (1) patients with a-γ-globulinemia but with normal numbers of circulating B lymphocytes and (2) a few patients with absent serum immunoglobulins but with a small number of circulating B lymphocytes.

Dys-γ-globulinemias

This term is used to describe those conditions which are characterized by abnormal concentrations of one or several, but not all, of the major classes of serum immunoglobulins. With only one exception, the dys-γ-globulinemias are quite uncommon disorders. The major exception, selective IgA deficiency, needs to be discussed in some detail.

Selective IgA Deficiency. This term is applied to those patients who have serum IgA levels less than 5 mg/100 ml and lack secretory IgA, without evidence of deficiency of other immunoglobulins or of impaired antibody production or cell-mediated immunity. Such patients were first reported in 1962 and there are a large number of subsequent reports of such patients. Selective IgA deficiency is by far the most common form of primary immunodeficiency, the best estimates of its incidence in the general population ranging from 1 in 500 to 1 in 700 individuals. While most cases are sporadic, there have been occasional reports of autosomal dominant and autosomal recessive inheritance patterns. A fascinating aspect of this disorder is the fact that many individuals with selective IgA deficiency are asymptomatic even though they lack the major immunoglobulin normally present on mucosal surfaces. The great majority of patients with selective IgA deficiency lack both serum and secretory IgA but have free secretory component present in their secretions. A few patients with deficiency of serum IgA but normal levels of secretory IgA have been reported but this clearly is the exception. Very recently, the first case of absent secretory IgA, normal serum IgA, and apparent inability to synthesize secretory component was reported. Many patients with selective IgA deficiency present a history of frequent respiratory infections, particularly in those patients with associated elevated IgE levels, suggesting that allergy may play a role in the frequent respiratory problems. The incidence of selective IgA deficiency in a population of allergic individuals is as high as 1 in 200, suggesting that this defect may predispose to allergy. Several groups have shown an increased incidence of precipitating and hemagglutinating milk antibodies in patients with selective IgA deficiency, although the significance of this observation is unclear. Such patients may develop chronic bronchitis or obstructive lung disease, and there have been several patients reported with selective IgA deficiency associated with pulmonary hemosiderosis.

A large variety of gastrointestinal disorders have been associated with selective IgA deficiency, including celiac disease, nodular lymphoid hyperplasia of the small bowel, lactase deficiency, ulcerative colitis, regional enteritis, and pernicious anemia. The clinical features of these disorders in IgA-deficient patients are very similar to those of patients without this condition. The most intriguing association of selective IgA deficiency with clinical disease is the apparent high incidence of autoimmune disorders. More than 50% of selective IgA-deficient patients have been reported in association with autoimmune diseases. The list of disorders associated with selective IgA deficiency is very long, including classic autoimmune disorders such as systemic lupus, rheumatoid arthritis, dermatomyositis, thyroiditis, Sjögren's syndrome, as well as chronic aggressive or lupoid hepatitis, regional enteritis, ulcerative colitis, pernicious anemia, and others. It is of some interest that two of the 10 children with chronic aggressive hepatitis that we are following, manifest selective

IgA deficiency as their only immunologic disorder. It is not clear why selective IgA-deficient patients should be predisposed to the development of these autoimmune disorders although there are several postulations: (1) IgA deficiency may lead to some form of immunologic imbalance which predisposes to these conditions; (2) absent IgA may be the result of a subtle thymic deficiency which predisposes to autoimmune disease; (3) absent secretory IgA may increase susceptibility to viral infections which could play a role in the pathogenesis of autoimmune disorders; and (4) lack of secretory IgA may allow antigens ordinarily excluded to gain access into the body.

An additional association with selective IgA deficiency has been with malignancies, including lymphoma and carcinoma of the esophagus, stomach, and lung. It has been pointed out that each of the malignancies which have been reported has occurred in a site where secretory antibodies are normally present.

Most available data suggest that patients who are IgA deficient have normal numbers of circulating lymphocytes which bear IgA on their surface but that IgA is clearly not being released by such lymphocytes. In vitro pokeweed mitogen stimulation of lymphocytes from IgA deficient patients induces IgA secretion. This finding suggests that in vivo there is failure of terminal differentiation or initiation of immunoglobulin secretion by IgA-bearing lymphocytes. It has been suggested that this may reflect a deficiency in a T cell subpopulation essential for the triggering of IgA-bearing lymphocytes. It is clear that further detailed study of patients with selective IgA deficiency may yield valuable insight into the mechanisms of antibody synthesis and secretion as well as into the role of IgA in the protection of normal individuals against the development of a variety of disease states, including malignancies.

Therapy of selective IgA deficiency must be directed toward the associated disease which is present. There are no data to suggest that patients with selective IgA deficiency respond differently to therapy than do other patients with similar disorders, with the exception of the allergies which may be a bit more resistant to standard therapy. Commercial preparations of γ globulin contain insufficient IgA to boost the patient's serum IgA levels and indeed may induce the development of anti-IgA antibodies because of the trace amounts of IgA present in commercial γ globulin preparations. γ Globulin, therefore, should be avoided. No effective means of supplementing the IgA levels of such patients exists at this time, and the prognosis relates directly to the severity of any associated illnesses.

Selective IgM Deficiency. This is a very rare dys-γ-globulinemia which has been reported in several cases. Most patients have had low but not absent levels of IgM, with repeated determinations less than 20 mg/100 ml. A few patients have manifested autoimmune or allergic disorders, while others have had an apparent predisposition to meningococcal infection, recurrent bacterial infection, or generalized vaccinia. The true significance or incidence of this disorder is not yet established.

Immunodeficiency with Normal or Hyperimmunoglobulinemia. There have been several reports of individuals who are unable to synthesize antibody after antigenic stimulation despite normal or elevated levels of serum immunoglobulins. Patients such as these emphasize the importance of establishing that an individual undergoing evaluation for possible immunodeficiency produces functional antibody in response to antigenic stimulation. This can be established in a number of ways, including performing a Schick test, measuring serum isohemagglutinins, polio or tetanus titers, etc.

X-linked Immunodeficiency with Hyper-IgM. This disorder was first described in 1961 and may be found in siblings of patients with Bruton's a-γ-globulinemia. Patients have low IgG and IgA levels, normal or increased IgM, and impaired production of antibody. Patients manifest recurrent pyogenic infections, especially of the respiratory tract, skin, and cervical lymph nodes. Persistent, cyclic, or recurrent neutropenia or other hematologic abnormalities may be seen. Hepatosplenomegaly and lymphadenopathy are frequently present. Cell-mediated immune parameters are intact, and lymph node histology generally reveals disorganization and lack of follicles, germinal centers, and significant numbers of plasma cells.

This group of patients appears to benefit from injections of γ globulin, with fall in IgM levels sometimes observed. Prognosis is probably better than that of Bruton's a-γ-globulinemia.

Deficient IgA and IgM with Normal IgG. In this form of dys-γ-globulinemia, the quantitatively normal IgG is nonfunctional in some cases. Males predominate although the inheritance patterns are poorly characterized. Two characteristic presentations have been observed: (1) infections beginning early in life (especially with nonfunctional IgG) and (2) adult patients with malabsorption and evidence of nodular lymphoid hyperplasia (associated with functional IgG). The former patients benefit from γ globulin therapy while the latter do not.

Selective IgG Deficiency. This quite rare dys-γ-globulinemia is characterized by normal IgA and IgM levels with low to absent IgG. Both familial and sporadic cases have been reported. The clinical picture resembles that of Bruton's a-γ-globulinemia, and patients respond to γ globulin injections. Prognosis is somewhat better than in Bruton's, presumably because of the presence of secretory immunoglobulin and the other serum immunoglobulin classes.

Extreme Elevation of Serum IgA Associated with Low IgM and IgG Levels. We have recently treated a 4 year-old white boy with this unusual form of immune deficiency. He had been diagnosed as having hypo-γ-globulinemia (IgG = 100 mg/100 ml, IgM = 10 mg/100 ml, IgA

= 0) at 3 months of life and began to receive monthly γ globulin injections. Chronic sinopulmonary infections developed and subsequent immunoglobulin determinations showed IgA levels which rose to 4500 mg/100 ml, IgM remaining about 10 mg/100 ml, and IgG levels consistent with exogenous administration. Serum protein electrophoresis failed to reveal a monoclonal spike as might be seen in myeloma. Rheumatoid factor was present in high titer. This child developed a refractory sprue-like disorder and succumbed to malnutrition, Pseudomonas sepsis, and *P. carinii* pneumonitis. Previously reported patients with this disorder have been boys with recurrent respiratory infection. In this patient and in the previously described patients, the IgA present seemed to have little or no function.

Common Variable Immunodeficiency

This term, which is synonymous with "acquired a-γ-globulinemia" or "adult antibody deficiency syndrome" has been applied to a very heterogeneous group of disorders. The patients with this disease have low immunoglobulin levels (frequently being a-γ-globulinemic), have the onset of their disease after the first several years of life, lack evidence of X-linked inheritance, and are unable to produce antibody in response to antigenic stimulation.

The symptoms manifested by these patients resemble those of patients with X-linked a-γ-globulinemia, with recurrent respiratory infections, bronchiectasis, and chronic gastrointestinal difficulties. Lymph nodes of such patients lack plasma cells and germinal centers.

The heterogeneity of this disorder becomes apparent from review of recent immunologic studies of these patients. Several groups of investigators have found that normal, markedly reduced, or even increased numbers of B cells can be found in the circulation of such patients. Among those with normal or elevated numbers of B cells, some failed to synthesize immunoglobulin when stimulated by T cell-derived mitogens, while others showed evidence of immunoglobulin synthesis but failure of secretion. This recent work demonstrates that common variable immunodeficiency is a very heterogeneous disorder resulting from blocks at various stages in the maturation of B cells into antibody-producing cells. Recently, Waldmann and colleagues at the National Institutes of Health presented data that suppressor T cells of these patients are responsible for the impaired synthesis and/or release of immunoglobulin by B cells in common variable hypo-γ-globulinemia.

Acquired (Secondary) Humoral Immunodeficiencies

Secondary immunoglobulin deficiencies occur as the result of a primary disease process. Decreased levels of serum immunoglobulins result from impaired synthesis, excessive external loss, or increased catabolism.

Impaired Synthesis

A number of disease states have been found to result in secondary humoral immunodeficiency as a consequence of impairment in the synthesis of immunoglobulin. These include malnutrition, malignancies of the lymphoreticular system, multiple myeloma, aging, and the postsplenectomy state. In each of these conditions, impaired antibody response to antigenic stimulation is present.

Malnutrition. Among patients with primary protein-calorie malnutrition, as seen in developing areas of the world, severe bacterial, viral, and other infections are frequent and are a major source of mortality. While serum immunoglobulin levels are generally not significantly abnormal, the ability of malnourished patients to mount an appropriate primary antibody response after antigenic stimulation is impaired. Similarly impaired antibody responses have been observed in experimental animals fed diets moderately deficient in protein or in essential amino acids.

Lymphoreticular Malignancy. Lymphoproliferative malignancies have long been associated with both a high incidence of infection and a variety of immunologic defects. In untreated Hodgkin's disease, humoral immunity appears relatively intact, with generally normal serum immunoglobulin levels, primary antibody response, and number of circulating B lymphocytes. In other forms of lymphoma, the humoral immune response may be significantly impaired. In leukemia, humoral responses are relatively intact except terminally. Multiple myeloma patients generally exhibit decreased levels of nonmyeloma immunoglobulin and distinct impairment of the primary antibody response after antigenic stimulation.

Postsplenectomy. The spleen has a number of functions and its removal would be expected to have a number of consequences. Schulkind et al. showed that the spleen was the most efficient organ for clearing particulate antigens in the nonimmune animal. There is additional evidence that the spleen is essential for the optimal primary antibody response to intravenous immunization with particulate antigens, e.g., bacteria. In contrast, splenectomized patients appear to respond normally to immunization by other routes and to soluble antigens. These findings explain in part the susceptibility of splenectomized patients to overwhelming pneumococcal infection.

Aging. The effect of increasing age upon the immune system has been the subject of recent investigations. It is clear that humoral immune activity declines with age from its peak in early adult life. With increasing age in humans, levels of isoantibodies decline, while in experimental animals decrease in primary and secondary humoral immune responses to both thymus-dependent and thymus-independent antigens has been documented. Nevertheless, conflicting data exist regarding serum immunoglobulin concentrations in aged individuals. Total numbers of circulating B cells remain fairly constant throughout adult life, even though antibody responses are somewhat feeble in the aged.

Excessive Losses of Immunoglobulins

Several diseases are associated with excessive losses of serum immunoglobulins, including the nephrotic syndrome, exudative enteropathy, and extensive skin diseases, especially burns. In general, such losses are not of sufficient magnitude to predispose patients to infection seriously but on occasion may be.

Nephrotic Syndrome. Hypoproteinemia occurs in nephrosis, and albumin and β and γ globulin levels are frequently depressed. In those patients with selective proteinuria, smaller immunoglobulins such as IgG and IgA may be lost while IgM is retained, resulting in relatively normal IgM concentrations. In addition, it was demonstrated that an impaired antibody response to pneumococcal antigens is present in nephrotic children although response to influenza vaccine is normal. Nephrotics manifest an increased incidence of bacterial peritonitis as well as soft tissue infection, although the role of deficient serum immunoglobulin levels has not been clearly defined. Predisposition to other infections, such as viral and fungal diseases, seems to be a consequence of T cell dysfunction induced by immunosuppressant drugs.

Exudative Enteropathy. A large variety of gastrointestinal disorders, as well as chronic congestive heart failure and constrictive pericarditis, may be associated with significant loss of protein into the intestinal tract. Turnover studies suggest that such protein losses are relatively independent of protein size and that resultant serum concentrations primarily reflect synthetic rates. In these patients, low serum immunoglobulins are found, although antibody responses to antigen are intact and predisposition to infection rarely occurs. Therapy in this condition is directed toward the primary disease which commonly includes inflammatory bowel disease, intestinal lymphangiectasia, and celiac disease.

Burns. A variety of defects in host immunity are present after major thermal injury, and infection is a prominent cause of morbidity and mortality. Among the immune defects, serum immunoglobulin levels fall, particularly IgG. Little or no impairment in the ability to respond to antigenic stimulation by the synthesis of antibody is present, for burned patients respond to Pseudomonas colonization and/or immunization and can mount other humoral immune responses.

Excessive Catabolism. Rarely, hypo-γ-globulinemia results from an increased catabolic rate of some or all immunoglobulin classes. In myotonic dystrophy, specific hypercatabolism of IgG has been demonstrated, with normal survival of immunoglobulins of other classes. In one patient with a mixed IgM-IgG cryoglobulinemia, survival of those IgG subclasses to which a monoclonal IgM anti-IgG was directed was markedly reduced.

Several other patients have been described to have increased catabolism of a number of classes of immunoglobulin, including patients with the Wiskott-Aldrich syndrome and those with a newly described familial hypercatabolic hypoproteinemia.

In summary, it is clear that humoral immunodeficiency may have multiple etiologies. While the therapeutic measures available at this time are somewhat limited, continued detailed investigation of this group of patients offers the best hope for the development of more effective forms of therapy and for furthering our understanding of the basic workings of the immune system.

SELECTED REFERENCES

Alexander, J. W., and Moncrief, J. A.: Alterations of the immune response following severe thermal injury. Arch. Surg., *93:* 75, 1966.

Ammann, A. J., and Hong, R.: Selective IgA deficiency and autoimmunity. Clin. Exp. Immunol., *7:* 833, 1970.

Ammann, A. J., and Hong, R.: Selective IgA deficiency—presentation of 30 cases and a review of the literature. Medicine, *50:* 223, 1971.

Ammann, A. J., and Hong, R.: Selective IgA deficiency. In *Immunologic Disorders in Infants and Children,* edited by E. R. Stiehm and V. Fulginiti. Philadelphia: W. B. Saunders, 1973, pp. 199–214.

Barandun, S., Morell, A., Skvaril, F., and Keller, H.: Immunopertubation in paraproteinemia. Birth Defects, *11:* 95, 1975.

Barr, M., and Fairley, G. H.: Circulating antibodies in reticuloses. Lancet, *1:* 1305, 1961.

Bachmann, R.: Studies on the serum γ-A-globulin level. III. The frequency of A-γ-A-globulinemia. Scand. J. Clin. Lab. Invest., *17:* 316, 1965.

Buckley, R. H., and Dees, S.: Correlation of milk precipitins with IgA deficiency. N. Engl. J. Med., *281:* 485, 1969.

Bruton, O. C.: Agammaglobulinemia. Pediatrics, *9:* 722, 1952.

Cooper, M. D., Faulk, W. P. Fudenberg, H. H., Good, R. A., Hitzig, W., Kunkel, H., Rosen, F. S., Seligmann, M., Soothill, J., and Wedgwood, R. J.: Classification of primary immunodeficiencies. N. Engl. J. Med., *288:* 966, 1973.

Cooper, M. D., Lawton, A. R., and Bockman, D. E.: Agammaglobulinaemia with B lymphocytes. Specific defect of plasma-cell differentiation. Lancet, *2:* 791, 1971.

Ellis, E. F., and Smith, R. T.: The role of the spleen in immunity. With special reference to the post-splenectomy problem in infants. Pediatrics, *37:* 111, 1966.

Gajl-Peczalska, K., Lim, S. D. and Good, R. A.: Birth Defects, *11:* 33, 1975.

Geha, R. S., Schneeberger, E., Merler, E., and Rosen, F. S.: Heterogeneity of "acquired" or common variable agammaglobulinaemia. N. Engl. J. Med., *291:* 1, 1974

Goldberg, L. S., Barnett, E. V., and Fudenberg, H. H.: Selective absence of IgA: a family study. J. Lab. Clin. Med., *72:* 204, 1968.

Good, R. A., and Jose, D.: Immunodeficiency secondary to nutritional deprivation: Clinical and laboratory observations. Birth Defects, *11:* 219, 1975.

Gotoff, S.: Acquired and Transient Immunodeficiency Disorders. In *Immunologic Disorders in Infants and Children,* edited by E. R. Stiehm and V. Fulginiti. Philadelphia: W. B. Saunders, 1971.

Kunin, C., Schwartz, R., Yaffe, S., Knapp, J., Fellers, F. X., Janeway, C. A., and Finland, M.: Antibody response to influenza-virus vaccine in children with nephrosis: effect of cortisone. Pediatrics, *23:* 54, 1959.

Lawton, A. R., Self, K. S., Royal, S. A., and Cooper, M. D.: Ontogeny of B-lymphocytes in the human fetus. Clin. Immun. Immunopathol., *1:* 104, 1972.

Lawton, A. R., Wu, L. Y. F., and Cooper, M. D.: Birth Defects, *11:* 28, 1975.

Medical Research Council Working Party. Hypogammaglobulinaemia in the United Kingdom. Lancet, *1:* 163, 1969.

Miller, M. E.: The immunodeficiencies of immaturity. In *Immunologic Disorders in Infants and Children,* edited by E. R. Stiehm and V. Fulginiti. Philadelphia: W. B. Saunders, 1973, p. 168.

Munster, A. M., and Hoagland, H. C.: Surg. Forum, *20:* 76, 1969.

Price, G. B., and Makinodan, T.: Immunologic deficiencies in senescence. I. Characterization of intrinsic deficiencies. J. Immunol., *108:* 403, 1972.

Rosen, F. S., and Janeway, C. A.: The gamma globulins. II. The antibody deficiency syndromes. N. Engl. J. Med., *275:* 709, 1966.

Rosen, F. S., Kevy, S. V., Merler, E., Janeway, C. A., and Gitlin, D.: Recurrent bacterial infections and dysgammaglobulinemia: deficiency of 7S gamma-globulins in the presence of elevated 19S gamma-globulins. Report of two cases. Pediatrics, *28:* 182, 1961.

Schulkind, M. L., Ellis, E. F., and Smith, R. T.: Effect of antibody upon clearance of I^{125}-labelled pneumococci by the spleen and liver. Pediat. Res., *1:* 178, 1967.

Smith, R. T., Eitzman, D. V., Catlin, M. E., Wirtz, E. O., and Miller, B. E.: The development of the immune response. Characterization of the response of the human infant and adult to immunization with Salmonella vaccines. Pediatrics, *33:* 163, 1964.

Sterzl, J., and Silverstein, A. M.: Developmental aspects of immunity. Adv. Immunol., *6:* 337, 1967.

Stiehm, E. R., Ammann, A. J., and Cherry, J.: Elevated cord macroglobulins in the diagnosis of intrauterine infections. N. Engl. J. Med., *275:* 971, 1966.

Stocker, F., Ammann, P., and Rossi, E.: Selective γ-A-globulin deficiency, with dominant autosomal inheritance in a Swiss family. Arch. Dis. Child., *43:* 585, 1968.

VanFurth, R., Schuit, H. R. E., and Hijmans, W.: The immunological development of the human fetus. J. Exp. Med., *122:* 1173, 1965.

Waldmann, T. A., Durm, M., Broder, S., Blackman, M., Blaese, R. M., and Strober, W.: Role of suppressor T cells in pathogenesis of common variable hypogammaglobulinaemia. Lancet *2:* 609, 1974.

Waldmann, T. A., and Schwab, P. J.: IgG (7S gamma globulin) metabolism in hypogammaglobulinemia: studies in patients with defective gamma globulin synthesis, gastrointestinal protein loss, or both. J. Clin. Invest., *44:* 1523, 1965.

Waldmann, T. A., Strober, W., Blaese, R. M., and Terry, W. D.: Immunoglobulin metabolism in disease. Birth Defects, *11:* 87, 1975.

West, C. D., Hong, R., and Holland, N. H.: Immunoglobulin levels from the newborn period to adulthood and in immunoglobulin deficiency states. J. Clin. Invest., *41:* 2054, 1962.

Chapter 12

PASSIVE ENHANCEMENT OF HUMORAL IMMUNITY

M. Lee, M.D. and Robert H. Waldman, M.D.

The passive enhancement of humoral immunity became practical in the mid 1940's, when Cohn and his colleagues developed a method for fractionating serum proteins by precipitation with ethanol under carefully controlled conditions in the cold. This process proved feasible on a large scale and the so-called "Cohn Fraction II," which contains γ globulins devoid of most other serum proteins, is the major source of γ globulin used today. Three types of such preparations are used in the passive transfer of immunity: (1) standard human immune serum globulin, used primarily in the treatment of antibody deficiency disorders and for prevention or modification of hepatitis A (Table 12.1) (2) special human immune globulins with known high antibody content for specific disease (Table 12.2); (3) animal antisera and antitoxins (Table 12.3) of which horse serum is the most common. When available, human γ globulin is preferable because of the risk of serum sickness and the shorter half-life of animal antisera.

There are certain characteristics of commercial human γ globulin which are useful to know before using this biologic product: (1) it is known officially as immune serum globulin (human) or as poliomyelitis immune globulin (human) in the case of serum which meets certain standards with regard to titers of antibody to poliovirus; (2) its source is either outdated whole blood or from placental blood; each pool must be obtained from at least 500 donors; (3) it is marketed as a 16.5% protein solution (165 mg/ml) with IgG accounting for 94–99% of the protein. There are trace amounts of IgA and IgM. Preparations of IgM and IgA are undergoing trials, but the short half-life of these immunoglobulins makes frequent injection necessary. Variable amounts of other serum proteins such as albumin, C3, and transferrin have been found, and

TABLE 12.1. *Use of Immune Serum Globulin (Human)*

Treatment of antibody deficiency disorders
Prevention or modification of measles
Prevention or modification of hepatitis A
Prevention or modification of hepatitis B
Prevention of rubella in pregnancy[a]
Modification of varicella[a]

[a] Efficacy unproven.

TABLE 12.2. *Special Human Immune Globulins*

Licensed
Mumps immune globulin
Pertussis immune globulin
Rabies immune globulin
Tetanus immune globulin
Vaccinia immune globulin
Hepatatis B immune globulin
Under development
Rubella immune globulin
Zoster immune globulin
Pseudomonas immune globulin
Western equine encephalitis immune globulin

TABLE 12.3. *Animal Antisera and Antitoxins*

Antirabies serum
Boltulism antitoxin
Diphtheria antitoxin
Gas gangrene antitoxin
Black widow spider antivenin
Antisnake bite antivenin

nonserum proteins of placental origin have been identified in lots derived from placental blood; (4) injected γ globulin has a half-life of about 3 weeks if there is no excessive loss, such as through gastrointestinal tract, or kidney, or a hypercatabolic state. The maximum plasma level is reached in 2–4 days after injection; (5) standard preparations must be given intramuscularly. Aggregation of IgG occurs as a result of the fractionation process and storage. These aggregates are strongly anticomplementary and may cause anaphylactic-type reactions if given intravenously. Several different methods for preventing or removing aggregates have been developed, and special preparations for intravenous use may soon be available; (6) γ globulin may be stored indefinitely at 4°C, although some aggregation and denaturation of protein does occur which may reduce its effectiveness slightly; (7) it has never been known to transmit hepatitis A or B; (8) γ globulin produced by different manufacturers and from different areas of the country appears to have great uniformity in effectiveness.

The indications for passive humoral immune enhancement by gamma globulin are: (1) antibody-deficiency syndromes such as congenital or acquired a-γ-globulinemia; and (2) prophylaxis or therapy of diseases in otherwise immunologically competent individuals under certain circumstances: (a) when there is insufficient time for active immunization in an unvaccinated individual exposed to a serious disease such as tetanus or rabies; (b) when there is no vaccine commercially available for persons at high risk, such as in the case of hepatitis; (c) when there is potential exposure but vaccination with live virus is contraindicated, such as with eczema or pregnancy. Obviously, γ globulin therapy is useful in the second instance only when the disease is preventable with effective serum antibody and when the γ globulin is given early in the incubation period.

Despite its usefulness, there are certain disadvantages of γ globulin therapy: (1) protection is of short duration because of the 3-week half-life of injected γ globulin; (2) in severe infections, large doses cannot easily be given; (3) there is unpredictable and unsteady uptake from the injection site; (4) immunoglobulins are themselves potentially immunogenic. Although this may not be clinically significant in a-γ-globulinemic patients, an immunologically competent individual might become sensitized to antigenic determinants on the injected immunoglobulin different from his own. This could later lead to a transfusion reaction.

There is also a theoretical hazard that sensitization to placental proteins present in some lots might endanger later pregnancy. IgA-deficient individuals may develop anti-IgA antibodies, leading to later transfusion reactions; (5) exogenous γ globulin may theoretically inhibit endogenous antibody synthesis; (6) although γ globulin is one of the safest biologic products available and no long-term side effects are known, there are potential short-term side effects such as tenderness at the injection site, sterile abscesses, fibrosis, and rare anaphylactic-type reactions; (7) γ globulin injections are painful and expensive.

The two most common uses of standard γ globulin are in antibody-deficiency disorders and the prevention or modification of hepatitis.

Standard γ globulin preparations are effective in preventing the acute, recurrent pyogenic infections in a-γ-globulinemic patients. It has been determined empirically that if the serum level is raised to approximately 200 mg/100 ml, invasive bacterial infections can be prevented. Initial therapy in children should be begun with 1.8 ml/kg (Table 12.4). If symptoms such as cough, conjunctivitis, arthralgias, or purulent nasal discharge occur near the end of the injection period, then more frequent

TABLE 12.4. *Replacement Therapy in Immunodeficiency*

Initial: 1.8 ml/kg (300 mg/kg)
Maintenance: 0.6 ml/kg (100 mg/kg) monthly
Adults: 10 ml weekly

injections are necessary. Older children and adults usually require 10 ml per week. Serial immunoglobulin determinations are probably unnecessary if the patients are followed clinically, and the necessity for increasing the frequency of injections may vary from patient to patient. During acute infection, more rapid catabolism of γ globulin occurs, which will necessitate extra injections.

An alternative to the use of standard γ globulin preparations is the use of whole plasma, which has certain advantages, but carries the risks of volume overload and hepatitis. Plasma therapy is particularly useful: (1) when there are contraindications to intramuscular therapy, such as thrombocytopenia in a patient with Wiskott-Aldrich syndrome, or when an antibody-deficient individual has extensive skin lesions or becomes markedly cachectic; (2) when an antibody-deficiency syndrome is refractory to intramuscular therapy; and (3) in severe, life-threatening infections when large doses of antibody must be given rapidly.

There are certain precautions which must be taken when plasma therapy is used: (1) the donor should be a relative with the same blood type as the patient or whose plasma antibodies do not react with the patient's red blood cells; (2) the donor should be hepatitis B surface antigen negative; (3) plasma obtained via plasmapheresis should be fresh-frozen or irradiated to kill immunocompetent lymphocytes; and (4) plasma must be given very slowly to small children. Plasma usually has an IgG content to 0.6 ml/kg of standard γ globulin. The half-life of IgG given in plasma is longer than that of standard γ globulin, with a mean of 32 days.

The effectiveness of γ globulin in preventing or modifying hepatitis A virus infections was established 30 years ago and was based on the assumptions that hepatitis A is a common viral infection of childhood in which second attacks are rare, suggesting that circulating antibody might mediate immunity. Recently, identification of an antigen associated with hepatitis A infection and the development of serologic techniques for the measurement of this antigen and of antibodies to it have borne out the validity of these assumptions. Of 42 patients recently reported with epidemiologically confirmed hepatitis A infection, 100% were shown to develop antihepatitis A antibody, while none of those with hepatitis B developed the antibody. This antibody was detectable in 20 patients 5–10 years after infection. In a preliminary study of the general population, frequency of antibody to HA antigen was found to increase with age. Presumably, it is these antibodies to hepatitis A antigen which explain why immune serum globulin administered either before exposure or within 1 to 2 weeks prevents clinical illness in 80–90% of those treated. Its value decreases with time after exposure, and its use more than 6 weeks later or after the onset of clinical illness is not warranted. Current recommendations are that household contacts, institutional contacts, those exposed to contaminated needles and common-source outbreaks, and travelers planning to stay 3 or more months in tropical areas or developing countries receive γ globulin according to the schedule noted in Table 12.5.

The use of γ globulin in the prevention or modification of hepatitis B infection has been more controversial and γ globulin has not generally been recommended for use after hepatitis B virus exposure. However, with recent advances in the detection of hepatitis B antigen and antibody and some newer clinical studies, this is changing. In the past 30 years, there have been 10–12 studies which attempted to evaluate the effectiveness of standard γ globulin preparations in preventing or modifying posttransfusion hepatitis, the majority of which was probably hepatitis B. The results of the studies are conflicting, some showing protection and others not. Plasma containing HB surface antigen may be infectious in a 1:10,000,000 dilution; therefore, patients in those studies, most of whom received multiple blood transfusions, were probably receiving massive doses of virus. Also, there are marked variations in the anti-HB surface antigen titers of different γ globulin preparations. Variations in the infective dose of virus received by the patients in these studies and the amount of specific anti-HB surface antigen antibody in the γ globulin may account for the conflicting results.

Standard γ globulin may be useful in preventing hepatitis B infection. Most sporadic cases of contact-type hepatitis B are due to low-dose exposure, such as fecal-oral contamination or inoculation from a contaminated needle. In addition, the titer of antihepatitis B surface antigen in commercial preparations is increasing. An explanation for this phenomenon may be that routine screening of donors for HB Ag has eliminated much of the antigen from pooled blood, antigen which would otherwise have complexed with antibody and lowered the effective antibody titer. In 1972, Ginsberg and his colleagues demonstrated that gammaglobulin from paid donors, when given in 5 or 10 ml doses before exposure,

TABLE 12.5. *Guidelines for ISG Prophylaxis of Hepatitis A*[a]

Weight of person (lb)	Dose (ml)
Most exposure situations	
<50	0.5
50–100	1.0
>100	2.0
Institutional contacts or foreign travel	
<50	1.0
50–100	2.5
>100	5.0

[a] Modified from Immune serum globulin for protection against viral hepatitis. Recommendation of the Public Health Service Advisory Committee on Immunization Practices. Ann. Intern. Med., *77:* 427, 1972.

conferred significant protection against nonparenterally acquired hepatitis B infection in United States army personnel stationed in Korea (Table 12.6). In 1974, children admitted to three large institutions for the mentally retarded were given either hepatitis B immune globulin with high-titer antibody, standard globulin, or no prophylaxis (Table 12.7). Those receiving treatment were given injections every 4 months. Of patients 8% treated with standard γ globulin, compared with 25% receiving placebo, developed either hepatitis B antigen or anicteric hepatitis. No patients treated with γ globulin became chronic carriers, while 13% of the placebo-treated group did.

There are still questions to be answered concerning the use of standard γ globulin after hepatitis B exposure. First, we do not know whether antibody to HB surface antigen actually prevents the disease or merely modifies it so that it is clinically inapparent. The seroconversion seen in many patients suggests subclinical infection. Second, will exogenous antibody suppress the immune response and lead to an increased risk of the carrier state. Finally, the inadvertent administration of antibody to a carrier of large amounts of antigen might lead to immune complex disease. Despite these unanswered questions, it does appear that standard human immune globulin may be efficacious in preventing or at least modifying hepatitis B infection.

Commercially available high titer antihepatitis B γ globulin has recently become available. It has been shown to be effective in preventing serious illness when given within a few days of nontransfusion exposure. However, it is very expensive, and there is not convincing evidence that it is more effective than recent standard γ globulin preparations.

TABLE 12.6. *Nonparenteral Exposure, Therapy Prophylactic, Follow-up 1 Year*

Group I	Group II
5–10 ml ISG Titer 1:1280 (radioimmunoassay)	No ISG
11/20,000	29/20,000

[a] Modified from: A. L. Ginsberg, M. E. Conrad, W. H. Bancroft, C. M. Ling, and L. R. Overby. Prevention of endemic HAA-positive hepatitis with gamma globulin. Use of a simple radioimmune assay to detect HAA. N. Engl. J. Med., *286:* 562, 1972.

TABLE 12.7. *Nonparenteral Exposure, Therapy Prophylactic, and q 4 Months Follow-up 1½ to 2 Years*

	ISG (1:262,144)	ISG (1:16)	Placebo
1. Ag only or anicteric hep.	6/44	3/37	13/53
2. Ab seroconv only	8/44	18/37	20/53
3. Persistant Ag	0	0	7/53

[a] Modified from: W. Szmuness, A. M. Prince, M. Goodman, C. Enrich, R. Pick, and M. Ansari. Hepatitis B immune serum globulin in prevention of nonparenterally transmitted hepatitis B. N. Engl. J. Med., *290:* 701, 1974.

SELECTED REFERENCES

Dosik, H. and Jhaveri, R.: Prevention of neonatal hepatitis B infection by high-dose hepatitis B immune globulin. N. Eng. J. Med., *298:* 602, 1978.

Ellis, E. F., and Henney, C. S.: Adverse reactions following administration of human gamma globulin. J. Allergy, *43:* 45, 1969.

Ginsberg, A. L., Conrad, M. E., Bancroft, W. H., Ling, C. M., and Overby, L. R.: Prevention of endemic HAA-positive hepatitis with gamma globulin. Use of a simple radioimmune assay to detect HAA. N. Engl. J. Med., *286:* 562, 1972.

Grady, G. F.: Passive immunization against viral hepatitis—status and prospects. Am. J. Med. Sci., *270:* 369, 1975.

Havens, W. P., Jr., and Paul, J. R.: Prevention of infectious hepatitis with gamma globulin. J.A.M.A., *129:* 270, 1945.

Heiner, D. C., and Evans, L.: Immunoglobulins and other proteins in commercial preparations of gamma globulin. J. Pediatr., *70:* 820, 1967.

Janeway, C. A., and Rosen, F. S.: The gamma globulins. IV. Therapeutic uses of gamma globulin. N. Engl. J. Med., *275:* 826, 1966.

Kohler, P. F., Dubois, R. S., Merrill, D. A., and Bowes, W. A.: Prevention of chronic neonatal hepatitis B virus infection with antibody to the hepatitis B surface antigen. N. Engl. J. Med., *291:* 1378, 1974.

Krugman, S., Friedman, H., and Lattimer, C.: Viral hepatitis, type A, Identification by specific complement fixation and immune adherence tests. N. Engl. J. Med., *292:* 1141, 1975.

Prince, A. M., Szmuness, W., Brotman, B., Ikram, H., Lippin, A., Stryker, M., Ehrich, C., and Finlayson, N. C. D. C.: Hepatitis B immune globulin. In *Hepatitis and Blood Transfusion,* edited by G. N. Vyas, H. A. Perkins, and R. Schmid. New York: Grune and Stratton, 1972, pp. 335–347.

Prince, A. M., Szmuness, W., Woods, K. R., and Grady, F. G.: Antibody against serum-hepatitis antigen. Prevalence and potential use as immune serum globulin in prevention of serum hepatitis infections. N. Engl. J. Med., *285:* 933, 1971.

Purcell, R. H., Dienstag, J. L., Feinstone, S. M., Kapikan, A. Z.: Relationship of hepatitis A antigen to viral hepatitis. Am. J. Med. Sci., *270:* 61, 1975.

Smith, G. N., Griffiths, B., Mollison, D., and Mollison, P. L.: Uptake of IgG after intramuscular and subcutaneous injection. Lancet, *1:* 1208, 1972.

Szmuness, W., Prince, A. M., Goodman, M., Ehrich, C., Pick, R., and Ansari, M.: Hepatitis B immune serum globulin in prevention of nonparenterally transmitted hepatitis B. N. Engl. J. Med., *290:* 701, 1974.

Villarejos, V. M., Visona, K. A., Kutierrez, A., and Rodriguez, A.: The role of saliva, urine and feces in the transmission of type B hepatitis. N. Engl. J. Med., *291:* 1375, 1974.

Veterans Administration Cooperative Study: Type B hepatitis after needle-stick exposure: prevention with type B immune globulin. Ann. Int. Med., *88:* 285, 1978.

Chapter 13

ACTIVE IMMUNIZATION

Robert H. Waldman, M.D. and Rama Ganguly, Ph.D.

Immunization is derived from the Latin "immunis," meaning "exempt from public burden." The purpose of immunization is to enhance the host's immune system, so that infectious diseases (and possibly, in the near future, other diseases which are protected against by immune mechanisms, e.g., cancer) are prevented or treated, leading to reduced morbidity and mortality. Immunization procedures can be conveniently divided into two types, passive and active. The former was covered in the preceding chapter.

The purpose of active immunization is to stimulate the individual's own protective mechanisms. In order to do this in a rational manner, the protective mechanisms must be known. Unfortunately, there are few instances in infectious diseases where the protective mechanisms have been elucidated. Despite this fact, from a practical point of view, the central question is whether a vaccine works or not. Thus, the most important aspect with regard to a vaccine development is efficacy. Some vaccines were introduced into general use before they were critically assessed, and at about the same time that great advances were being made in other general public health measures. When the diseases for which some vaccines were given decreased in incidence, the vaccines were widely accepted as being efficacious, although the improvement in hygienic conditions in this country in the early part of this century may have been responsible.

Vaccines can be evaluated indirectly by measuring the immune mechanism thought to play a role in protection. Despite the fact that this is usually unknown, serum antibody has often been assumed to correlate with vaccine efficacy. This is the easiest parameter to measure, but serum antibody has not been shown to play a protective role in very many infectious diseases. Thus, a potent and prolonged serum antibody response when vaccines with adjuvants are used, is not necessarily a good indication of vaccine effectiveness. A second indirect measure of vaccine efficacy is the development of secretory antibody. But once again, it must be emphasized that there are even fewer infectious diseases in which secretory antibody has been proven to play an important role.

Although indirect measurements of vaccine efficacy are much easier and less expensive, the only definite way to define vaccine effectiveness is its ability to protect against illness. This is most accurately done in a field trial. Obviously, to be worthwhile, the field trial must have an adequate control group with assurance that it is identical to the vaccine group in all respects. While field trials are valuable in indicating protective efficacy, they are difficult to carry out and are expensive. A second direct means of assessing the vaccine's effectiveness is the use of challenge studies. A challenge study has the advantage of being more convenient, since much smaller populations need to be involved, but have two disadvantages: one scientific, the other ethical. The dose of the challenge organism used in a study may not be equivalent to that which occurs naturally, e.g., in challenge studies with influenza virus, most investigators try to cause illness in about 50% of the control group. During an epidemic, however, only 10–20% of susceptibles become ill. Thus it would appear that in many challenge studies, volunteers receive a much higher dose and, therefore, the results might erroneously indicate that a vaccine is ineffective. The ethical question regards the sources of the volunteers. In the past, most challenge studies in the United States used prisoner volunteers. It is questionable whether they can be considered to be true volunteers.

A recent area of interest with respect to immunization is the route of vaccine administration. The most common method of vaccine administration has been the parenteral route, although alternate routes have been used for many years. In the Middle Ages, the Turks used intranasal immunization with crusts from smallpox lesions, believed to be the first example of immunization. Since the most common method for assessing a vaccine's effectiveness has been the measurement of serum antibody, the most common route for immunization has been the parenteral one. However, one recent highly successful immunization has been given by an alternate route, i.e., the oral attenuated polio vaccine. The route of immunization should depend upon the immune host defense mechanism that is responsible or is thought to be responsible for protection. If the stimulation of serum antibody is the aim of immunization, then subcutaneous, intramuscular, or intradermal immunization would be most efficient. However, if secretory antibody is the aim of the immunization, then local application of antigen such as by nose drops, aerosol, oral ingestion, intravaginal, or eye drops would be most efficient.

A very important phenomenon in the epidemiology of infectious diseases, which relates to immunization, is the phenomenon of "herd immunity." It has been observed that immunization of a certain proportion of people in a community achieves the protection of the unimmunized remainer. This depends on the degree of transmissibility of the communicable disease. Transmission of diphtheria depends on the presence of a relatively large proportion of susceptibles, and, therefore, herd immunity is relatively easy to establish. On the other hand, herd immunity to measles is very difficult to establish, since measles may continue to spread with 90% of the population immune. In order to eradicate an infectious disease, using the example of the only one which has been eradicated, i.e., smallpox, the spread of the disease is controlled by seeking out the source of the agent and immunizing all contacts. It is obvious that this requires that humans be the only reservoir of infection. Smallpox has been eradicated, but can we look forward to any other infectious diseases following this pathway? The two best possibilities would be polio and measles. However, there are significant problems with respect to both of these. With polio, there are probably too many asymptomatic or subclinical cases to determine effectively the source of the agent and thereby immunize all contacts. With measles, there is a different problem, and that is the potential difficulty with latent virus infection. Thus, we might presume that we have eradicated the disease, only to have the infection pop up later because the virus has remained latent for many, many years in a high percentage of the population.

Another important consideration in evaluating vaccines is the duration of protection. In most instances, it would be very desirable to give a vaccine once and obtain lifelong immunity. This is not an unrealistic aim, since many infectious diseases, e.g., measles infection, render the individual immune for life. It is generally felt that live attenuated organisms give longer immunity than do killed organisms. The evidence for this is not good. There have been no controlled studies in which a live attenuated vaccine has been compared with the comparable killed vaccine. Live attenuated oral polio vaccine as compared with the killed injected vaccine is an invalid comparison since more than one variable has been changed; i.e., in addition to the difference in live versus killed organisms, the route of administration of vaccine is different. Although there have been no direct studies comparing the two, the general results with the live attenuated measles vaccine have been superior to that of the killed measles vaccine. However, this is probably not due to a difference in the duration of protection but due to the poorly understood hypersensitivity reaction which is induced by the killed measles vaccine.

In some studies, higher titers of antibody result from live vaccines as compared to killed vaccines. This is probably due to a larger antigenic mass, since the organisms replicate, and also due to longer contact with immunocompetent cells, since again with replication, the antigens are present in the body for a longer period of time. Theoretically, the same result would be obtained by administering killed organisms repeatedly

TABLE 13.1

Vaccine	Type of vaccine	Suggested use	Comment
Cholera	Killed whole organism.	For travel to some countries in South and Southeast Asia, Africa, Middle East. Dose 1, 0.5 ml subcutaneously or intramuscularly; dose 2, 1.0 ml, about 1 month later.	High incidence of local and general reactions of "nuisance" type. Effectiveness marginal and of short duration. Because of rarity of cholera in westerners, vaccine not recommended except for fulfilling requirements of International Certificate of Vaccination.
Diphtheria Tetanus Pertussis	Toxoid-adsorbed Toxoid-absorbed Killed bacteria or bacterial fraction.	DPT, Td, or T alone. DPT at 6 weeks-3 months 3X at 4–8 weeks intervals, booster 1 year later. Booster at time of entrance to school. Td thereafter and 10 years, unless used as part of wound management. Wound: previous dose 3 years before, give T booster. No previous, give TX2 4–6 weeks interval, booster 1 year later.	Tetanus is almost an ideal immunizing agent: sensitization a slight problem. Pertussis: rare side-effects of severe central nervous system reaction occasionally leading to permanent sequelae and death.
Influenza	Egg-grown virus, formalin inactivated, highly purified by zonal ultracentrifugation.	1 dose subcutaneously in "high risk" groups in October or November.	(1) local and general reactions of "nuisance" types; (2) no evidence that ID is effective; (3) some indication that everyone should be immunized every year.
Measles (rubeola)	Live attenuated virus, chick embryo or canine tissue culture grown.	At 15 months; susceptibles any time thereafter.	Very common febrile reaction day 6–11, but more severe reactions very rare. Use should be postponed in children with acute febrile illness. Should not be used in children with severe underlying diseases that are associated with lowered resistance or in pregnant women. Duration of protection unknown.

TABLE 13.1—*Continued*

Vaccine	Type of vaccine	Suggested use	Comment
Mumps	Live attenuated chick embryo cell culture.	At 1 year or later.	Untoward reactions very rare. Duration of protection unknown. Only warranted use probably in males approaching puberty who have not had mumps parotitis, either unilateral or bilateral (Mumps skin test too unreliable to warrant use as test, for immunity).
Rabies	Active: β-propiolactone inactivated virus grown in embryonated duck eggs.	Postexposure: 14 daily doses subcutaneously, 21 doses in cases of severe exposure. Boosters given 10–20 days after completion of primary course. Preexposure: in high risk groups (e.g., vets) 3 doses for primary immunization; booster at 2 years.	Effectiveness of postexposure prophylaxis unproved. Local and systemic reactions common, especially late in course of immunization. Rationale of treatment: (1) species of animal; (2) circumstances of biting incident; (3) extent and location of bite wound; (4) vaccination status of biting animal; (5) presence of rabies in area.
Rubella	Live attenuated.	All children 1 year to puberty. Routine immunization of adolescent girls not indicated because of danger of inadvertently administering vaccine during pregnancy. Each case considered individually. Alternative: test serum antibody titers of girls age 8–10 and immunize only susceptibles.	Purpose: preventing infection of fetus; accomplished by eliminating transmission among source of infection for pregnant women, i.e., among children. Risk of vaccine virus for fetus is unknown. Side-effects: arthritis 2–4 weeks after vaccination. Duration of protection unknown.
Plague	Formaldehyde inactivated *Pasteurella pestis.*	Persons travelling to Indochina, persons in contact with wild rodents in endemic areas and laboratory personnel	Unknown effectiveness. Local and systemic reactions mild, but tend to become more severe with repeated doses.

TABLE 13.1—*Continued*

Vaccine	Type of vaccine	Suggested use	Comment
		working with the disease. 0.5 ml × 2, 4 weeks apart, then 0.2 ml 4–12 weeks later, 0.2 ml booster at 6–12 months.	
Polio	Inactivated virus.	Beginning at any age from 6 weeks–3 times at 1 month intervals, 4th dose 12 months later. Booster at 6–12 months.	
	Attenuated virus monovalent or trivalent.	Convenient to give at same time as DTP doses.	Not suggested for adults not immunized previously. Duration of protection not known. Easier to give, stimulates local immunity thereby decreasing circulation of virus, immunity may be longer duration.
Smallpox	Live vaccinia virus: glycerated or lyophilized; latter more stable.	Not recommended.	
Typhoid	Whole organism killed by several different techniques.	Intimate exposure to carrier or case or travel to endemic area. 0.5 ml subcutaneously 2 times, 4 weeks apart.	Immunization: has probably played no role in the decline of typhoid fever in the U.S. in the last 60 years. Recent field trials have demonstrated slight, but definite, protective effect of vaccine, for short period of time; however, best prophylaxis is careful selection of food and water in endemic area. Immunization for foreign travel, when balanced against side-effects and tendency to relax hygiene, probably not worthwhile.
Paratyphoid A and B	TAB vaccine combined with typhoid.	Not suggested—TAB should not be used.	Not effective.
Typhus	Formaldehyde inactivated *Rickettsia prowazekii* grown in embryonated	May be used prior to travel to remote highland areas of Ethiopia, Rwanda,	Effective in North Africa during World War II. Local reactions

TABLE 13.1—*Continued*

Vaccine	Type of vaccine	Suggested use	Comment
	eggs.	Burundi, Mexico, Ecuador, Chile, Bolivia, Peru, and mountainous areas of Asia. Suggested for field workers in close contact with natives, medical personnel providing patient care and lab workers. Two subcutaneous doses 4 weeks apart followed by a 6–12 month booster.	common—general reactions uncommon.
Yellow fever	Live attenuated virus prepared in chick embryo Dakar strain or 17D strain.	Persons traveling to or living in area where the infection exists (Africa and South America); lab personnel, revaccination at 10 years.	Dakar strain—0.5% incidence of meningencephalitic reactions—not recommended. For international travel, vaccination must be certified on International Certificate of Vaccination (yellow card) at a Yellow Fever Vaccination Center listed with WHO. Mild systemic reactions 5–10 days after vaccination.
Pneumococcal	Capsular polysacccharides of 14 pneumococcal types	In patients with a high risk of serious pneumococcal infection: 0.5 ml, containing 50 μg of each of 14 serotypes	Duration of protection probably 3–5 years, therefore booster should be given no more often than every 3 years.

and in larger doses. This may be impractical in many cases, and thus a real advantage of live vaccines is that fewer doses may be given and less material must be prepared. The disadvantages of live vaccines are that they necessitate more care in handling, and the ever present danger of administration of an adventitious agent along with the live organism. This is especially important with respect to viral vaccines in which viruses are grown in a living cellular milieu; it is virtually impossible to rule out the presence of another agent.

Another consideration with respect to duration of protection is the question of booster immunization. There are very little data on the timing, number, or necessity of booster immunizations. One reason for "booster" immunizations is "insurance," i.e., if there is a 90% "take" with a particular vaccine, with two doses the susceptibles decrease from 10% to 1%. Boosters give added insurance when the primary immunization is given early in life, since maternal IgG antibody may still be present and inhibit the infant's antibody response. A second reason for booster immunizations is to induce memory, resulting in a secondary antibody response with respect to serum IgG antibody. Immunity may be greatly prolonged and on reexposure to the antigen, protection may be effected much more rapidly. Specific immunization suggestions are shown in Table 13.1.

In ending a discussion of immunizations, it is imperative that the dangers and potential dangers of immunizations be emphasized. We must be aware of the risk to not only the recipient but also to contacts, since a live vaccine organism may be spread to others. Obviously, one must always balance the risks of the procedure with the benefit. This is nowhere better exemplified than with the smallpox immunization. There are well-documented dangers associated with vaccination. This must be balanced with the danger of introduction of smallpox into the United States. It is obvious that for several years the balance has been on the side of a greater danger from immunization than the risk of disease.

Another example of the dangers of immunization is the polio virus vaccine. The danger of immunization is less clear, but it would appear that cases of polio with residual paralysis occur as a result of the vaccine virus becoming more virulent on passage through the gut (in about 1 in 4,000,000 recipients). At the present time, most of the workers in the area would agree that the dangers of polio immunization are far less than the danger of the disease.

There are many potential dangers with respect to the rubella virus vaccine, particularly the danger of the vaccine being administered or being transmitted to a pregnant woman. With some of the vaccines currently in use, it has been shown that the vaccine strain, although attenuated, can infect the placenta. Thus, there is a real danger that fetal abnormalities could be induced by the vaccine. The second potential danger of the rubella vaccine is that if duration of protection is not lifelong, and we continue the procedure of immunizing young children, we could be producing an adult population which is completely unprotected 20 years from now.

The age at which a vaccine should be administered depends not only on the age at which the dangers from immunization are minimal, but also the age at which the vaccinees are most at risk from the infectious disease.

These two considerations often work in opposite directions. After measles immunization, convulsions are occasionally seen, occurring 4½ times more commonly in infants immunized before 1 year of age than in children immunized between 1 and 2 years. On the other hand, the frequency is much, much less than following naturally occurring measles. It would thus seem reasonable to be flexible on the timing of administration of measles vaccine: earlier in life where natural measles is occurring but later (e.g., about year 2) in communities where measles has been nearly eradicated.

Pertussis is a very severe illness in young babies, therefore, the first dose of the vaccine is administered at about the age of 2 months, despite the fact that reactions are more severe in younger babies, and despite the probable presence of maternal antibody. However, the severeness of the infection warrants a more aggressive immunization practice. An alternative approach would be to insure that all mothers are well immunized, have high titers of antibody, resulting in newborns with protective levels of antibodies for the first several months of life. If this were the case, then immunization of babies could be postponed until about 6 months of age.

Another aspect of timing is to ensure that immunity is solid on entrance to school, whether this is nursery school or kindergarten, because of the heavy exposure at that point.

With the widespread use of a vaccine, the disease often becomes much less prevalent. When the prevalence decreases, the population very rapidly becomes lax about obtaining immunization. This can lead to a very large adult susceptible population. Many diseases, which are fairly benign in childhood become much more virulent when they affect adult populations, e.g., poliomyelitis.

A final theoretical danger of immunizations is the development of new strains of the organism. It has been postulated that immunization simply hastens the evolution of new strains, as for example, with influenza virus, in which new strains develop periodically, possibly as a result of population immunity.

SELECTED REFERENCES

Cluff, L. E., and Allen, J. C.: Principles of active immunization for prevention of infection. J. Chronic Dis., *15:* 575, 1962.

Hornick, R. B., Woodward, T. E., McCrumb, F. R., Snyder, M. J., Dawkins, A. T., Bulkeley, J. T., de la Macorra, F., and Corozza, F. A.: Typhoid fever vaccine—yes or no? Med. Clin. North Am., *51:* 617, 1967.

Krugman, S., and Katz, S. L.: Childhood immunization procedures. J. Am. Med. Assoc., *237:* 2228, 1977.

Lauteria, S. F., Kantzler, B. C., High, P. C., Lee, J. D., and Waldman, R. H.: An attenuated influenza virus vaccine: reactogenecity, transmissibility, immunogeneicity and protective efficacy. J. Infect. Dis., *130:* 380, 1974.

Meiklejohn, G.: Smallpox: is the end in sight. J. Infect. Dis., *133:* 347, 1976.

Meyer, H. M., and Parkman, P. D.: Rubella vaccination, a review of practical experience. J. Am. Med. Assoc., *215:* 613, 1971.

Perkins, J. C., Tucker, D. N., Knopf, H. L. S., Wenzel, R. P., Hornick, R. B., Kapikian, A. Z., and Chanock, R. M.: Evidence for the protective effect of an inactivated rhinovirus vaccine administered by the nasal route. Am. J. Epidemiol., *90:* 319, 1969.

Pollock, T. M.: Assessing immunization procedures. Proc. Roy. Soc. Med., *63:* 811, 1970.

Stuart-Harris, C.: The principles and practice of immunization. Practitioner, *215:* 285, 1975.

Wilson, G. S.: *The Hazards of Immunization.* London: The Athlone Press, 1967.

Chapter 14

IMMUNE COMPLEX DISEASES

Gerald Blandford, M.B.

After an immunogenic stimulus, antibodies are produced which combine with the evoking antigenic determinants wherever they are encountered. These specific antibody responses are generally beneficial as the combination of antigen with antibody usually facilitates antigen elimination. This is achieved by a variety of means including amplification of nonspecific inflammatory responses. The antigen involved in these inflammatory reactions may itself be relatively noninflammatory, so that tissue damage and clinical disease may be mainly attributed to the host response. Some clinical examples involving inert antigens include penicillin hypersensitivity, serum sickness, and hepatitis B virus antigenemia.

The following discussion will review briefly the basic mechanism of immune complex-mediated tissue damage, consider certain prototypic clinical entities with some examples, suggest clinical presentations which could indicate an underlying immune complex etiology, indicate laboratory diagnostic techniques, and finally summarize the logical but currently limited therapeutic possibilities.

Immune Complex-Mediated Tissue Damage

The mechanisms by which immune responses may cause tissue damage have been subdivided into four types. In type I, antibody is bound to a cell containing an effector system and reacts with passing antigen; in type II, antibody reacts with antigen on or in a cell membrane; in type III, antibody reacts with antigen in fluid phase in the tissues or blood; and in type IV, specifically sensitized lymphocytes trigger or mediate effector systems directly on contact with antigen.

Immune complex diseases are mediated by the type III reaction. In order to understand this mechanism clearly it is necessary to know the component parts and to appreciate the importance of the quantity and quality of the response and of time. In the primary humoral response to an antigen there are moments in time when antigen is in excess, when antigen and antibody are at equivalence and finally, if the response is adequate, when antibody is in excess (Fig. 14.1a). The type III reaction occurs when there is a slight antigen excess and when the antibody concerned can trigger the complement system. It is evident that if the antibody response is slow (Fig. 14.1b) or the antigen is replicating (Fig. 14.1c and d), then the duration and the amount of immune complexes can vary. The size of the complexes is generally inversely proportional to the amount of antigen. Large complexes are rapidly cleared by reticulo-endothelial cells, while small complexes are associated with the Arthus reaction. The greater the mass of damaging complexes that are present at any moment in time the greater the amount of tissue damage. The site of formation of potentially damaging complexes is important to the resulting clinical picture. The tissue hallmark of an immune complex-mediated event is the finding of IgG antibody, complement components

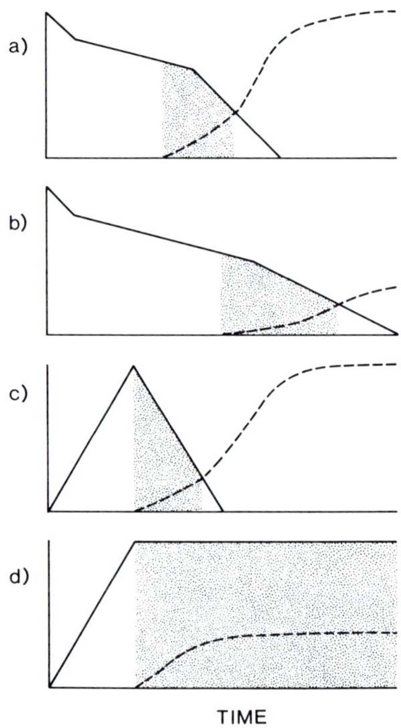

FIG. 14.1. The duration of immune complexes following primary challenge. (a), single injection of non-replicating antigen in normal host; (b), single injection of non-replicating antigen in a slow responder; (c), acute infection—replicating antigen in normal host; (d), chronic infection—replicating antigen with inadequate response. Antigen concentration (——); antibody titer (-----). Shaded area indicates presence of complexes in antigen excess.

and antigen at the reaction site. Nonreplicating antigens are rarely detectable after the first 24 hours as they are rapidly phagocytosed and cleared. Localized antigen results in a localized Arthus reaction and circulating immune complexes result in a generalized serum sickness-like syndrome or glomerulonephritis. There are, therefore, two prototypic entities which can be ascribed to immune complex formation.

The Arthus Reaction

This is a localized event in which antigen in the tissues combines with potentially precipitating antibodies either formed locally or diffused from the blood as originally described by Arthus (Fig. 14.2). The reaction is associated with local histamine release, complement activation, lysosomal enzyme release, anaphylatoxin formation, entrapment of leucocytes (mostly polymorphonuclear leucocytes in the first 24 hours and lymphocytes later), platelet activation, and local hemorrhage and thrombus formation. Experimentally, previous antihistamines or heparin, or depletion of platelets, polymorphonuclear leucocytes or complement, diminish the inflammatory results. The inflammatory reaction may also be suppressed before or after the event by steroid administration.

Serum Sickness

The rabbit model of serum sickness using spontaneous and preformed circulating immune complexes has greatly clarified our understanding of the pathogenesis of this condition. The basic model is illustrated in Figure 14.1a. A single injection of bovine serum albumin is given. It is eliminated from the blood in three phases. Initially there is intra- and extravascular

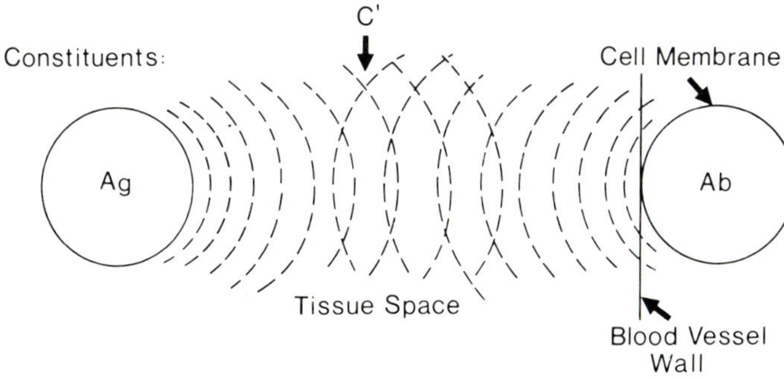

FIG. 14.2. Diagrammatic representation of a localized type III (Arthus) reaction. A packet of antigen (Ag) on the left allows diffusion through the tissue space. IgG antibody (Ab) from either a cell or from the blood diffuses through the tissue space towards the antigen. At a point in the concentration gradient formed in the tissue fluids antigen is present in moderate excess and complement (C′) is activated. This results in histamine and lysosomal enzyme release, anaphylatoxin formation, entrapment of leucocytes and platelets, and fibrinogenesis activated. Local thrombosis or hemorrhage may occur.

equilibration, then slow catabolization and, finally, a phase of rapid clearing. During the last phase immune complexes are detectable in the blood, there is a generalized vasculitis effecting the heart, joints, and glomeruli, and total hemolytic complement in the blood is reduced. The lesions contain IgG antibody, antigen, and complement. This acute disease may also be modulated by previous antihistamine or heparin, or by complement, platelet or polymorphonuclear leucocyte depletion. The disease resolves without residua.

After repeated administration of antigen chronic disease may follow. If rabbits are given daily injections of bovine serum albumin most animals clear the antigen promptly, a few are tolerant and fail to clear antigen by means of antibody, and neither develops disease. A third small group of animals mount an inadequate antibody response which fails to clear antigen and they develop an immune complex mediated glomerulonephritis similar to the consequences of chronic viral infection (Fig. 14.1d). The generalized acute vasculitis of acute serum sickness is absent. It has been postulated that the reason for this is that, in the acute disease, antigen is widely distributed in the interstitial tissues, including blood vessel walls, before antibody is produced. When antibody finally appears the tissue reaction occurs within the vessel walls. After repeated doses the complexes are formed intravascularly, not in vessel walls, and are concentrated and/or trapped in glomeruli.

Clinical Prototypes of Immune Complex Disease

There are three groups of clinical disease in man which appear to be closely analogous to the experimental models described above. These are (1) Arthus-like reactions (such as erythema nodosum leprosum and extrinsic allergic alveolitis), (2) multifocal vasculitis, and (3) isolated glomerulonephritis. Each group will be discussed separately. It is important to realize that in many of the disorders the ultimate proof for the presence of immune complexes is lacking because relevant antigens have not so far been detected in lesions or in circulating immune complexes. It must be emphasized that, (1) even where there is proof of the presence of immune complexes and complement components in a lesion they may be passively deposited at a site of increased capillary permeability and not have caused the lesion and (2) where evidence for immune complex deposition in a lesion is absent the triggering complexes may have been removed by the time of biopsy. Nevertheless, search for an antigen is imperative where immune complex-mediated tissue damage is the possible pathogenic mechanism, since removal of the antigen is the key therapeutic maneuver. In some conditions alternative and additional immunopathologic mechanism may also be active, particularly types I and IV.

Localized Immune Complex Reactions in Man

Classical Arthus reactions may occur in the skin after skin tests with *Aspergillus fumigatus*, *Candida albicans*, avian serum proteins, and thyroid extracts when serum-precipitating antibodies are present in the blood. An acute wheal and flare reaction in 10–20 min followed by a boggy edematous reaction at 6–8 hours is characteristic. Similar reactions used to be common after repeated antitoxin or antibacterial serum administration and more recently have followed insulin injections. In all of these conditions antigen is deposited in the skin and combines with antibody in the local tissue fluids in previously sensitized individuals (Fig. 14.2).

The spontaneous clinical lesion most analagous to the experimental Arthus reaction is that of erythema nodosum leprosum. The lesions contain antibody, antigen, and complement components and are predominantly infiltrated with neutrophil polymorphs. Lesions, either of erythema nodosum, nodular vasculitis, or a multiform erythema have been associated with many bacterial, viral, and fungal infections. Some associations of vasculitic lesions of the skin which may have a local immune complex pathogenesis are listed in Table 14.1 and have been reviewed in detail. Recovery without residua is the general rule and follows removal of the antigen by normal physiologic processes or appropriate medical

TABLE 14.1. *Some Possible Causes of Immune Complex Cutaneous Vasculitis (Erythema Nodosum, Nodular Vasculitis, Multiform Erythema)*

Infections	Neoplasms
Mycobacteria[a]	Hodgkin's disease
Streptococci[a]	Leukemias
Staphylococci[a]	
Gonococci	Granulomata
Meningococci	Sarcoidosis
Pasteurella pseudotuberculosis	Regional enteritis
Typhoid	
Diphtheria	Drug sensitivities
Syphilis[a]	Sulphonamides
Mycoplasma	Salicylates
Psittacosis	Iodides
Lymphogranuloma venerium	"The pill" (high estrogen types)
Mumps	
Measles	
Polio	
Candida albicans	
Coccidiomycosis	
Histoplasmosis	
Upper respiratory tract infections (unspecified causes)	

[a] Indicates definitive proof of association available.

TABLE 14.2. *Diseases Associated with Inhaled Organic Dusts*

Fungal spores	Mammalian proteins
Farmer's lung	Bird fancier's lung
Ventilation pneumonitis	Pituitary snuff worker's lung
Fog fever in cattle	Fish-meal worker's lung
Bagassosis	
Mushroom worker's lung	Antigens not identified
Maple-bark pneumonitis	New Guinea thatch disease
Malt worker's lung	Smallpox handler's lung
Cheeseworker's lung	Paprika-splitter's lung
Suberosis	Furrier's lung
Sequoisis	Coffee worker's lung
Insect antigens	
Wheat weavil	

intervention. Occasionally repeated or more chronic symptoms may require steroid therapy. This should only follow a careful and complete work-up of the case.

Extrinsic allergic alveolitis, a condition causally related to inhalation of organic dusts, appears to be a form of localized type III reaction occurring in alveoli. All are characterized by late (5–8 hours) respiratory reactions after provocation tests with appropriate antigens. There is often accompanying fever, leucocytosis, and wheezing which is incompletely and temporarily reversed by inhaled bronchodilators. Where antigens have been clearly identified, precipitating antibodies are present in the blood and skin tests may reveal a classic type III Arthus response. Occasionally, early reactions occur on provocation challenge of the respiratory tract or in the skin, similar in timing and character to type I reactions. Sometimes the clinical history will also reveal a bimodal response. The mechanism of the early reaction is not clear. It has been suggested that it is mediated by reaginic IgG or IgE antibodies. The beneficial effects of inhalation of disodium chromoglycate before respiratory provocation is thought to be due to inhibition of the early reaction suggesting that it is a requirement for the later response. There is also recent evidence in an experimental model that a type IV allergic reaction may be involved. A list of diseases which have been associated with inhalation of "organic dusts" is given in Table 14.2. The condition is self-limiting if antigen withdrawal occurs early. Later, pulmonary fibrosis may occur and persist.

There is evidence which suggests that a type III allergic mechanism is involved in the pathogenesis of severe respiratory syncytial virus infection in neonates or in recipients of killed respiratory syncytial virus vaccine. There is little doubt that a transient immune complex-mediated mechanism is involved during normal recovery in the microenvironment of

TABLE 14.3. *Clinical Indicators of Circulating Immune Complex Disease (Multifocal Vasculitis)*

Fever
Arthralgia
Rash (urticaria, erythema, purpura, and necrosis)
Renal disease (nephrotic syndrome, glomerulonephritis)
Abdominal pain
Raynaud's phenomenon
Mononeuritis
Central nervous system abnormalities (dementia)
Serositis

myxovirus infections of the lung. It seems likely that such a mechanism is also involved in other primary infections (Fig. 14.1c).

Circulating Immune Complex Diseases

Multifocal Vasculitis

Multifocal vasculitis as the name implies is essentially a diagnosis based upon histologic evidence of inflamed blood vessels at different sites and/or in several organs. The condition may be acute or chronic. Although diagnostic clinical criteria have not been formalized there are clearly patterns of symptoms and signs which suggest to the aware physician that a disease, probably associated with circulating immune complexes, is present. These are set out in Table 14.3.

There are three recognizable circumstances in which multifocal vasculitis occurs; (1) iatrogenic, (2) infections, and (3) associated with several rheumatic diseases.

Iatrogenic. Penicillin hypersensitivity may cause a condition resembling classical "serum sickness" (Fig. 14.1a) and is now probably the most common cause of this syndrome. The onset is usually 8–12 days after a primary exposure but may be much more rapid (4–6 hours) in an already sensitized patient. An acute wheal and flare (type I reaction) often occurs at the injection site followed by fever, rash, arthralgia, nephritis, and lymphadenopathy. The condition is usually self-limiting but early appropriate treatment is needed for severe acute anaphylaxis or renal failure. The provoking agent should not knowingly be given again and the patient should be clearly informed and told to warn medical attendants. A "Medicalert" bracelet is a worthwhile precaution.

Infections. A fairly common prodromal illness in serum hepatitis consists of fever, urticaria, and arthralgia. Jaundice may be absent but free hepatitis-associated antigen (HAA) is detected in the serum often with hypocomplementemia. The onset of hepatic involvement usually accompanies the disappearance of both the symptoms and HAA from the blood. This clinical entity is similar to the diagrammatic presentation of an acute infection depicted in Figure 14.1c. An alternative outcome with chronic HAA antigenemia is well recognized, however, indicating a host response similar to that presented in Figure 14.1d. It is, therefore, not surprising that HAA's have now been well documented in chronic vasculitic lesions, particularly in polyarteritis nodosum and in some glomerulonephritic kidneys.

Subacute bacterial endocarditis is frequently associated with an immune complex type of glomerulonephritis. Although bacterial antigens have not been detected in glomeruli there is considerable data which indicate the presence of immune complexes and hypocomplementemia in the serum of such patients. The circulating immune complexes in subacute bacterial endocarditis have frequently been shown to contain rheumatoid factor and to be cryoprecipitable. Cryoprecipitable immune complexes are discussed in more detail below.

Secondary syphilis is often associated with fever, a skin eruption, and lymphadenopathy and may present with an acute nephritis or a nephrotic syndrome. The renal lesions have all the hallmarks of an immune complex disease with immunoglobulin and complement components present in granular deposits in the glomeruli. Specific antitreponema antibody has been isolated from the renal lesion of a single patient but treponema antigens have yet to be found.

Rheumatic Diseases. Various manifestations of vasculitis are quite common in the more severe cases of rheumatoid arthritis and Sjögren's syndrome, in systemic lupus erythematosus (SLE), dermatomyositis, and rheumatic fever. In the first three, circulating immune complexes have been identified with certainty.

In rheumatoid arthritis and Sjögren's syndrome the complexes detected have been rheumatoid factors (IgM, IgG) complexed to circulating IgG. These complexes are often cryoprecipitable and usually activate complement in vitro. They have also been detected in rheumatoid synovial fluid in the presence of low complement levels. There is histologic evidence that renal and dermal lesions contain rheumatoid factors, IgG, and complement. In SLE, anti-DNA/DNA complexes have been detected in the serum and histologic lesions as discussed in Chapter 15. Cryoglobulinemia in immune complex disease is discussed in more detail below.

Isolated Glomerulonephritis

The indication that a renal lesion may be attributed to an immune complex mediated mechanism is the presence of demonstrable immunoglobulin, complement components, and sometimes antigens in a granular distribution in glomeruli. Detailed studies of experimental models have clearly shown that such complexes may cause nephropathy. However, circulating complexes may be present without deposition in glomeruli and complexes may certainly occur and be deposited without apparent renal pathology.

There is clear evidence in acute nonlethal respiratory virus infections in rodents that transient immune complex deposition of immunoglobulin and viral antigen occur. This has not been documented in man but the close association of preceding nonbacterial upper respiratory tract infection with acute nephritis, nephrotic syndrome and exacerbations of both suggest that such a mechanism may be responsible. These patients could be pictured as having a slow response (Fig. 14.1b) after acute infection (Fig. 14.1c) with a result close to that seen in chronic infection (Fig. 14.1d).

Chronic virus infections in animals are associated with an immune complex mediated glomerulopathy. Protracted viral and bacterial infection in man have been associated with similar findings. Antigen has been detected in the kidney in serum hepatitis, salmonellosis, and malaria. Tumor antigens have been detected in the kidney of a patient with colonic carcinoma and, of course, DNA has been found in the kidneys of patients with SLE, which may be a disease associated with chronic virus infection (see Chapter 15).

The picture of an immune complex nephropathy has also accompanied other conditions in which chronic antigenic challenge is present or likely (e.g., narcotic addicts) but in which the specific antigens have not yet been identified in the renal lesions. The deposits have sometimes been shown to contain rheumatoid factors and IgG which in turn have been present as circulating complexes. When carefully studied these complexes are often cryoprecipitable. Some isolated cryoprecipitates have been carefully studied and relevant antigens have sometimes been found. Thus, circulating antigen-antibody complexes are sometimes present in the blood as a triple complex of antiantibody (rheumatoid factor)/specific antibody/antigen. The conditions in which this has been shown to occur are listed in Table 14.4.

TABLE 14.4. *Clinical Associations of Cryoglobulinemia*

Lymphocyte neoplasia	Infections
Myeloma	Subacute bacterial endocarditis
Macroglobulinemia	Syphilis
Chronic lymphatic leukemia	Leprosy
Lymphoma	Tuberculosis
	Infectious mononucleosis
Reticuloendothelial, granuloma	Cytomegalovirus mononucleosis
Reticulosis	Trypanosomiasis
Sarcoidosis	
	Chronic antigenic challenge
Rheumatic	Cirrhosis
Systemic lupus erythematosus	Narcotic addiction
Rheumatoid arthritis	Hemolytic anemia
Sjögren's syndrome	Acute glomerulonephritis
Ankylosing spondylitis	"Essential" cryoglobulinemia

Cryoglobulinemia

Cryoglobulins are globular serum proteins which precipitate or gel on cooling and redissolve on warming. Cryoglobulins contain immunoglobulins and other serum proteins. They may be characterized according to the type of immunoglobulins present. Type I contain monoclonal immunoglobulins; type II contain mixed immunoglobulins which include a monoclonal component, most frequently monoclonal IgM with rheumatoid factor activity; type III contain a mixture of polyclonal immunoglobulins and also frequently polyclonal rheumatoid factors.

Cryoglobulins have been detected in the serum of patients with what appear to be either primary lymphocyte-derived neoplasia or diseases characterized by polyclonal hyper-γ-globulinemia or chronic antigenic stimulus (Table 14.4). The most frequent symptom complex in cryoglobulinemia is Raynaud's phenomenon, dependent vascular purpura, and arthralgia or arthritis, and the most frequent lethal complication is nephritis. Peripheral neuropathy, acute abdominal pain and cold urticaria also occur. Histologically the lesions show a vasculitis, often with all components of the cryoglobulin present. There is clearly a great clinical and pathologic similarity between patients with circulating immune complexes and cryoglobulinemia (particularly types II and III), and cryoglobulins can often be shown to contain immune complexes.

Laboratory Investigations

The presence of circulating immune complexes has been correlated with disease prognosis and shown to be an excellent parameter of disease activity. An additional reason for searching exhaustively for the presence of immune complexes in body fluids or tissues relates to the possibility of identifying associated antigens which is vital information for the formulation of specific therapy. Although history and physical examination may provide important clues to the nature of the antigen (e.g., drug exposure, specific infection, rheumatoid disease), investigation for specific antigens may be negative. A plan for further investigation is then needed. Unfortunately this often requires the help of a sophisticated and often research-oriented laboratory. The bare bones of such a plan are presented in Table 14.5.

Immune Complexes

A great variety of methods has been described which are claimed to be able to detect the presence of immune complexes in serum or other body fluids (Table 14.6). Many are sophisticated techniques beyond the capabilities of routine laboratories, quite expensive, and not entirely reliable. The most recent variant involves the adherence of IgG and C′ components in the complexes to receptors on a lymphoblastoid B cell line (Raji cells) and subsequent radioimmunoassay to quantitate IgG bound to the cells. This technique has been successfully used in a recent detailed study of infective endocarditis. Its promise relates to (1) extreme sensitivity and the ability to quantify the amount of complexes and (2) the potential for use in isolating and concentrating the complexes and subsequent search for contained antigens.

Cryoglobulins

Few laboratories are efficient in their techniques for collecting blood (warm syringe), separating serum (clotting and spinning at 37°C), and examining the sera, stored at 4°C, daily for 48–96 hours. As a result it is certain that many cryoglobulins have been missed. However, there are laboratory clues which may indicate the presence of cryoglobulins. Essentially one should look for unexpected variations in total γ globulin determinations, quantitation of immunoglobulins, and in specific antibody titers (e.g., R.F. or A.N.F.) between successive serum samples. The implication is that if one serum had greatly reduced levels then a

TABLE 14.5. *Laboratory Investigations in Immune Complex Disease*

Serum/serous fluid (e.g., synovial, pleural aspirates)
1. Immune complexes
2. Cryoglobulins
3. Suspected antigen(s)
4. Reduced complement components
5. Culture for suspected organisms

Tissue biopsies
1. Conventional histology
2. Studies for deposition of immunoglobulins, complement components and suspected antigen(s)
3. Elution of antibodies and/or antigen(s)
4. Culture for suspected organisms

TABLE 14.6. *Some Methods for Detecting Circulating Complexes*

1. Precipitation with Clq in agarose gel
2. Precipitation with monoclonal rheumatoid factor
3. Precipitation with polyethylene glycol
4. Precipitation with polyethylene glycol of ^{125}I-Clq bound to complexes
5. Agglutination of latex particles
6. Competitive inhibition of uptake of ^{125}I-complexes by guinea pig macrophages
7. Microcomplement consumption
8. Inhibition of antibody dependent cytotoxicity
9. Platelet aggregation
10. Cryoprecipitation
11. Alternate free antibody, free antigen
12. Analytical ultracentrifuge

cryoglobulin may have been lost between taking the blood and testing the serum. Not all technicians look at the serum taken from the refrigerator and may ignore the presence of a cryoprecipitate. Cruder clues are the presence of rouleaux formation and an unexpectedly high sedimentation rate.

In fact it is not necessary to use a special laboratory or any expensive equipment to detect the presence of cryoglobulins, as this could easily be done in most doctor's offices. The only requirements are a thermometer, warm water, a refrigerator, and a clinical centrifuge. The details have been outlined above. Once detected further study is indicated including repeats of serum protein, immunoglobulin, and complement estimations and antibody titers on serum at 37°C and similar studies of the isolated and washed cryoprecipitate. Various more sophisticated studies of the latter are possible including culture of organisms, elution procedures for specific antibodies, electronmicroscopic studies for virus particles, and special studies for specific suspected antigens.

Complement Assays

The complement system has been discussed in Chapter 10. In the context of immune complex diseases suffice to say that the complement system is activated and is the principal mechanism for causing and amplifying tissue damage. Thus total hemolytic complement may be greatly diminished as may various individual complement components. Of these, C3 and C4 are readily measured by immunodiffusion in clinical laboratories. Reduced C3 and normal C4 would indicate activation of the complement sequence from C3 onwards (the bypass mechanism) and, therefore, suggest that antibody was not involved. In immune complex diseases total hemolytic complement, C3 and C4 may all be reduced in the active stage indicating activation of the antibody-dependent part of the sequence, and may be helpful laboratory parameters of disease activity. It is of great importance to recognize that false laboratory results are frequent if serum is not fresh (<1 day at 4°C, >2 days at −20°C).

Free Antigen

In certain clear-cut immune complex diseases antigens circulate freely and may be detected by fairly simple means. Thus, in SLE free DNA may be present, in serum hepatitis free HAA, and in subacute bacterial endocarditis the causative organism. In apparent chronic clinical immune complex disease DNA and HAA should always be looked for and blood cultured. Other specific antigens should also be sought in both acute and chronic disease states if a technique is available for the antigen suspected (Table 14.1).

Histology

The pathognomonic lesion in immune complex disease is a vasculitis in which immunoglobulins, preferably with proven specific antibody activity, specific antigen(s), and complement components are deposited. The lesion biopsied should preferably be in an early phase. Skin and kidney are the most rewarding tissues.

Therapeutic Approaches

Unfortunately critical information (i.e., the specific causative antigen(s)) is frequently lacking. A simple and logical approach is offered in Table 14.7.

The obvious practicalities of avoidance of a known antigen or appropriate therapy for a treatable cause need no amplification. In acute conditions the disease is self-limiting and only symptomatic and supportive measures are needed. In chronic disorders the need for nonspecific antiinflammatory measures must be determined by clinical judgment. The complications of therapy must be weighed against the effects of the disease on the patient or on the patient in relation to his or her environment. Vasculitic involvement of a vital organ, in particular the kidneys, is a clear indication for urgent active therapeutic intervention. All patients with suspected or proven immune complex disease should have regular urine microscopy looking for hemegranular casts as evidence of glomerulitis, as most deaths are attributable to renal failure. Parameters for therapeutic efficacy include clinical judgment, correction of anemia, fall of sedimentation rate, fall of immunoglobulin levels, rise of complement components, and the disappearance of cryoglobulins or demonstrated immune complexes.

Special measures in cryoglobulinemia include avoidance of cold exposure, antihistamine for cold urticaria, and avoidance of prolonged stand-

TABLE 14.7. *Therapeutic Approaches to Immune Complex Diseases*

Practical

1. Known extrinsic antigen
   —Avoid
2. Known intrinsic antigen and treatable (e.g., infection)
   —Appropriate therapy
3. Unknown antigen or known and untreatable
   a) Nonspecific antiinflammatory agents (steroids, azathioprine, cyclophosphamide, hydroxychloroquine)
   b) Plasmaphoresis
   c) Appropriate cytotoxic therapy for macroglobulinemia or multiple myeloma

Experimental

—Actively or passively improve host response to eradicate antigen physiologically
—Administer inert harmless antigen in excess

ing to reduce dependent purpura. In quantitatively impressive cryoglobulinemia in which complexes, because of their size, are largely intravascular (e.g., type I, monoclonal IgM, or type II, monoclonal rheumatoid factor IgM with polyclonal IgG) plasmaphoresis may be lifesaving. Plasmaphoresis may also be worth trying in other forms of life threatening nonresponsive immune complex disease.

The choice of antiinflammatory, cytotoxic, and often incorrectly called "immunosuppressive" drugs must still be left largely to the clinicians' own discretion. Unfortunately, as with so many chronic or relapsing disorders of unknown etiology, convincing, controlled drug trials are conspicuously absent from the literature, so proven regimens are not available. In patients with serious active disease one approach is to start steroids, and later to add azathioprine, as much for its steroid sparing effect as for its own antiinflammatory properties. If renal involvement is present then the combination is used from the start. In more indolent conditions in which renal involvement is absent, a trial of hydroxychloroquine with ophthalmologic surveillance may be worthwhile. As a last resort in nonresponsive premorbid states plasmaphoresis has met with some limited immediate success.

Experimental Approaches

In theory, active or passive improvement of host responses to a given antigen should accelerate removal of all damaging complexes. Neither possibility has been tried in humans. Indeed, one might well be reluctant to induce or provide higher immunoglobulin levels in patients with rheumatoid factors. On the other hand, the passive administration of rheumatoid factors if absent could improve macrophage handling of complexes.

Some of the modest therapeutic success achieved with cytotoxic and antiinflammatory drugs may be theoretically attributed to allowing larger amounts of antigen to circulate, thus reducing the size of circulating complexes to below that which will trigger the type III response. Passive administration of high dose of antigen in chronic immune complex disease has been beneficial in animal experiments.

Summary

There is little doubt that potentially damaging immune complexes occur at least transiently in any specific antibody response to any antigen. Immune complex disease occurs when a sufficient concentration of complexes at the critical antigen/complement fixing antibody ratio occurs in the circulation or tissues. Localized and circulating complexes cause clinical states which have distinct symptom profiles. A condition characterized by fever, rash, and arthralgia is highly suspicious of an immune complex pathogenesis. Glomerulonephritis is the single most lethal complication. Laboratory proof of the presence of complexes in serum may be difficult but an approach is offered. Lesion histology may be of great help. The single most important and least satisfactorily solved problem is the identification of the provoking antigen(s). Cryoglobulins are often present in immune complex diseases and may contain all elements of the circulating complexes. An ordered therapeutic approach is offered.

SELECTED REFERENCES

Bayer, A. S., Theofilopoulos, A. N., Eisenberg, R., Dixon, F. J., and Guze, L. B.: Circulating immune complexes in infective endocarditis. N. Engl. J. Med., *295:* 1500, 1976.

Bhorade, M. S., Carag, H. B., Lee, H. J., Potter, U. P., and Dunea, G.: Nephropathy of secondary syphilis. A clinical and pathological spectrum. JAMA, *216:* 1158, 1971.

Blandford, G., and Charlton, C.: Studies of pulmonary and renal immunopathology after non-lethal primary Sendai virus infection in normal and cyclophosphamide treated hamsters. Am. Rev. Resp. Dis., *115:* 305, 1977.

Brouet, J. C., Clavvel, J. P., Danon, F., Klein, M., and Seligman, M.: Biologic and clinical significance of cryoglobulins. Am. J. Med., *57:* 775, 1974.

Cochrane, C. G., and Koffler, D.: Immune complex disease in experimental animals and man. Adv. Immunol., *16:* 185, 1973.

Christian, C. L., and Sergent, J. S.: Vasculitis syndromes: clinical and experimental models. Am. J. Med., *61:* 385, 1976.

Couser, W. G., Wagonfeld, J. B., Spargo, B. H., and Lewis, E. J.: Glomerular deposition of tumor antigen in membranous nephropathy associated with colonic carcinoma. Am. J. Med., *57:* 962, 1974.

Cream, J. J., and Turk, J. L.: A review of the evidence for immune complex deposition as cause of skin disease in man. Clin. Allergy, *1:* 235, 1971.

Gamble, C. N., and Reardan, J. B.: Immunopathogenesis of syphilitic glomerulonephritis. Elution of anti-treponemal antibody from glomerular immune complex deposits. N. Engl. J. Med., *292:* 449, 1975.

Gocke, D. J., Hsu, K., and Morgan, G.: Association between polyarteritis and Australia antigen. Lancet, *2:* 1149, 1970.

Gutman, R. A., Striker, G. E., Gilliland, B. C., and Cutler, R. E.: The immune complex glomerulonephritis of bacterial endocarditis. Medicine, *51:* 1, 1972.

McIntosh, R. M., Griswold, W. R., Chernack, W. B., Williams, G. Strauss, J., Kaufman, D. B., Koss, M. N., McIntosh, J. R., Cohen, R., and Weil, R.: Cryoglobulins. III. Further studies on the nature, incidence, clinical, diagnostic, prognostic and immuno-pathologic significance of cryoproteins in renal disease. J. Med., *44:* 285, 1975.

Nicholson, D.P.: Extrinsic allergic pneumonias. Am. J. Med., *53:* 131, 1972.

Parish, W. E.: Studies on vasculitis. IV. The low incidence of antibacterial anaphylactic antibodies in the sera of persons with cutaneous vasculitis following bacterial infection. Clin. Allergy, *1:* 433, 1971.

Richerson, H. B., Cheng, F. H., and Bauserman, S. C.: Acute experimental hypersensitivity pneumonitis in rabbits. Am. Rev. Resp. Dis., *104:* 568, 1971.

Sutherland, J. C., Markham, R. V., and Mardiney, M. R.: Subclinical immune complexes in the glomeruli of kidneys post mortem. Am. J. Med., *57:* 536, 1974.

Theofilopoulos, A. N., Wilson, C. B., and Dixon, F. J.: The Raji cell radioimmune assay for detecting immune complexes in human sera. J. Clin. Invest., *57:* 168, 1976.

Chapter 15

AUTOANTIBODIES AND HUMAN DISEASE

Richard S. Panush, M.D.

Autoantigens and Autoantibodies

A great variety of autoantibodies, directed to virtually all organ systems, occurs in patients with many different diseases. They may also be found in some normal persons. Some of the antigens against which antibodies have been recognized—including cellular, subcellular, protein, or other antigens—are listed in Table 15.1. It is beyond the scope of this discussion to review all of these situations in detail. Rather, the mechanisms by which autoantibodies may be produced and their role in certain immunologic diseases will be examined. In these examples, autoantibodies have been particularly well studied and their role in disease clarified.

The old concept of "horror autotoxicus" implied that autoantibodies were autodestructive. This has now been extensively modified. The possible relationships of autoantibodies to disease are outlined in Table 15.2. First, autoantibodies may occur without any clear relationship to pathogenesis of disease or diagnostic specificity. Certain antibodies to normal tissue antigens occur in normal persons without evident harmful effects. For example, some individuals have rheumatoid factors demonstrable in their serum but never develop arthritis or other immunologic disease. The same antibodies may occur with disease but without demonstrable biologic effects or diagnostic specificity, such as rheumatoid factor in hyperglobulinemic purpura. Second, autoantibodies may occur without being related to the pathogenesis of the disease. Autoantibodies, such as Wasserman antibodies in syphilis, may be demonstrated to have diagnostic specificity but have no biologic importance. Antibodies may be directly involved in pathogenesis of disease, such as antibodies to erythrocyte antigens which mediate hemolysis. Autoantibodies may be present in disease and have biologic activities, but not be harmful. They may sometimes prove beneficial—the same rheumatoid factors that may be innocuous in normal people and injurious in patients with rheumatoid arthritis may actually facilitate clearance of antigen-antibody complexes in systemic lupus erythematosus (SLE) or subacute bacterial endocarditis. Autoantibodies may occur with and potentiate disease without being directly involved in pathogenesis, such as blocking antibodies in patients with neoplasms. Last, antibodies may have nothing to do with the pathogenesis, but may actually be the result of a disease process, i.e., tissue damage may lead to changes in structure of substances such that the body no longer recognizes them as "self".

TABLE 15.1. *Antigens Against Which Antibodies Have Been Recognized*

Cellular	Subcellular	Protein—other
Neutrophils	DNA	Myelin
Lymphocytes	RNA	Basement membrane
Erythrocytes	Extractable nuclear antigen	Enzymes
Platelets	Histone	Clotting factors
Smooth muscle	Nucleoprotein	Thyroglobulin
Salivary duct	Other nuclear antigens	Hormones
Muscle	Ribosomes	Complement
Endothelium	Lysosomes	Immunoglobulin (IgG, IgA, IgM, IgD, IgE)
Neurons	Mitochondria	
Renal tubular epithelium	Cytoplasm	
Oncofetal antigens		
Histocompatibility antigens		
Blood group antigens		

TABLE 15.2. *Possible Relationships of Autoantibodies to Disease*

1. Unrelated
   a. Occurrence in normal individuals without development of symptoms (e.g., rheumatoid factors in normals)
   b. Occurrence in disease without demonstrable biologic effects or diagnostic specificity (e.g., rheumatoid factors in hyperglobulinemic purpura)

2. Related
   a. Occurrence with disease without biologic effects but with diagnostic specificity (e.g., Wasserman antibody in syphilis)
   b. Occurrence with disease and contributing to pathogenesis (e.g., erythrocyte antibodies in hemolytic anemias)
   c. Occurrence with disease and potentiating disease (blocking antibodies with neoplasms)
   d. Occurrence with disease with possible beneficial effects (e.g., rheumatoid factors in systemic lupus erythematosus or subacute bacterial endocarditis)

Autoimmunity

It should be apparent that the presence of autoantibodies alone does not necessarily imply that a disease is autoimmune. An autoimmune etiology for an illness should fulfill the following criteria (Table 15.3): (1a) circulating or tissue-bound antibodies, active under physiologic conditions, should be demonstrated; or (1b) circulating or localized populations of sensitized lymphocytes or their products should be present and active under physiologic conditions. (2) The sensitizing antigen should be identified. (3) Production of antibodies or sensitized lymphocytes to the same antigen should be demonstrated in vitro or in animals. (4) Pathologic events in vitro or changes in the experimental animal should correspond to those in human disease. (5) The disease should be transferred from immunized to normal animals by either competent lymphocytes or immune serum. It is important that these or comparable criteria be carefully applied to diseases so that loose characterization is avoided and roles of possible immunoreactants remain clear.

How is it that "self" may become "nonself" and result in formation of autoantibodies? The answers are not yet clear. Two general mechanisms are listed in Table 15.4. (1) The first of these mechanisms presupposes that autoantibodies may be produced as part of a normal immune response. This antibody response may be elicited by five possible stimuli. (a) This response may be to modified tissue antigens, as in syphilis where spirochete infection may alter a normal tissue antigen and stimulate production of the Wasserman antibody. Similarly, drugs such as procainamide can modify nuclear antigens so that antinuclear antibodies are made. (b) A second stimulus results from cross-reactivity between extrinsic antigens and normal structures in host tissue. For example, streptococcal infections may induce antibodies that cross-react with heart or glomerular basement membrane (GBM) in patients with rheumatic heart disease or glomerulonephritis. (c) A third stimulus arises from neoplastically altered tissue rendering the tissue antigenic. Antibodies to tumor antigens have been found in many patients with malignancies. (d) Fourth,

TABLE 15.3. *Criteria for Autoimmune Disease*

1. a. Circulating or tissue-bound antibodies, active under physiological conditions, should be demonstrated; or
   b. Circulating or localized populations of cells sensitized to antigen, or products of immunologically activated cells, active under physiological conditions, should be present.
2. Sensitizing antigen should be identified and characterized.
3. Antibodies or sensitized lymphocytes should be produced in vitro or in animals against the same antigen.
4. Pathological events in vitro or in the experimental animal should correspond to those in human disease.
5. Transfer of disease from immunized to normal animal by cells or serum.

TABLE 15.4. *Possible Mechanisms of Autoantibody Production*

1. Normal immune response
   a. To modified tissue antigens (e.g., Wasserman antibody, drug-induced antinuclear antibodies)
   b. To extrinsic antigens cross-reacting with normal tissue antigens (e.g., ? post-streptococcal rheumatic heart disease or glomerulonephritis)
   c. To neoplastically altered tissue antigens (e.g., tumor-specific antibody)
   d. To ontogenically late-developing antigens (e.g., anti-I)
   e. To normally "protected" antigens (e.g., lens of the eye)

2. Abnormal immune response
   a. By mutant clones (e.g., monoclonal rheumatoid factors)
   b. By loss of normal suppressor mechanisms (e.g., ? systemic lupus erythematosus)
   c. By breakdown of tolerance (? antithyroglobulin)

structural substances appearing relatively late in ontogeny may be more autoantigenic than others. Erythrocyte I antigen develops late in ontogeny, and cold agglutinins frequently are directed to it. (e) Fifth, substances that are relatively sequestered, such as in the lens of the eye, or, possibly, thyroid colloidal proteins, may provoke autoantibody formation; but these circumstances are poorly understood. These five mechanisms all envision antibody formation as a normal response of an intact immune system; it is to new, altered, or cross-reacting antigens that they are made.

(2) The second general mechanism of autoantibody production supposes that the immunologic responses are inappropriate. Three possible abnormal responses have been proposed: (a) An abnormal clone of antibody-producing cells may evolve to produce autoantibodies. This may be the case for such monoclonal antibodies as rare rheumatoid factors or possibly for diseases characterized by antibodies of restricted heterogeneity. Since most autoantibodies, however, are polyclonal and since many diseases feature a variety of disparate autoantibodies, it is difficult to imagine all the necessary mutations occurring to form all the clones needed to explain autoantibodies solely on this basis. (b) The second abnormal immune response is receiving increasing attention. This is abnormal immunoregulation. T lymphocytes are thought to exert a suppressor function over B lymphocytes, thereby preventing abnormal cell proliferation or abnormal antibody production. If T cell suppressor function is impaired, then autoantibody production could occur by unregulated antibody-forming B cells. This may be the case in SLE. Animals with lupus were shown to have abnormal suppressor T cell function and high levels of autoantibodies; antibody levels fell when their suppressor T cell function was restored. (c) A third abnormal immune response appears when tolerance to autoantigens fails and antibody formation results. This has not been well characterized in man. Antibodies to thyroglobulin may occur when hapten-linked thyroglobulin may stimu-

late T helper cells to cause otherwise tolerant B cells to elaborate antibody.

Autoantibodies appear commonly, may or may not relate to disease pathogenesis, and may occur via normal responses to altered antigens or by abnormal responses to normal (or altered) antigens.

Mechanisms by Which Autoantibodies Participate in Disease

Autoantibodies mediate tissue injury by two major pathways. They can either form circulating immune complexes (with antigen) or affix to antigens on target cells. Circulating complexes can deposit in tissues, activate complement, and elicit a local inflammatory response. Autoantibodies affixed to tissue antigens can destroy the target cell by complement-mediated lysis or antibody-dependent lymphotoxicity. The immune complex mechanism is important in diseases like SLE, whereas tissue-bound antibodies are important in Goodpasture's syndrome. Thus, to participate in the inflammatory response, according to conventional schemes, autoantibodies interacting with these antigens must be capable of fixing complement or reacting with lymphocytes. It is generally thought that antigens plus IgG—subclasses IgG_1, IgG_2, and IgG_3, but not IgG_4—or IgM are able to activate the classic complement pathway. For this reason patients with circulating anticoagulant (autoantibodies) to clotting factor VIII, which are often IgG_4 antibodies, can be treated with massive infusions of factor VIII (antigen) without inducing immune-complex disease or serum sickness. It may be for similar reasons that many autoantibodies are innocuous in many individuals. Many factors contribute to determining the pathogenicity of a given autoantibody—the nature of the inducing antigen, the integrity of the host's immune system, the antibody concentration, the Ig class, the affinity of antibody for antigen, and capacity of the host's reticuloendothelial system to remove formed complexes.

Autoantibodies may affect cell-mediated immune mechanisms. Antibodies to tumor or other tissue antigens occur in many patients with neoplasms, allografts, or autoimmune diseases. These antibodies may alter host immune responses to antigen-bearing cells and have important clinical implications. For example, "blocking" antibodies to cell-bound tumor antigens may cover antigenic sites and prevent recognition and destruction of cancer cells by immunocompetent lymphocytes. Reduction of blocking antibodies in cancer patients or induction of such antibodies in transplant recipients or certain patients with autoimmune disease might be beneficial.

Another area in cellular immunology where autoantibodies may be of biologic importance is antibody-dependent lymphocytotoxicity. In this reaction, sensitized lymphocytes attack target cells coated with antigen to which antibody is attached. Lymphocytes function much like complement: together with antibody they mediate cytolysis. Studies of this reaction indicate that: (1) the antigen may naturally reside on the target cell or be passively adherent; (2) low concentrations of antibody are effective; (3) antibodies are IgG subclasses 1 through 4; (4) complement is not required; (5) cytolysis is probably produced by direct contact between cells and not by release of soluble substances; (6) effector cells recognize the Fc portion of antibody; and (7) effector cells are probably heterogeneous, and in man seem to be largely null lymphocytes, sometimes called K cells. The biologic importance of antibody-dependent lymphocytotoxicity is undergoing clarification. Antibody-dependent lymphocytotoxicity has been shown against tumor cells, myeloblasts, virus-infected cells, and normal lymphocytes. Percentages of null cells in blood are elevated in autoimmune diseases, neoplasia, or immunodeficiency syndromes. It seems possible that autoantibodies, of the appropriate type, might mediate or modulate lymphocyte-mediated cytolytic tissue injury in autoimmune and other diseases.

Autoimmune Diseases

With this general discussion in mind, Goodpasture's syndrome, SLE, and rheumatoid arthritis will be examined in detail. Autoantibodies are characteristic of these diseases and are intimately related to the pathogenetic events. Review of these concepts will, therefore, illustrate how autoantibodies may be involved in disease.

Goodpasture's Syndrome: Antiglomerular Basement Membrane-Mediated Nephritis

Certain types of glomerulonephritis have long been known to have immunologic features and are thought to be mediated by immunologic

TABLE 15.5. *Immune Complex-Mediated Glomerulonephritis*

Exogenous antigens
Foreign serum proteins
Drugs
Bacterial—streptococcal, staphylococcal, syphilis
Plasmodial
Viral—hepatitis-associated antigen, experimental viruses
Other unidentified
Endogenous antigens
Nuclear—systemic lupus erythematosus
Renal tubular
Tumor antigens
? IgG—cryoglobulinemia
? Other unidentified

mechanisms. The majority (> 90%) of immunologic renal diseases are generally thought to be caused by formation and deposition of immune complexes (Table 15.5). Usually the antibodies produced are to foreign (exogenous) antigens (heterologous proteins, drugs, or infectious agents) although autoantibodies to endogenous antigens may also participate in immune complex disease. These include antibodies to DNA, tubular antigens, basement membrane antigens, tumor antigens, or IgG. Immune complex deposition is characterized by granular-type fluorescent staining with antisera to immunoglobulin and complement.

The clearest example of autoantibody-mediated glomerulonephritis is nephritis caused by antibody to GBM. Linear GBM deposition of Ig and complement are uncommon in human disease, probably occurring in less than 10% of renal biopsy material. This immunofluorescent staining pattern classically reflects disease mediated by anti-GBM antibody, although similar findings have occasionally been described in other nephritides. When anti-GBM nephritis is associated with lung purpura, it has been termed Goodpasture's syndrome. Goodpasture's syndrome was originally described in 1919 as a febrile, hemorrhagic pneumonia, with hemosiderin-laden sputum macrophages, accompanied by glomerulonephritis in young males. The nephritis is often a necrotizing progressive glomerulitis characterized by linear fluorescent staining. This illness is believed to be the human analogue of animal models of well-studied anti-GBM disease. Similar clinical syndromes can, however, be caused by other immunopathologic mechanisms and have been described with cryoglobulinemia and granular immunofluorescent staining. Evidence that anti-GBM antibodies mediate disease in most patients whose illness is called Goodpasture's syndrome derives from the following observations: (1) similarity of immunopathologic lesions to those in animal models, (2) in vitro reactions of serum and renal eluates with GBM antigen, (3) fixation of antibodies to animal GBM in similar staining patterns, (4) production of glomerulonephritis upon injection into animals, and (5) fixation of circulating antibodies in an anephric patient to a subsequent renal allograft with development of nephritis. This evidence indicates that Goodpasture's syndrome fulfills the criteria discussed for autoimmune disease mediated by autoantibody to GBM.

However, just as the pulmonary-renal disease termed Goodpasture's syndrome has been seen without anti-GBM antibodies, anti-GBM antibodies are not always restricted to this condition. Assays for serum anti-GBM antibodies have been carried out by diffusion in gel, indirect immunofluorescence, or passive hemagglutination. By these techniques, circulating antibodies have been detected in many patients with focal, diffuse, subacute, chronic, membranous, poststreptococcal, posttransplantation, lupus, or polyarteritis nodosa nephritis. The role of anti-GBM antibodies in nephritides not characterized by linear fluorescent staining (presumed antigen-antibody deposition) remains to be clarified.

Although the mechanism by which anti-GBM produced nephritis seems clear, it is not known what events lead to autoimmunization by GBM. Possibilities include (1) alterations in renal handling of normal small amounts of filtered antigen leading to immunogenicity, (2) alterations in antigen after environmental (microbial) exposure, (3) or cross-reaction of antigen with environmental antigens. For example, Goodpasture's syndrome has been associated with influenza infection, which is consistent with these speculations.

Systemic Lupus Erythematosus: Anti-DNA:DNA Immune-Complex-Mediated Systemic Disease and Nephritis

SLE is a multisystem disease of unknown cause and presumed immunologic pathogenesis. To facilitate recognition, classification, and study of patients with SLE, a set of preliminary diagnostic criteria was suggested by the American Rheumatism Association. These were (1) facial erythema; (2) discoid lupus erythematosus (LE); (3) Raynaud's phenomenon; (4) alopecia; (5) photosensitivity; (6) oral or nasopharyngeal ulceration; (7) nondeforming arthritis; (3) lupus erythematosus cells; (9) false-positive serologic test for syphilis; (10) profuse proteinuria; (11) cellular casts; (12) pleuritis or pericarditis; (13) psychosis or seizures; and (14) hemolytic anemia, leukopenia, or thrombocytopenia. Fulfillment of four or more criteria serially or simultaneously was 90% sensitive and 98–99% specific for the diagnosis of SLE. These criteria summarize prominent clinical features of SLE. Incidence of constitutional symptoms is approximately 80%; skin, 77%; cardiac, 40%; pulmonary, 50%; articular, 90%; neurologic, 50%; and renal, 50%.

Antibodies to a variety of antigens have been described in patients with SLE—namely, nuclear, cytoplasmic, lysozymes, ribosomes, mitochondria, cells (red cells, neutrophils, lymphocytes, platelets), tissues (thyroid, neuronal, muscle, liver, kidney, joint, capillaries), treponemes (serologic test for syphilis, fluorescent treponemal-absorbed), human IgG, bovine γ globulin, basement membrane, clotting factors, enzymes, and others. Many of these antibodies, when present, are related to pathogenesis. Of these, antinuclear antibodies are most pertinent to our current understanding of SLE.

The discovery of LE cells in 1948 was followed by the subsequent recognition of antibodies to multiple nuclear antigens in patients with SLE. The LE-cell phenomenon occurs in vitro (rarely in vivo in pathologic effusions). It is caused by IgG antibody to nucleoprotein (LE factor) reaching cell nuclei, fixation of complement, and engulfment of homogeneous nuclear material by phagocytic cells. The LE-cell test is rather specific for SLE, occurring infrequently in other disease, but not very sensitive (60–90%). For these reasons and because of technical and interpretive difficulties for the routine laboratory, LE-cell testing has been largely supplanted by antinuclear antibody determinations.

"Antinuclear antibodies" is a term designating antibodies to a variety of nuclear constituents, not all of which have been well characterized (Table 15.6). These constituents include native, or double-stranded, DNA (DS-DNA); denatured, or single-stranded, DNA (SS-DNA); soluble or insoluble DNA:histone (nucleoprotein); nuclear (RNA):protein (Mo); acidic nuclear proteins (Sm); extractable nuclear antigen (ENA) (composite of Sm and Mo); and histone and nucleolar antigens. Antibodies to these antigens have now been well studied. As expected, the antibodies are distributed among all immunoglobulin classes—IgG, IgA, IgM, IgD, or IgE.

Many methods have been developed for detecting antinuclear antibodies, including antiglobulin consumption tests, complement fixation tests, precipitin reactions in gel, hemagglutination reactions (sheep red blood cells, latex, or bentonite particles), hemagglutination inhibition, horseradish peroxidase-conjugated antibody, DNA-binding assays, counterimmunoelectrophoresis, and immunofluorescence techniques. Of these, indirect immunofluorescence using tissue substrate as a source of nuclear antigen is most widely used (Fig. 15.1). By this method, titers of antinuclear antibodies can be determined and certain patterns of immunofluorescence recognized (Table 15.7). The homogeneous, or diffuse, pattern is produced by antibodies to deoxyribonucleoprotein. The peripheral (rim or shaggy) pattern is produced by antibodies to DS-DNA. The speckled pattern results from antibodies to extractable ribonucleoprotein antigens. Nucleolar pattern reflects antibodies to nucleolar antigens, possibly RNA-protein. Additional patterns have also been described. The incidence of antinuclear antibodies in certain clinical states is listed in Table 15.8. It can be seen that positive test results occur in some normal individuals (approximately 5%), virtually all patients with SLE, approximately 15–35% of patients with discoid lupus erythematosus, most patients with drug-induced lupus erythematosus, 15–40% of patients with juvenile or adult rheumatoid arthritis, 60% of patients with scleroderma, 68% of patients with Sjögren's syndrome, all reported patients with

TABLE 15.6. *Nuclear Antigens*

1. DNA
   a. Native or double-stranded (DS-DNA)
   b. Denatured or single-stranded (SS-DNA)
2. DNA:Histone
   a. Soluble
   b. Insoluble
3. Nuclear RNA:protein (Mo)
4. Acidic nuclear protein (Sm)
5. Extractable nuclear antigen (ENA) (composite of Mo and Sm)
6. Histone
7. Nucleolar

"mixed connective tissue disease," and infrequently in patients with vasculitis and poly/dermatomyositis. The titers and patterns of positive antinuclear antibody tests are helpful clinically. High titer-positive test results are seen most commonly in patients with SLE, or drug-induced lupus erythematosus, and mixed connective tissue disease, but have also been noted in some patients with scleroderma or Sjögren's syndrome. The peripheral pattern (anti-DS-DNA) is seen almost exclusively in patients with SLE and is considered to be virtually diagnostic for lupus. Speckled patterns are common in scleroderma and mixed connective tissue disease.

It is also possible to test specifically for antibodies to DNA, in addition to fluorescent antinuclear antibodies. Antibodies to double-stranded native DNA, present in most patients with SLE at some time during the disease process, are almost always diagnostic of SLE and are rarely seen in other instances. It is generally thought that antinuclear antibodies are present in sera of all patients with SLE. However, antinuclear antibodies are not diagnostic for SLE, because positive test results frequently occur in other disease states (Table 15.8). A positive test for anti-DS-DNA is usually diagnostic for SLE, but is not necessarily found in all patients. A properly performed and consistently negative antinuclear antibody in a patient suspected of having SLE is very unusual and suggests several possibilities. Excluding laboratory error, a serum might conceivably give

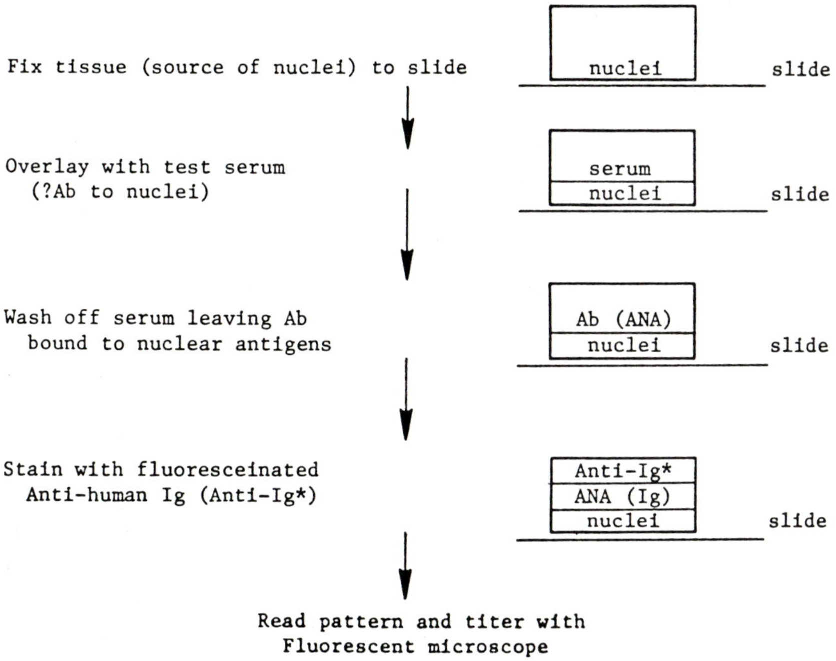

FIG. 15.1. Indirect immunofluorescent detection of antinuclear antibodies (ANA).

TABLE 15.7. *Correlation of Antinuclear Antibody Fluorescent Staining Patterns and Disease*

Pattern	Antigen	Disease
1. Peripheral	DS-DNA	SLE
2. Speckled	Acidic nuclear protein	Rheumatoid arthritis
	Ribonucleoprotein	SLE
	Extractable nuclear antigen	Scleroderma
		Mixed connective tissue disease
3. Homogeneous	Desoxyribonucleoprotein	Rheumatoid arthritis
		SLE
		Other
4. Nucleolar	Nucleolar RNA	Progressive systemic sclerosis
		Other

TABLE 15.8. *Antinuclear Antibodies (ANA) in Health and Disease*

Condition	Percent Positive ANA	Titer	Pattern[a]
Normals	5	Low	
SLE	99–100	High	P, D, S, N
Discoid LE	15–35	Low	S, D
Drug-induced LE	68–100	Low–high	
Rheumatoid arthritis	20–40	Low	D
Juvenile rheumatoid arthritis	15	Low	D, S
Scleroderma	60	Low–high	S, N, D
Sjögren's syndrome	68	Low–high	P, S, N
Mixed connective tissue disease	99–100	High	S
Vasculitis	25	Low	
Poly/dermatomyositis	30	Low	

[a] P, peripheral; D, diffuse; S, speckled; N, nucleolar.

a negative test at low dilutions but be positive in higher dilutions; hemolysis during venipuncture might liberate leukocyte nuclear antigens to bind antibodies; or antigen excess or therapeutic immunosuppression might also give rise to negative test results. Alternatively, other diagnoses should be carefully considered in a patient with a test negative for antinuclear antibodies and with multisystem disease—systemic Weber-Christian disease, vasculitis, cryoglobulinemia, polychondritis, atypical infection, lymphoma, malignancy, Whipple's disease, sarcoidosis, periodic syndromes, adult Still's disease, etc.

Antinuclear antibodies not only have diagnostic use but also are of clinical value in following patients with SLE. Anti-DS-DNA tends to be detectable in increasing titers in sera of patients with disease exacerbations. Titers also correlate with lowered serum complement levels, increased levels of circulating DNA, active nephritis, or active nonrenal SLE. Anti-DS-DNA, together with other such serologic abnormalities as serum complement levels, can be followed to facilitate the management of patients with SLE.

Little evidence exists that antinuclear antibodies alone are phlogistic in patients with SLE. Rather, the immune complexes of circulating antigen-antibody appear to lead to tissue injury through deposition and activation of complement. Immune complexes have been demonstrated in serum and tissues of patients with SLE by a variety of techniques. The evidence that DNA:anti-DNA is the principal recognized antigen-antibody system involved in SLE is as follows: (1) detection of DNA, anti-DNA, and complexes in serum; (2) detection of complexes and complement in tissues and elution of immunoreactants from tissues; (3) correlation of levels with depressed complement and clinical symptoms; and (4) similarity to murine SLE.

Recent observations concerning other antigen-antibody systems in lupus patients are of interest. Recall that a variety of nuclear and cytoplasmic antigens can induce autoantibody formation. These do not appear to occur randomly in patients with SLE. There have been definite positive and negative associations suggesting that the immune responses in patients maintain selectivity at the level of immunogen. Moreover, these differences among patients may have clinical importance. For example, anti-Mo (anti-ENA) and anti-DS-DNA rarely occur together. Thus, patients with anti-ENA (mixed connective-tissue disease) infrequently develop nephritis or cerebritis.

Possibly, extractable nuclear antigen exerts a protective effect, perhaps by reacting with DNA and preventing DNA:anti-DNA complex formation. Lymphocytotoxic antibodies occur in SLE patients and related and unrelated household contacts of patients with SLE. Family members had anti-DS-RNA but not anti-DS-DNA. Patients with SLE had anti-DS-DNA and anti-SS-RNA. Household contacts did not have anti-RNA or anti-DNA. These data were interpreted as showing (1) the importance of both genetic and environmental factors in SLE, (2) selective and perhaps specific immunization of SLE patients, and (3) possible exposure to an infectious pathogenic agent—handled successfully by contacts, but unsuccessfully by probands who developed SLE.

A scheme of the possible pathogenesis of human SLE is shown in Figure 15.2. There is evidence that hereditary factors are important. Environmental factors are also critical. There is much evidence compatible with, but not final proof of, viral influences. Host immune responses are clearly abnormal. Humoral immune responses are exaggerated, which may reflect immunoregulatory defects. Patients make antibodies to many antigens that may form circulating immune complexes. The factors leading to immune complex deposition in certain tissues are not well understood. DS-DNA and anti-DS-DNA have been clearly shown to deposit in certain tissues. Possibly, other antigen-antibody systems—bovine IgG, RNA, cell-surface antigen, IgG, etc.—behave similarly. Once localized to tissue, complexes activate and consume comple-

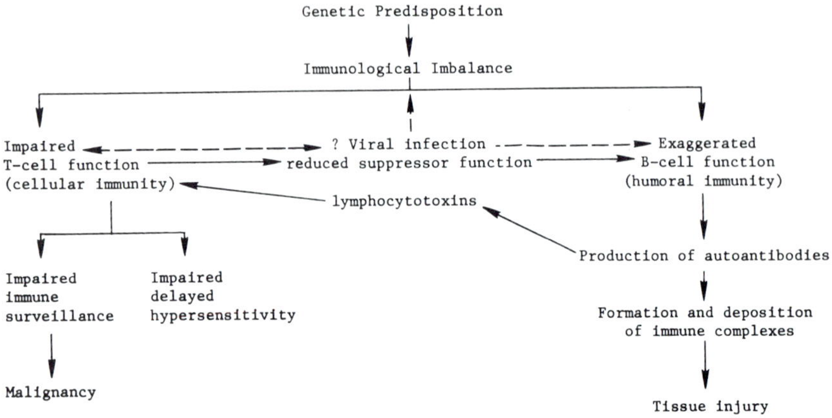

FIG. 15.2. Possible pathogenesis of SLE.

ment and lead to production of biologically active substances, provoking immunologic inflammation. Neutrophils appear, ingest complexes, and release enzymes. In addition, cell-mediated immunity seems diminished in patients. Whether human SLE is characterized by loss of T cell regulatory function, whether cellular responses to antigen are inappropriately blunted or unusually exaggerated, and the possible role of lymphocytes as effector cells at the site of tissue injury remain to be clarified.

Rheumatoid Arthritis: Anti-IgG:IgG-Mediated Synovitis and Systemic Disease

Rheumatoid arthritis is another well-studied autoantibody-mediated disease. In this illness, for reasons that are not clear, immunologic injury is focused in the synovial cavity.

Since no single feature is pathognomonic of rheumatoid arthritis, diagnostic criteria are used, including:(1) morning stiffness; (2) pain or tenderness in one joint; (3) swelling in one joint; (4) swelling in a second joint within 3 months; (5) symmetrical swelling; (6) subcutaneous nodules; (7) typical radiologic changes; (8) positive rheumatoid factors test; (9) poor synovial fluid mucin clot test; (10) characteristic synovial histology; and (11) characteristic nodule histology. Patients meeting seven criteria have "classical" rheumatoid arthritis; patients fulfilling five have "definite" rheumatoid arthritis, whereas others have probable or possible disease. Certainly the most prominent clinical manifestation of disease is the symmetrical polyarthritis. Occasionally, however, initial presentation may be atypical with oligo-, mono-, or an-articular rheumatoid disease. Extraarticular disease can also occur and is becoming increasingly recognized.

A number of autoantibodies occur frequently in patients with rheumatoid arthritis. The antibody most often encountered is rheumatoid factor. An appreciation of its role focuses on many clinical and immunologic considerations in rheumatoid arthritis. Its nature, methods of detection, diagnostic applications, biologic properties, and pathogenetic role will be briefly considered.

The ability of sera from patients with rheumatoid arthritis to agglutinate sensitized sheep red blood cells was first recognized in 1922. By the late 1950's this phenomenon was widely appreciated and was adapted for use in serologic diagnosis of this condition. It has now been clearly established that rheumatoid factors were anti-γ-globulins—IgG, IgA, IgD, 7S, and 19S IgM antibodies to IgG.

Many test systems for the detection of anti-γ-globulins have been developed, most of which use the agglutinating capacity of the high-molecular-weight 19S IgM rheumatoid factors. The most commonly used tests have been sensitized sheep cell agglutination and latex fixation. Several additional methods of testing for rheumatoid factor have recently been devised, but these are currently limited to the research laboratory (radioimmunoassay, immunoabsorption, immunofluorescence, and lymphocyte rosette formation).

The sensitivity and specificity of clinical test methods differ. As yet, no method will detect only those antibodies present in patients with rheumatoid arthritis. Thus, rheumatoid factor testing remains but one of many diagnostic criteria for evaluating rheumatoid arthritis. Of the tests available for routine clinical use, the sheep cell test is believed to be more specific but less sensitive than latex agglutination tests. The latex tests, and particularly slide tests, appear to be more sensitive but less specific. These latter tests have the added advantage of being easily performed.

Although rheumatoid factors are common in patients with rheumatoid arthritis, they are by no means specific for this disease. Rheumatoid factors are found in many other clinical circumstances (Table 15.9). The incidence of positive tests in disease is difficult to assess accurately because of the variability of different test methods and study populations. Estimates are listed in Table 15.9. High-titered rheumatoid factors are usually seen in patients with rheumatoid arthritis or Sjögren's syndrome.

Determining the presence or absence of rheumatoid factor in patients with rheumatoid arthritis provides useful clinical, as well as diagnostic, information. The presence of rheumatoid factor has been associated with poor prognosis; progressive and unremitting disease course; significant functional impairment; presence of subcutaneous nodules; high erythrocyte sedimentation rate; many actively inflamed joints; radiologic evidence of joint destruction; cryoglobulinemia; low synovial fluid complement; and frequent extraarticular complications, such as vasculitis, pleuropulmonary disease, pericarditis, or episcleritis. Tests for rheumatoid factor that are positive usually remain so during the course of the disease.

Titers do not tend to fluctuate with disease activity. Titers may decrease with sustained remission; plasmapheresis; or treatment with corticosteroids, penicillamine, gold, antimalarials, or immunosuppressive drugs. Conversely, many patients in long-term remission retain high rheumatoid factor titers in their serum.

Once it was recognized that rheumatoid factors were prevalent in high titers among most patients with rheumatoid arthritis, attempts to define their biologic role were undertaken in hopes of clarifying mechanisms of disease production. In vitro studies have shown that rheumatoid factors possessed many diverse properties that could be either harmful or protective (Table 15.10). Many, but not all, of these biologic activities can fit into a pathogenetic scheme for rheumatoid arthritis. Some of these properties will be summarized and then the role of rheumatoid factor will be considered. IgM rheumatoid factor has been shown to neutralize infectivity of virus-antibody complexes. Both IgG and IgM rheumatoid factors, under appropriate conditions, are capable of interacting with

TABLE 15.9. *Incidence of Rheumatoid Factors in Various Diseases*

Disease	Incidence positive rheumatoid factor test (%)	Titer
Rheumatoid arthritis	60–95	High
Sjögren's syndrome	80–95	Low–high
Poly/dermatomyositis	50	Low
Subacute bacterial endocarditis	50	Low
Progressive systemic sclerosis	25–30	Low
SLE	20–30	Low
Hepatic diseases	20–30	Low
Juvenile rheumatoid arthritis	20	Low
Chronic infectious diseases	15–25	Low
Sarcoidosis	15–20	Low
Aged individuals (>65 years)	10–20	Low
Osteoarthritis	5–20	Low
Spondylitides	<5	Low
Normal individuals	<5	Low

TABLE 15.10. *Biological Activities of Rheumatoid Factors*

Neutralize infectivity of virus-antibody complexes
Interact with IgG to activate complement
Serum and synovial fluid IgG anti-IgG, IgM anti-IgG, and IgG anti-IgG:IgG are inversely proportional to complement levels
Facilitate immune complex phagocytosis
Enhance elimination of immune complexes
Influence Ig catabolism and antibody responses
? activate kinin system
? mitogenic for lymphocytes

aggregated γ-globulin and of activating the classical complement system and generating complement-derived chemotactic activity. Levels of serum and synovial fluid IgG and IgM anti-γ-globulins are, in fact, inversely proportional to serum and synovial fluid complement levels. In addition, IgG:anti-IgG complexes have been identified in rheumatoid joints and, similarly, are inversely proportional to joint fluid complement concentrations. Rheumatoid factor may block IgG opsonins and impair phagocytosis, may actually inhibit complement activation under certain conditions, and impair complement-dependent phagocytosis. Rheumatoid factor may attach to circulating immune complexes and facilitate immune elimination—or tissue deposition—of complexes. Rheumatoid factor may be capable of activating the kinin system, which may also be important in the inflammatory response. Rheumatoid factors are weak stimulants for lymphocytes. In vivo, injected rheumatoid factor or antigen-antibody complexes induced mesenteric vasculitis in rats. Transfusions of rheumatoid factor-positive plasma did not produce disease in recipients. Autologous IgG (antigen) injected into knees of patients with rheumatoid arthritis (usually rheumatoid factor-positive) provoked inflammation. Passive administration of human rheumatoid factor reduced mouse antibody responses to subsequent immunization with human IgG. Rheumatoid factor has also influenced Ig catabolism.

Present conceptualization of the immunopathology of rheumatoid arthritis is as follows (Fig. 15.3). An inciting event occurs, which initiates disease. This event may be more likely to result in disease in certain environmental circumstances or in certain individuals than in others and could result from exposure to microorganisms. Antigen may localize to articular and periarticular collagenous tissue and be protected from rapid immune elimination. A series of intraarticular immune events follows.

Immunoglobulin G may undergo alteration ($\overline{\text{IgG}}$)—as a result of lysosomal enzyme degradation, aggregation, or interaction with putative infectious antigen—and itself become antigenic. Rheumatoid factor, anti-$\overline{\text{IgG}}$, is produced against the $\overline{\text{IgG}}$. Immunoglobulins G and M anti-$\overline{\text{IgG}}$, together with $\overline{\text{IgG}}$, activate the classical complement sequence and begin to generate the necessary ingredients of an inflammatory reaction—vasoactive substances, chemotactic factors, anaphylatoxins, and adherence- and phagocytosis-promoting activities. Polymorphonuclear leukocytes are recruited into the joint space and phagocytize immune complexes of RF-$\overline{\text{IgG}}$-C. Leukocytes then release lysosomal enzymes and collagenase, which contribute to synovitis and joint destruction. Lysosomes are capable of partially degrading IgG which may increase its antigenicity. The rheumatoid synovium can synthesize IgG and complement, thereby providing immunoreactants needed to perpetuate inflammatory events. Inflamed synovium also produces an "activator peptide," which is thought to promote transition of exudative to proliferative

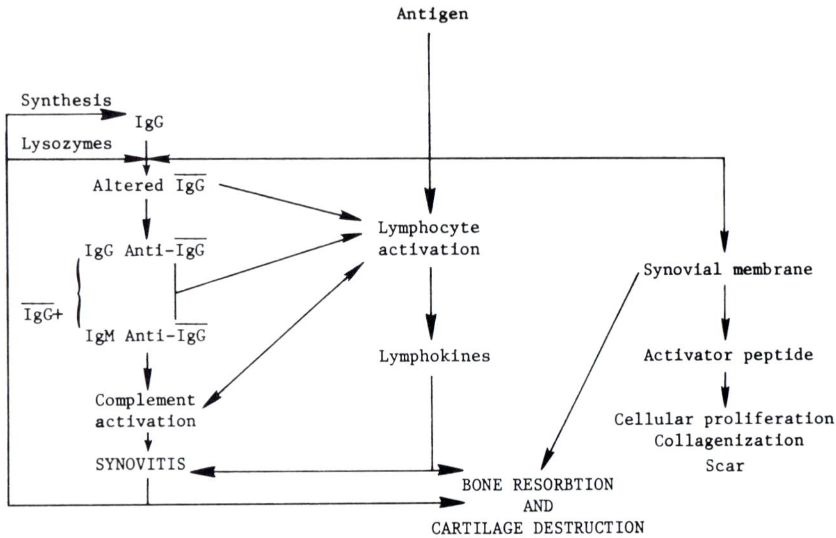

FIG. 15.3. Possible pathogenesis of rheumatoid arthritis.

synovial fluid and synovial membrane. Lymphocytes are activated—perhaps by hypothetical antigen, altered Ig, rheumatoid factor, complement, or complexes—to produce lymphokines. These substances probably also participate in rheumatoid synovitis, and their precise role is undergoing investigation. It seems likely that humoral and cell-mediated pathways interact. Lymphocytes contain a substance (complement-activating factor) capable of activating the classical complement sequence. Complement molecules, in turn, can modulate lymphocyte reactivity. Thus, inciting events initiate self-perpetrating intraarticular inflammation, involving actions and interactions between humoral and cellular systems. Elucidation of these events offer the possibilities of therapy to eradicate initiating event(s) or to modify specific abnormal immune responses.

Most observers agree that rheumatoid factors do participate in these immunologic events. The principal supporting evidence is: clinical observations associating the presence of large quantities of rheumatoid factors with severe joint disease, the demonstration of an inverse relationship of anti-γ-globulins and complement levels, and the in vitro capacity of rheumatoid factors to produce inflammation or activate mediators of inflammation. The precise role of rheumatoid factors in rheumatoid inflammation is still not clear. It is thought that IgG and IgM rheumatoid factors, combined with $\overline{\text{IgG}}$, may themselves activate the complement pathway. Alternatively, rheumatoid factors may enhance the interaction of other immune complexes with phagocytic cells. But the possibility that rheumatoid factors are merely produced as a result of tissue damage cannot be completely excluded.

SELECTED REFERENCES

Bartfield, H., and Epstein, W. V.: Rheumatoid factors and their biological significance. Ann. N.Y. Acad. Sci., *168:* 1, 1969.

Bianco, N., Panush, R. S., Stillman, J., and Schur, P. H.: Immunologic studies of juvenile rheumatoid arthritis. Arthritis Rheum., *14:* 685, 1971.

Blau, R., and Caldwell, J. R.: Complement activating factor (CAF). A new mediator of rheumatoid inflammation. Arthritis Rheum., *18:* 387, 1975.

Block, S. R., and Christian, C. L.: The pathogenesis of systemic lupus erythematosus. Am. J. Med., *59:* 453, 1975.

Blomgren, S. E., Condemi, J. J., Vaughan, J. H.: Procainamide-induced lupus erythematosus. Clinical and laboratory observations. Am. J. Med., *52:* 338, 1972.

Brier, A. M., Chess, L., and Schlossman, S. F.: Human antibody-dependent cellular cytotoxicity. J. Clin. Invest., *56:* 1580, 1975.

Capra, J. D., Winchester, R. J., and Kunkel, H. G.: Hypergammaglobulinemic purpura. Studies on the unusual anti-gamma-globulins characteristic of the sera of these patients. Medicine, *50:* 125, 1971.

Cochrane, C. G., and Koffler, D.: Immune complex disease in experimental animals and man. Adv. Immunol., *16:* 185, 1973.

DeHoratius, R. I., and Messner, R. P.: Lymphocytotoxic antibodies in family members of patients with systemic lupus erythematosus. J. Clin. Invest. *55:* 1254, 1975.

DeHoratius, R. J., Pillarisetty, R., Messner, R. P., and Talal, N.: Anti-nucleic acid antibodies in systemic lupus erythematosus patients and their families. Incidence and correlation with lymphocytotoxic antibodies. J. Clin. Invest., *56:* 1149, 1975.

Feldman, J. D.: Immunological enhancement: a study of blocking antibodies. Adv. Immunol., *15:* 167, 1972.

Fries, J. F., Weyl, S., and Holman, H. R.: Estimating prognosis in systemic lupus erythematosus. Am. J. Med., *57:* 561, 1974.

Gordon, D. A., Stein, J. L., and Broder, I.: The extra-articular features of rheumatoid arthritis. A systemic analysis of 127 cases. Am. J. Med., *54:* 445, 1973.

Koffler, D., Agnello, V., Thoburn, R., and Kunkel, H. G.: Systemic lupus erythematosus: prototype of immune complex nephritis in man. J. Exp. Med., *134:* 169s, 1971.

Laham, N. M., Panush, R. S., and Caldwell, J. R.: Modulation of peripheral blood lymphocyte responses by complement. Arthritis Rheum., *19:* 907, 1976.

Lehman, D. H., Wilson, C. B., and Dixon, F. J.: Extraglomerular immunoglobulin deposits in human nephritis. Am. J. Med., *58:* 765, 1975.

McCluskey, R. T., and Klassen, J.: Immunologically mediated glomerular, tubular and interstitial renal disease. N. Engl. J. Med., *288:* 564, 1973.

Merrill, J. P.: Glomerulonephritis. N. Engl. J. Med., *240:* 257, 313, 374, 1974.

Panush, R. S., Bianco, N. E., and Schur, P. H.: Serum and synovial fluid IgG, IgA and IgM antigammaglobulins in rheumatoid arthritis. Arthritis Rheum., *14:* 737, 1971.

Panush, R. S., Bianco, N. E., Schur, P. H., Rocklin, R. E., David, J. R., and Stillman, J. S.: Juvenile rheumatoid arthritis. Cellular hypersensitivity and selective IgA deficiency Clin. Exp. Immunol., *10:* 103, 1972.

Reichlin, M., and Mattioli, M.: Antigens and antibodies characteristic of systemic lupus erythematosus. Bull. Rheum. Dis., *24:* 756, 1974.

Rosenthal, C. J., and Franklin, E. C.: Depression of cellular-mediated immunity in systemic lupus erythematosus. Arthritis Rheum., *18:* 207, 1975.

Rubin, B. S., and Winkelstein, A.: Theories of autoimmunity. Bull. Rheum. Dis., *26:* 842, 1975–1976.

Sharp, G. C.: Mixed connective tissue disease. Bull. Rheum. Dis., *25:* 828, 1974–1975.

Stage, D. E., and Mannik, M.: Rheumatoid factors in rheumatoid arthritis. Bull. Rheum. Dis., *23:* 720, 1972–1973.

Tanimoto, K., Cooper, N. R., Johnson, J. S., and Vaughan, J. H.: Complement fixation by rheumatoid factor. J. Clin. Invest., *55:* 347, 1975.

Tannenbaum, H., and Schur, P. H.: The role of lymphocytes in rheumatic diseases. J. Rheum., *1:* 392, 1974.

UCLA Symposium: Immunopathology of nucleic acids in rheumatic diseases. Los Angeles, Calif. J. Rheum., *2:* 125, 1975.

Weisman, M., and Zvaifler, N.: Cryoimmunoglobulinemia in rheumatoid arthritis. Significance in serum of patients with rheumatoid vasculitis. J. Clin. Invest., *56:* 725, 1975.

Wilson, C. B., and Dixon, F. J.: Anti-glomerular basement membrane antibody-induced glomerulonephritis. Kidney Int., *3:* 74, 1973.

Wilson, C. B., and Smith, R. C.: Goodpasture's syndrome associated with influenza A2 virus infection. Ann. Intern. Med., *76:* 91, 1972.

Winfield, J. B., Winchester, R. J., Wernet, P., and Kunkel, H. G.: Specific concentration of antilymphocyte antibodies in the serum of cryoprecipitates of patients with systemic lupus erythematosus. Clin. Exp. Immunol., *19:* 399, 1975.

Chapter

16

THE ACUTE ALLERGIC RESPONSE: MEDIATORS OF ACUTE INFLAMMATION

Jacques Caldwell, M.D.

The acute inflammatory response results from the recruitment of several biochemical pathways which interact in ways incompletely understood. Activation of each pathway results in the elaboration of several low molecular weight substances which act on blood vessels, smooth muscle, and inflammatory cells to produce an inflammatory reaction. This chapter will cover three of these systems—the acute allergic response, the prostaglandin system, and the Hageman factor-kallikrein-bradykinin system.

The Acute Allergic Response

The anaphylactic or immediate allergic reaction is mediated by a group of chemical substances from the mast cells. To date, four mediators have been described: histamine, slow reacting substance of anaphylaxis (SRS-A), eosinophilic chemotactic factor (ECF-A), and platelet-activating factor. Release of these substances is initiated by the interaction of two adjacent IgE molecules on the mast cell membrane with antigen.

Histamine, β-imidazoylethylamine, is produced in body tissues by decarboxylation of the amino acid histidine by the enzyme L-histidine decarboxylase. The chief site of histamine storage is the mast cell in most tissues and the blood basophil in the circulation. These cells synthesize histamine and couple it to heparin stored within the secretory granule. Mast cells and basophils are not the only tissue source of histamine; it also is found in the central nervous system, in the epidermis of human skin, and in the gastrointestinal mucosa.

Histamine has multiple functions. In general it constricts the smooth muscles of larger blood vessels such as arteries and veins but dilates minute blood vessels such as capillaries and venules. Additionally, it promotes capillary permeability which facilitates the efflux of proteins and fluid from the intravascular to the extravascular space. Increased capillary permeability results from the direct action of histamine on postcapillary venules 20–30 micra in diameter. Histamine causes endothelial cells to shrink in size, to separate at their adjacent boundaries and thus to produce a gap between contiguous cells. The exposed underlying basement membrane is freely permeable to the plasma proteins and intravascular fluids and permits passage of particles such as platelets through the vascular wall. The "naked" basement membrane is a highly charged structure which readily entraps immune complexes onto its surface.

Histamine, in small doses, produces intense bronchoconstriction in humans with bronchial asthma, but its effect is much less pronounced in normal individuals. It has varying effects on other extravascular smooth muscles of man and animals. It is a powerful stimulant of gastric secretion and elicits secretions of gastric juice of high acidity and high pepsin content. Part of this effect on pepsin secretion is mediated through the vagus nerves.

When injected into the skin, histamine produces the classic triple response of Lewis which includes: (1) the appearance of a small localized area of erythema at the injection site which appears immediately after the injection and which is caused by vasodilatation of the local capillaries; (2) a large erythematous flush which results from an axon reflex which produces a widespread vasodilatation; (3) the development of a wheal at the injection site characterized by the appearance of a pale, localized collection of edema fluid which arises from the increased small venule permeability.

It has been recognized that histamine mediates its various biologic functions through at least two receptors termed the H1 and H2 receptors. Actions on the H1 receptor are responsible for the constrictor action of histamine on bronchial smooth muscle and for the increased capillary permeability seen in venules. Vasodilatation is mediated by both H1 and H2 receptors. Increased gastric secretion is mediated by H2 receptors alone.

Histamine has other biologic activities. In small amounts it appears to be chemotactic for eosinophils; in large amounts it has the reverse effect—it inhibits eosinophilic chemotactic activity. Histamine has the ability of increasing intracellular cyclic adenosine monophosphate (AMP) of the mast cell and thereby may inhibit further release of additional histamine from the mast cell.

Slow Reacting Substance of Anaphalaxis

The ability of antihistamines to reverse the symptoms of allergic rhinitis but their failure to reverse the bronchospasm of allergic asthma has been recognized for decades. It became apparent that mediators, other than histamine, must be involved in the acute allergic asthmatic attack. A second substance called SRS-A, was found in extracts of asthmatic lung. It is capable of producing a slow, sustained contraction of antihistamine-treated, atropinized guinea pig ileum. The slow, sustained contraction markedly differs from the rapid contraction-relaxation response which occurs when the guinea pig ileum is treated with histamine—and thus the name slow reacting substance has been applied to this mediator. SRS-A is a powerful constrictor of human bronchial muscle and is active in nanogram quantities or less. It is an acidic, hydrophilic lipid with a molecular weight of about 400. It appears to be distinct from prostaglandins and contains no amino acid or peptide residues. Unlike histamine, SRS-A is not stored in tissues but rather is synthesized, de novo, and is subsequently released as a result of antigen-antibody interaction in the lung.

Eosinophilic Chemotactic Factor of Anaphalaxis

ECF-A is one of several substances which evoke the accumulation of the eosinophils at the site of an acute inflammatory response. Two tetrapeptides, val-gly-ser-glu and ala-gly-ser-glu have ECF-A activity. It is stored, preformed, in human lung, in leukemic human basophils, and in rat mast cells. It can be released from human lung tissue slices, and from nasal polyps which have been passively sensitized with reaginic antibody. It is released from mast cells in the same manner as histamine and this release is modulated both by adrenergic and cholinergic stimuli. The role of the eosinophil in the acute allergic response is unknown. During phagocytosis eosinophils release arylsulfatase, an enzyme which can inactivate SRS-A. It has been proposed that inactivation of SRS-A is one of the prime functions of the eosinophil.

Platelet Activating Factor

Platelet activating factor is a substance which, in rabbits, is released from basophils and mast cells and has the capacity to stimulate release of serotonin and histamine from platelets. Recently Kaplan and his group have demonstrated release of platelet activating factor from human basophils obtained from patients with chronic myelogenous leukemia. Its role in human disease remains to be demonstrated.

Modulation of Release of Mediators from Mast Cells and Basophils

The mechanism by which mediators of the acute allergic response are released from mast cells and blood basophils has been studied in some detail in recent years. Mediator release is initiated by the bridging by antigen of two adjacent IgE antibodies on the surface of the mast cell. This bridging alters the cell membrane structure so as to permit influx of calcium ions. Release of mediators proceeds in two steps: the first is antigen dependent and calcium independent; the second is calcium dependent and antigen independent. Calcium ionophores (drugs that promote transmembrane fluxes of calcium ion) can replace antibody interaction in the mediator release process.

The release process requires the activation of a serine esterase enzyme system within the cytoplasm and an intact glycolytic pathway. After activation and the influx of calcium ion, granule membranes coalesce, and microtubules appear and align themselves perpendicular to the cytoplasmic membrane. Subsequently, the granule contents are extruded, by way of the microtubules, to the exterior of the cell. Significantly the cell is not lysed during this entire process.

Mediator release from mast cells can be inhibited by increasing intracellular cyclic AMP. An increase in intracellular cyclic AMP is accomplished by increasing the synthesis of cyclic AMP by stimulation of membrane adenyl cyclase (β adrenergic drugs such as isuprel and adrenalin work by stimulating membrane adenyl cyclase); or by impeding its degradation. Normally, intracellular cyclic AMP is catabolized by cyclic nucleotide phosphodiesterase which catalyzes the conversion of cyclic AMP to 5′-AMP. The methylxanthine group of drugs, such as the theophylline derivatives, are competitive inhibitors of the phosphodiesterases.

Prostaglandin E_1 can also increase levels of intracellular cyclic AMP within the mast cell by stimulating a membrane adenyl cyclase receptor different from that through which the β adrenergic drugs, such as isuprel, work.

In recent years it has been shown that cholinergic agents such as acetylcholine or carbachol enhance antigen-induced release of mediators from lung tissue fragments or peripheral blood basophils, but do so without affecting tissue levels of cyclic AMP. The cholinergic agents evoke an increase in the levels of intracellular cyclic guanosine-5′-monophosphate. Cholinergic blocking agents such as atropine prevent the antigen-induced release of mediators that is augmented by the cholinergic drugs.

α-Adrenergic agents such as phenylephrine or norepinephrine, when given together with the β-blocking agent, propanalol, also enhance release of mediators from human lung tissue fragments by means of decreasing intracellular cyclic AMP.

The Prostaglandins

Prostaglandins are a family of unsaturated fatty acids widely distributed in biologic tissues. Unlike most mediators, these substances must be synthesized at the time of the inflammatory stimulus. This occurs by the action of the membrane enzyme phospholipase A_2 which induces the release of the essential fatty acid, arachidonic acid from the cell membrane. Arachidonic acid is converted by enzymes, collectively referred to as "cyclic oxygenase", to cyclic endoperoxides, PGG_2 and PGH_2. PGH_2 is converted into PGE_2 and PGF_{2a}, the major prostaglandins found in human lung tissue. The biologic activities of PGE and PGF_{2a} are highly dependent upon the target organ on which they act or in which they are produced. Prostaglandins E_1 and E_2 inhibit bronchial smooth muscle tone. Inhalation of PGE_2 by aerosol produces bronchial dilatation and inhibits the bronchoconstriction produced by histamine. The response to PGE_2 given by aerosol to asthmatic patients is very rapid; improvement in FEV_1 begins to occur 1 sec after administration of an inhaled dose of the drug. Unfortunately administration of prostaglandins E_1 or E_2 in their present form to patients with asthma produces a bronchial irritation which markedly compromises their therapeutic value.

Prostaglandin $F_2\alpha$ is a potent bronchoconstrictor of isolated human bronchial smooth muscle. Recent data by Hedquistd in Sweden demonstrate that asthmatics are 10^3 to 10^4-fold more sensitive to the bronchoconstrictive effects of $PGF_2\alpha$ than are normal individuals.

Piper and Vane described another mediator of the acute inflammatory response a few years ago which they called rabbit aorta contracting substance. Rabbit aortic contracting substance is highly unstable and has a half-life of only 30 sec. Recently it has been shown that this substance is probably thromboxane A_2, a major metabolic product of arachidonic acid.

The biologic effects of prostaglandins are dose related. Low dose PGE_1 and E_2 enhance mediator release from mast cells while large doses inhibit mediator release.

All tissues contain microsomal enzymes which are capable of synthesizing prostaglandins. Prostaglandins are released when cell membranes are perturbed by trauma or other injury; they must be synthesized de novo and are not stored in the cell. Inhibition of release may be effected by corticosteroids and it has been suggested that this is the mechanism of action of steroids.

Prostaglandins E and $F_1\alpha$ produce erythema in skin which is long lived—lasting 10 hours or more. They produce tissue edema both by directly increasing vascular permeability by inducing vascular leakage at the postcapillary and collecting venules, by directly contracting venular endothelial cells and potentiating the vascular permeability effects of other mediators such as histamine or bradykinin. PGE_1 induces hyperalgesia by "priming" pain receptors in such a way that pruritus or pain is produced by normally subthreshold doses of bradykinin or histamine. PGE_1 is the most powerful pyretic agent known.

Precursors of prostaglandins E and $F_2\alpha$, PGG_2, and PGH_2 are even more potent bronchoconstrictors than $PGF_2\alpha$.

Nonsteroidal antiinflammatory drugs such as indomethacin and aspirin act by inhibiting the cyclooxygenase enzyme system which converts arachidonic acid to the cyclic endoperoxide. It has been postulated that the antiinflammatory effect observed with these drugs in arthritis results from inhibition of intraarticular cyclic endoperoxide synthesis.

The role of the prostaglandins in human disease is largely unknown, but the characteristic of prostaglandins to interact with other mediators of inflammation in a potentiating or inhibitory fashion strongly implicates a major role for them in the inflammatory response.

The Hageman Factor-Kallikrein-Bradykinin System

The Hageman factor-kallikrein-bradykinin pathway of inflammation has received increasing attention in recent years and it has become apparent that there are definite interrelationships between this system, and the complement and clotting cascades. The central molecule in the pathway is Hageman factor-factor XII of the clotting system. Hageman factor is a β globulin which is activated by a large number of substances possessing a negative charge—such as collagen, vascular basement membrane, uric acid, and calcium pyrophosphate crystals, and endotoxin. Activation of Hageman factor is followed by its cleavage into fragments. These fragments are important in the generation of plasmin and in the release of bradykinin (Fig. 16.1).

Hageman factor fragments convert prekallikrein to kallikrein. Kallikrein has two functions; it is chemotactic for polymorphonuclear leukocytes and releases the nine-amino acid peptide bradykinin from its parent molecule kininogen. Bradykinin stimulates pain fibers, produces increased vascular permeability, dilates small blood vessels, and contracts some smooth muscle. Its role in human disease is unknown. Its biologic activities are enhanced by prostaglandins and by fibrinopeptide B.

Hageman factor fragments also convert the plasminogen proactivator into plasminogen activator; plasminogen activator is chemotactic for both

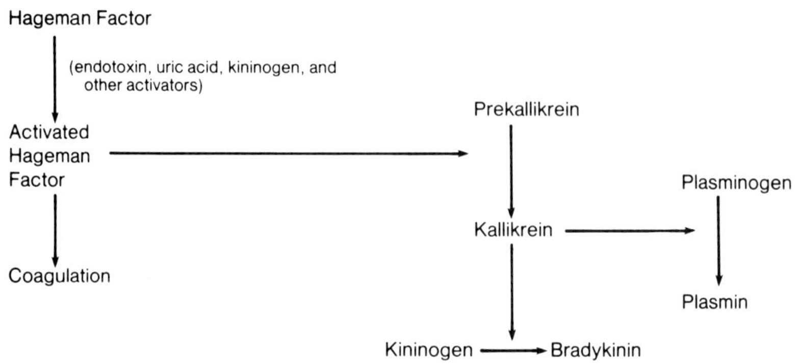

FIG. 16.1. The Hageman factor-kallikrein-bradykinin pathway.

polymorphonuclear and mononuclear cells and enzymatically cleaves the plaminogen molecule to release plasmin.

Plasmin has multiple biologic functions: it converts fibrin into biologically active fibrin split products; activates the first complement component; also cleaves activated Hageman factor into its fragments.

Activated Hageman factor also activates factor XI of the clotting sequences. Discharge of the clotting sequence results in the generation of fibrinopeptides A and B from fibrinogen; fibrinopeptide B is chemotactic for polymorphonuclear cells.

The clotting, Hageman factor-kallikrein-bradykinin and complement systems share at least one control protein—the inhibitor of the first complement component, the C1 esterase inhibitor. This one protein impedes the action of Hageman factor fragments on prekallikrein, blocks activated factor XI plasma thromboplastin antecedent (PTA) of the clotting system, and inhibits plasmin and kallikrein. These multiple inhibitory activities are important in the disease hereditary angioedema. This illness, inherited as an autosomal dominant trait is characterized by either an absent or an inactive C1 inhibitor. Patients with this illness develop periodic episodes of painless swelling of the limbs, oral cavity, upper respiratory tract of gastrointestinal tracts. Involvement of the larynx can cause asphyxiation. Swelling of the submucosa of the gut produces a cramp-like illness identical to that seen with intestinal obstruction due to any other cause. Trauma and surgery can precipitate an attack since tissue trauma activates Hageman factor which consequently results in the production of a multitude of factors which increase blood vessel permeability and promote accumulation of fluid in tissues. These factors are: kinin from the Hageman factor-kallikrein-bradykin system; C42 kinin; C3a and C5a from the complement system; and histamine released as a result of the anaphylatoxic activities of C3a and C5a; and vascular permeability substances derived from the prostaglandins (which are produced as a response to any tissue trauma). The C1 inhibitor blocks the vascular permeability factors derived from the Hageman factor-kinin and the complement systems and its absence or failure to function permits the unimpaired generation of these substances.

Summary

The biochemical pathways responsible for producing the swelling, erythema, heat, and cellular response characteristic of the acute inflammatory reaction do not act independently of one another; as knowledge from further research accumulates the interconnections between these diverse pathways become apparent. Therapeutic adventures directed toward inhibiting the inflammatory reaction and attempts to understand the pathophysiology of inflammatory diseases must acknowledge these complex relationships.

SELECTED REFERENCES

Kaliner, M.: Human lung tissue and anaphylaxis. I. The role of cyclic GMP as a modulator of the immunologically induced secretory process. J. Allergy Clin. Immunol., *60:* 204–211, 1977.

Kaliner, M., and Austen, K. F.: A sequence of biochemical events in the antigen-induced release of chemical mediators from sensitized human lung tissue. J. Exp. Med., *138:* 1077, 1973.

Kaplan, A. P.: Mediators of urticaria and angioedema. J. Allergy Clin. Immunol., *60:* 324–332, 1977.

Orange, R. P., Austen, W. G., and Austen, K. F.: The immunologic release of histamine and slow-reacting substance of anaphylaxis from human lung. I. Modulation by agents influencing cellular levels of cyclic 3′5′-adenosine monophosphate. J. Exp. Med. *134*(Suppl.)*:* 136, 1971.

Vane, J. R.: Prostaglandins as mediators of inflammation. Advances in Prostaglandin and Thromboxane Research *2:* 791–801, 1976.

Chapter 17

DRUG ALLERGY

Leighton E. Cluff, M.D.

The clinical manifestations of allergic reactions to drugs are like allergic reactions to other immunogens. They are distinguishable only by their etiologic relationship to drug administration. All four types of immunologically-induced hypersensitivity reactions have been caused by drug allergy, including type I reactions characterized by anaphylaxis, urticaria, and angioedema; type II reactions characterized by hemolysis, leukopenia, thrombocytopenia, and eosinophilia; type III reactions characterized by serum sickness, fever, arthralgia, lymphadenopathy, and skin eruption; as well as type IV reactions characterized by contact dermatitis.

The immunologic mechanism of most clinically suspected allergic drug reactions is difficult to prove. Most often an immunologic mechanism is inferred because the reaction occurs in temporal relationship to administration of a drug, subsides when use of the drug is discontinued, requires a latent period of several days after beginning administration of the drug before the reaction appears, is generally unrelated to the dose of the drug, may appear in an accelerated fashion when the drug is readministered, and resembles well established allergic clinical manifestations to other antigens. Only in a few instances, has it been possible to demonstrate an immunologic mechanism in drug allergy using skin tests or laboratory procedures.

Some drugs are more frequently responsible for allergic reactions than are other drugs. In addition, some persons seem to be more likely to develop allergic drug reactions. Fortunately, however, most of the allergic diseases caused by drugs are not serious or life threatening, subside promptly when use of the drug is discontinued, or their clinical manifestations can be suppressed. Anticipation and prompt recognition of serious reactions, however, is necessary to avoid a fatal outcome.

Epidemiologic studies of adverse reactions to drugs have shown that only about 15% of these reactions are attributable to drug allergy. Allergic reactions to drugs, however, are most often reported by physicians, even though drug toxicity attributable to pharmacologic rather than immunologic mechanisms is most common.

Immunologic mechanisms

Most drugs used today are simple chemicals, with molecular weights less than 1000. Substances of such low molecular weights do not generally induce an immunogenic response unless firmly bonded as haptens to a carrier protein. Experimentally, covalent bonding of haptenic simple chemicals to protein makes them immunogenic. Presumably, haptenic drugs which are immunogenic when given to human beings form covalent bonds with host protein. Drugs that are loosely or reversibly bound to protein are generally not immunogenic. For this reason, there is no apparent relationship between the reversible binding of a drug to serum albumin and the drug's immunogenic properties, although such binding may significantly affect the drug's pharmacologic action.

The drug or chemical hapten conjugated to a protein behaves like a partial or complete antigenic determinant. The amino acids in the protein to which the hapten is linked may be a part of the antigenic determinant. Specific antibody, however, can distinguish between structurally similar chemical haptens, although cross-reactions may occur. These immunologic reactions have shown that specific antibody recognizes the three dimensional shape of the antigenic determinant group rather than a specific chemical property of the hapten. Furthermore, antibodies directed against different haptens bonded to the same protein are specific for one or another of these antigenic determinants but not for both. Haptenic determinants with different charges, however, may result in antibodies recognizing not only a specific hapten but also the chemical bonds attaching the hapten to the carrier protein, as well as amino acids of the protein. Such antibodies may appear to cross-react with other haptens because of their reactivity with antigenic determinants partly constructed of the carrier protein.

Molecular size, electrical charge, covalent or irreversible bonding, and chemical complexity are factors influencing whether or not a drug can serve as a hapten and be immunogenic. In addition, such characteristics of degradation products of a drug will also influence their ability to be immunogenic. Even though the drug administered may not have properties enabling it to serve as a hapten and immunogen, its degradation products may have these properties and be responsible for drug allergy.

The dose of an immunogen and its mode of administration may influence the immunologic response. A dose of an immunogen which induces a considerable response when injected subcutaneously may induce no response when given intravenously. These differences may be attributable to distribution, dilution, and degradation of the immunogen.

They may also be attributable to the availability or accessability of a host protein or cell which will form a covalent or firm bond with the injected hapten. Epidemiologic and some experimental studies suggest that drugs given orally to individuals with ulcerative or inflammatory gastrointestinal disease may enhance the immunogenic properties of these drugs. Conceivably, this is associated with changes in drug absorption, drug binding, drug metabolism, or availability of immunologically responsive cells.

Type I allergic reactions are attributable to homocytotropic antibodies which have tissue binding properties and in man belong to the IgE class of immunoglobulin. The Fc region of IgE (reaginic) antibodies responsible for binding to cell membranes, is heat labile. Therefore, these antibodies lose their reactivity when heated. The IgE antibody response to an immunogen is T cell dependent and is under complex genetic control, as illustrated by its association with histocompatibility antigen HLA-B7.

Basophiles or mast cells have membrane receptors which bind the Fc region of IgE molecules. Bridging by specific antigen of adjacent IgE molecules attached to a cell membrane stimulates the release of biochemically reactive substances of mast cells and basophiles which are vasoactive. The cellular events initiated by the bridging of IgE molecules and antigen on cell membranes involve both activation and inhibition of cell enzymatic activity, often require Ca^{++} and intracellular cyclic adenosine monophosphate and cyclic guanosine monophosphate.

The biochemically active amines released by IgE and specific antigen include histamine, slow-reacting substance of anaphylaxis (SRS-A), eosinophil chemotactic factor of anaphylaxis (ECF-A), serotonin, heparin, kinins, and prostoglandins. These amines are responsible for most of the manifestations which are characteristic of type I allergic reactions mediated by IgE antibodies.

Type II allergic reactions are expressed by cell injury, most readily identified when affecting blood cells, but kidney, skin, and other tissues may also be affected. These cytotoxic reactions involve the combination of IgG or IgM antibodies with antigenic determinants on a cell membrane, which may be formed by binding of a hapten to cell membrane receptors. Complement fixation and activation, phagocytosis of target cells, or lysis and inactivation by lymphocytes lead to cell death. These phenomena can be studied in vitro, particularly when formed blood elements are the target cells.

IgG antibody may compete with IgE antibody directed against the same antigenic determinant and interfere with type I hypersensitivity reactions. These interfering IgG antibodies are called "blocking antibodies" and may be responsible for control of type I allergic reactions induced by "hyposensitization."

Type III allergic reactions characterized predominantly by inflamation, as observed in serum sickness, are attributable to antigen-antibody complexes. The inflammatory reaction develops at the site of deposition of these antigen-antibody complexes. When such complexes form in the blood with deposition at various sites the clinical manifestations may involve skin, joints, lymph nodes, spleen, kidney, serosal surfaces, and other organs or tissues. When complexes are formed at the site of antigen administration, inflammation may be dominant only at that site, for example in hypersensitivity pneumonitis. IgG and IgM antibodies are ordinarily involved in these so-called immune complex disorders. Complement plays an important role in producing inflammation and chemotaxis associated with immune complex disorders. Furthermore, attachment and release of immune complexes from lymphocytes and platelets maintains these complexes in a soluble form in plasma. Binding of complexes to platelets leads also to the release of vasoactive amines which increase vascular permeability, blood vessel injury, and deposition of immune complexes at the basement membrane. Binding of complexes to neutrophiles can release lysosomal hydrolases, which also contribute to acute inflammation.

Type IV allergic reactions result from interactions between actively sensitized lymphocytes and specific antigens, leading to the release of lymphokines or direct cytotoxicity. Antibody and complement are not involved. A delayed (24–48 hours) skin reaction characterized by inflammation and mononuclear cell infiltration, as typified by a positive tuberculin skin test, is the classical lesion of type IV hypersensitivity reactions. Antigen binds to receptors or specifically sensitized T lymphocyes, and this is followed by release of biologically active mediators of the allergic reaction. These mediators or lymphokines attract both T and B lymphocytes, induce mitogenesis in these cells, and attract neutrophiles and macrophages. The phagocytic properties of macrophages are activated. Contact skin reactivity, or contact dermatitis to simple chemicals is completely attributable to type IV allergic reactions.

Clinical Manifestations

Anaphylaxis is an acute, potentially fatal reaction which is more likely to occur if the immunogenic drug is given parenterally, but has also occurred when the specific drug is taken orally by exquisitely allergic individuals. Within 1–30 min after the drug is administered the allergic person rapidly develops weakness, dyspnea, cough, tightness in the chest, sweating, pallor, cyanosis, and hypotension which may lead to vascular collapse and death. Intense pruritus of the face, hands, and feet, which may be associated with erythema or urticaria occasionally precedes collapse.

Penicillin is most frequently incriminated as a cause of anaphylaxis, perhaps because it is so commonly prescribed and administered parenterally. Anaphylaxis to penicillin has been more common in individuals with a history of atopy and previous allergic drug reactions. Other drugs known to have been responsible for anaphylaxis include: chlortetracycline, nitrofurantoin, folic acid, salicylates, aminopyrine, iodinated contrast media, meprobamate, tripelennamine, dextrans, cephalosporins, streptomycin, and several other drugs.

A detailed and thorough drug history should be obtained from all patients to avoid administering or prescribing drugs which may induce adverse reactions. This is particularly important in prevention of anaphylaxis. Patients with atopy and a history of an allergic reaction to a drug should be given an alternate medication which is not likely to cause a reaction. Patients given a parenteral drug should remain under observation for several minutes before leaving. If symptoms such as severe pruritus, tightness in the chest, wheezing, or sweating develop, epinephrine should be given immediately before collapse occurs. If shock or collapse develop quickly, epinephrine must be available for prompt administration intravenously combined with cardiorespiratory support as needed. Corticosteroids are of no value in preventing or treating anaphylaxis.

Urticaria and angioedema are very common manifestations of allergic reactions to drugs which may last for a few hours or for several days, depending in part upon whether or not use of the responsible drug is discontinued or it persists in the body. The list of drugs which have caused urticaria and angioedema is long, but includes particularly penicillins, sulfonamides, barbiturates, morphine (opiate derivatives), bromides, iodides, hydantoin anticonvulsants, erythromycin, cephalosporins, and insulin. When the drug specifically responsible for urticaria is given subcutaneously urticaria may occur at the site of injection.

Identification and discontinuance of the offending drug is essential in control of urticaria and angioedema. Antihistamine drugs may relieve the symptoms if not severe. Manifestations which are not controlled by antihistamines, however, often require administration of corticosteroids.

Hemolytic anemia caused by immunologic reactions to drugs has been extensively studied. Four different immunologic mechanisms may be responsible for drug-induced immune hemolytic anemia. These mechanisms are classified as attributable to (1) immune complex formation, (2) hapten (drug) adsorption, (3) nonspecific protein adsorption, and (4) unknown.

Circulating immune complexes, composed of drug and specific antibody, can "sensitize" the erythrocyte as an "innocent bystander" and cause hemolysis, often associated with complement activation. Affected patients frequently have received the responsible immunogenic drug repeatedly and often in small doses. Acute hemolysis may produce renal failure, and occasionally thrombocytopenia develops concomitantly. IgG or IgM antibodies, and quinine, quinidine, phenacetin, and a few other drugs have been incriminated. There is considerable variability in the serologic findings in immune hemolytic anemia attributable to this mechanism, and the Coombs' test may or may not be positive.

Some drugs bound to red cell membranes function as immunogens and induce specific antibody which cause hemolysis only of erythrocytes to which the drug is adsorbed. Large doses of the responsible drug have usually been given, and when hemolysis occurs other allergic clinical manifestations also may develop. The Coombs' test is strongly positive when hemolysis occurs. Penicillins and the cephalosporins have often been incriminated.

Nonspecific adsorption of nonimmunologic serum protein upon erythrocytes has been caused by cephalothin, and other cephalosporins, which is associated with a positive Coombs' test. Seventy-five percent of patients receiving cephalothin, particularly those with azotemia, may have a positive direct Coombs' test. The nonspecific protein adsorption to red cells caused by cephalosporins can cause difficulty in cross-matching blood, but rarely leads to hemolytic anemia.

Methyldopa induces a positive Coombs' test in 20% of patients, particularly those receiving large doses of the drug, but hemolysis occurs less often. The antibody responsible for these events is not directed towards methyldopa, but reacts with erythrocyte antigens of the Rh system. The mechanism by which methyldopa induces this autosensitization is not known, but patients taking the drug may also develop antinuclear antibody. Occurence of a positive Coombs' test in persons given methyldopa is not an indication for discontinuance of the drug unless hemolysis develops. The erythrocyte antibodies slowly disappear when the drug is stopped. Corticosteroids may be effective in reducing hemolysis when it develops. Levadopa and mefenamic acid have produced reactions like those caused by methyldopa.

Neutropenia and thrombocytopenia may also be produced by immunologic reactions involving drugs. The mechanisms for their development are probably similar to those resulting in drug-induced hemolytic anemia. The clinical manifestations are those ordinarily associated with neutropenia and thrombocytopenia, and include infection and bleeding, respectively.

Eosinophilia and prominent eosinophilic tissue infiltration is particularly characteristic of some parasitic infestations, hay fever, and certain reactions to drugs that are immunologically mediated. The eosinophil chemotactic factor released by mast cells in type I hypersensitivity reactions involving IgE antibody is probably responsible for the eosinophilic reaction often observed in drug-induced urticaria and angioedema. The eosinophilic reaction associated with other forms of hypersensitivity, however, is less well explained. In some forms of immune complex disorders and in association with certain type IV hypersensitivity reactions eosinophils may be prominent. Eosinophils can phagocytose immune complexes and this may be their function in allergic reactions. Streptomycin and nirvanol may cause pronounced eosinophilia, but this is apparently not attributable to an immunologic mechanism.

Serum sickness, which is often associated with fever, arthralgia, lymphadenopathy, and rash is a common drug-induced allergic reaction, usually attributed to formation of circulating immune complexes. There are similarities between the features of serum sickness, systemic lupus erythematous, polyarteritis nodosa, erythema nodosum, and glomerulonephritis which also may be drug induced, and they also are probably caused by formation of immune complexes.

Fever is a particularly troublesome allergic drug reaction, particularly when it occurs without other allergic clinical manifestations in patients being treated for a febrile disease. When drug fever develops, however, it usually begins 7–10 days after the start of administration of the drug, unless the patient has previously been sensitized to the drug in which case the febrile reaction may be accelerated and appear very promptly, often with a chill. Not all drug fever is caused by an immunologic mechanism. Tissue injury caused by a drug, for example hemolysis in glucose-6-phosphate dehydrogenase deficiency, is often accompanied by fever. In addition, peripheral vasoconstriction induced by vasoactive drugs may reduce heat loss and cause elevation of body temperature. Other drugs such as amphetamines, atropine, caffeine, cocaine, and picrotoxin may cause fever by an effect upon central temperature regulation. The number of drugs which have been associated with allergic drug fever, however, is large, and includes penicillins, cephalosporins, streptomycin, antihistamines, barbiturates, diphenylhydantoin, and quinidine.

Contact dermatitis is the principal manifestation of type IV or delayed hypersensitivity reactions to drugs, developing as a result of topical application of drugs to the skin. If the antigenic drug is administered systemically to a patient who has developed contact dermatitis, however, a systemic reaction, particularly characterized by fever, may develop.

Immunologic Diagnosis

With a few exceptions, there are no laboratory procedures which serve to identify or establish the immunologic basis of a presumed allergic drug reaction. Therefore, routine screening of patients to avoid inducing an allergic drug reaction is very dependent upon a drug history. This history should include information on over-the-counter and prescription drugs the patient has taken. Possible adverse effects of drugs the patient has taken before must be ascertained and carefully dissected to characterize their clinical features and the circumstances under which they occurred.

Verification of the incriminated drug and the reaction is sometimes possible by enquiry to a previous physician or pharmacist. Recognition should be given to the fact that patients who have experienced reactions to drugs in the past are probably predisposed to development of reactions to other drugs now and in the future.

Skin tests to detect whether or not a patient is allergic to a particular drug are most valuable and reliable for recognizing predisposition to contact dermatitis or type IV hypersensitivity. Skin tests have been useful in detecting IgE-mediated allergic reactivity to pollen but have not been similarly useful in detection of type I drug hypersensitivity. This is probably explained by the inability to identify, in most instances, the reactive drug component for inoculation. Development of penicilloyl polylysine conjugates for skin testing have been useful in limited situations for detecting some forms of penicillin allergy, but their lack of general usefulness and reliability has restricted their wide application.

Serologic tests for allergic drug reactions have been deceptive and difficult to interpret, except for those used to study type II hypersensitivity reactions involving erythrocytes, and occasionally platelets and neutrophiles. As illustrated by the Coomb's test, however, the demonstration in vitro of an antibody reacting specifically with erythrocytes which have adsorbed a drug or been altered by drugs is not prima facie evidence of a drug induced or potential immunologic disease.

Management

Contrasted with adverse drug reactions caused by pharmacologic mechanisms which can usually be controlled by reducing drug dosage, reactions caused by immunologic mechanisms require elimination or complete discontinuation of drug administration. Rarely is it acceptable, desirable, or necessary to continue administering the responsible drug to a patient experiencing a specific allergic reaction. Infective endocarditis requiring treatment with one particular antimicrobial drug in a patient having an allergic reaction (e.g., exfoliative dermatitis) to this drug may necessitate administration of corticosteroid to suppress the allergic manifestations while continuing the antimicrobial drug. Similar life threatening diseases for which there is only one therapeutic drug available are unusual, as alternative drugs are most often available and should be used.

Antihistamine drugs may be useful in suppressing rash or itching resulting from allergic drug reactions, but, if these or more severe allergic manifestations persist after discontinuing the responsible drug, corticosteroids should be used. Corticosteroids applied topically to a few localized skin lesions may be helpful, but if the reaction is widespread or associated with systemic manifestations corticosteroids will have to be given systematically.

As discussed before, epinephrine is the only definitive drug useful in controlling or preventing death of patients developing anaphylaxis. Whenever drugs are given parenterally, therefore, epinephrine should be readily available for immediate use.

SELECTED REFERENCES

Butler, V. P., Jr., and Beiser, S. M.: Antibodies to small molecules: biological and clinical applications. Adv. Immunol., *17:* 255, 1973.

Cluff, L. E., Caranasos, G. J., and Stewart, R. B.: *Clinical Problems with Drugs.* Philadelphia: W. B. Saunders Co., 1975.

Cluff, L. E., and Johnson, J. E., III: Drug fever. Prog. Allergy, *8:* 149, 1964.

de Weck, A. L.: Immunochemical mechanisms in drug allergy. In *Mechanisms in Drug Allergy,* edited by C. H. Dash and E. H. Jones. London: Churchill Livingstone, 1972.

Fudenberg, H. H., Stites, D. P., Caldwell, J. C., and Wells, J. V.: *Basic and Clinical Immunology.* Los Altos, Calif.: Lange Medical Publications, 1976.

Levine, B. B., Immunochemical mechanisms in drug allergy. Ann. Rev. Med., *17:* 23, 1968.

SECTION THREE

THE PHAGOCYTIC SYSTEM AND OTHER TOPICS

Chapter 18

THE PHAGOCYTIC SYSTEM AND HOST RESISTANCE TO MICROBIAL DISEASE

Paul G. Quie, M.D.

Normal host resistance against microbial disease depends on an adequate phagocytic system. Clinical evidence for this is the remarkable susceptibility to severe infections of patients with deficient numbers of phagocytes or with phagocytes that do not function properly. Clinical examples are patients with cyclic neutropenia, asplenia, defective leukocyte chemotaxis, or defective phagocyte oxidative metabolism. Careful clinical observations and intense laboratory investigation of the phagocytes from these patients has provided important knowledge about the functions of phagocytic cells which are critical for adequate host resistance against infectious diseases.

Circulating Phagocytic Cells

Circulating phagocytic cells, i.e., neutrophils and monocytes, develop from the same pluripotent stem cells that under different influences differentiate into lymphocytes, erythrocytes, or megakaryocytes. Neutrophil precursors differentiate into cells with prominent cytoplasmic granules. As the cells mature, they become capable of phagocytosis, acquire oxidative metabolic capacity, and become mobile. It is this combination of microbicidal factors in granules, the capacity for rapid mobility, and unique oxidative response, which make these cells ideally suited for microbial defense.

Mononuclear leukocytes are released from the bone marrow as immature cells, which circulate for several hours and differentiate into specialized phagocytic macrophages depending upon organ or tissue localization.

The bone marrow produces approximately as many neutrophils each day as erythrocytes, but the neutrophils have a much shorter life (measured in hours instead of months) in the circulation, so there is approximately one circulating neutrophil for every 2000 erythrocytes. There are large stores of mature neutrophils marginating in capillaries and the bone marrow, so a "ready reserve" of neutrophils can be instantly mobilized when invasion of tissue by microbes occurs. During infection, there is mobilization of marginating cells, a release of reserve mature cells from the bone marrow, a shortening in maturation time, and increased activity in the mitotic pool. Circulating factors that stimulate increased production and rapid release of neutrophils are believed to be products of peripheral phagocytic cells which are actively engaged with microbial invaders.

Chemotaxis

Neutrophils in the circulation are concentrated in areas of inflammation because of increased stickiness of endothelial surfaces, attachment to capillary walls, and migration into the tissue. The kinin system (see Chapter 16) is involved in change of capillary permeability, but once in the tissues, chemotactic factors attract the cells in a unidirectional fashion toward the site of microbial invasion. This phenomenon is illustrated by Figure 18.1.

Chemotactic factors involved in the attraction of leukocytes include complement components, C3a, C5a, and C$\overline{567}$ and factors released from disrupted leukocytes and tissue cells. In addition, bacteria and fungi release potent chemotactic substances. It is the gradient of these chemotactic substances with highest concentration at the center of the inflammatory process which attracts unidirectional locomotion of neutrophils toward the site of inflammation.

In experimental animals, it has been demonstrated that a delay of influx of neutrophils into an inflammatory site of as little as 2 hours severely compromises the animal's ability to localize an infectious process. These experimental data and the finding of defective neutrophil chemotactic responsiveness in several clinical conditions characterized by recurrent bacterial infections, suggest a direct association between a rapid directional response of neutrophils to chemotactic stimulation, and normal host defense against bacterial disease.

Certain patients with eczema and extremely elevated levels of serum IgE have depressed neutrophil chemotaxis and suffer recurrent, severe disease from *Staphylococcus aureus*. These infections are usually subcutaneous abscesses, but may involve pulmonary tissue and septicemia as well. The association between allergic manifestations, extreme hyperimmunoglobulin E, and defective neutrophil chemotaxis, suggests that histamine or other circulating amines may be involved in regulation of neutrophil locomotion. Histamine stimulates the leukocyte membrane

Inflammation

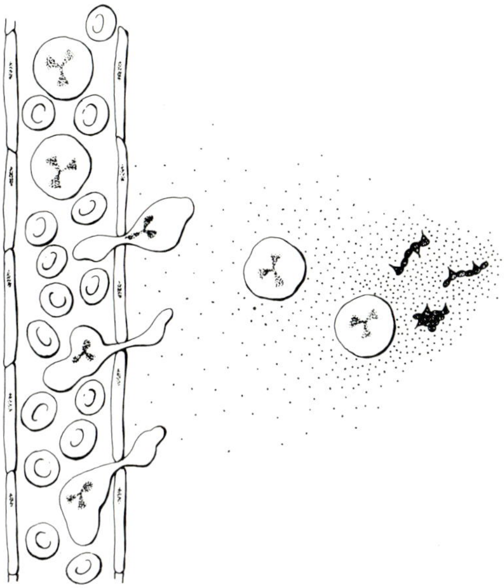

FIG. 18.1. A capillary in an area of inflammation. Neutrophils become sticky, attach to capillary endothelium, and diapedes between cells of the capillary wall. There is movement toward the area of bacterial invasion as a consequence of the gradient of chemotactic factors with highest concentration at the site of highest bacterial concentration.

ecoenzyme adenylate cyclase which increases intracellular cyclic adenosine monophosphate levels (cAMP). This cyclic nucleotide has a generally suppressive effect on neutrophil function. These increased levels of circulating histamine may depress neutrophil chemotaxis via a "second messenger" AMP and this neutrophil dysfunction may be related to recurrent infections in certain allergic patients.

Leukocyte locomotion is possible by contraction and relaxation of cytoplasm. This cellular activity is similar to that found in other contractile cells such as muscle cells. When viewed by phase contrast microscopy, migrating neutrophils have a leading edge of "hyaline ectoplasm" which appears to contract and relax and the rest of the cell contents are pulled along by this activity. Microfilaments can be seen with electron microscopic magnification, and it is believed that these filaments (composed of actin) together with microtubules are involved in cell locomotion.

Microtubules are composed of the protein tubulin which is also able to polymerize and depolymerize and may serve as a support for the contracting microfilaments. Receptors for chemotactically active substances are present on the surface membrane of neutrophils, and increased concentration of chemotactically active substances on one side of the cell may bring about increased microtubule activity on that side and hence directional movement.

Opsonization and Phagocytosis

Once neutrophils reach the microbial invaders, a complex interaction of humoral and cellular responses occur. In order for there to be attachment of microorganisms to phagocytes, potent antiphagocytic factors on the microbial surface must be neutralized. Examples of these microbial factors are: the M protein of group A streptococci, the polyribose phosphate of *Haemophilus influenzae* type b, and the capsular factors of *Escherichia coli.* The humoral factors that coat the microbial surfaces are termed opsonins. These include antibacterial antibodies which neutralize antiphagocytic factors on microbes and act as ligands between the microbe and the phagocyte, and complement components which greatly amplify the opsonic potential of specific antibodies.

There is a great variation in the opsonic requirement of different microbial species and of strains within species which are related to the virulence of the microbes, i.e., the more resistant to phagocytosis, the more virulent. Therefore, the availability of opsonins is critically important for rapid, efficient phagocytosis and adequate resistance against microbial disease.

Neutrophils have receptors for the Fc part of IgG antibodies and for the C3b component of complement on the surface of plasma membrane. If there are only a small number of opsonic configurations on the microbes which match receptors on the phagocyte plasma membrane, attachment alone occurs. However, when the microbe is thoroughly opsonized with antibody and C3b, the machinery of membrane locomotion is set into action and the neutrophil moves around microbes with an embrace that encloses the microbes inside a phagocytic pouch as illustrated in Figure 18.2

The energy for the neutrophil engulfment process involves adenosine triphosphate generated glycolysis and the movement of pseudopodia around microbes requires actin and myosin microfilament activity similar to that required for locomotion in response to chemotactic stimulation. When the neutrophil plasma membrane fuses, the "inside out" membrane which surrounds the engulfed microbes bud-off and becomes a new organelle in the cytoplasm. These new organelles are called phagosomes.

Intracellular Bactericidal Activity

Neutrophils contain a rich collection of granules in the cytoplasm that have specialized functions. During phagocytosis there is fusion of cytoplasmic granules with the newly formed phagosomes accompanied by vigorous "degranulation" and discharge of granule contents into the

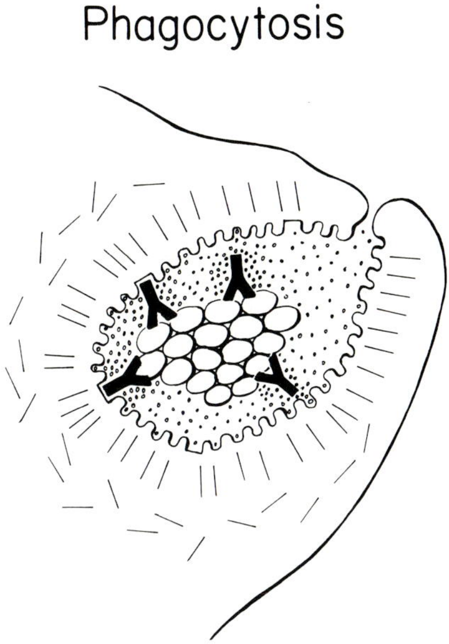

FIG. 18.2. A section of the neutrophil is shown engulfing a clump of opsonized bacteria. The neutrophil membrane is "activated" by antibody molecules and complement factor C3b. This causes contractile proteins in the cytoplasm to polymerize and become microfilaments and microtubules and the neutrophil engulfs the bacterial clump.

phagosomes until cytoplasmic vacuoles are formed. The environment within the vacuole is highly lethal for the microbes and most organisms are killed with nearly unbelieveable speed. Digestion of the killed organisms also proceeds with great rapidity. This is a result of factors present in the highly specialized granules of phagocytic cells. The two types that have been most carefully characterized are the azurophilic granules or lysosomes which contain acid phosphatase and other hydrolases, and specific granules which contain the antibacterial factors lysozyme and lactoferrin.

In addition to the fusion of membranes and discharge of granular contents into phagocytic vacuoles during phagocytosis, there is a sudden burst in the oxidative metabolic activity which is necessary for the microbicidal function of phagocytes. Intracellular microbes remain viable when phagocytes are incubated in anaerobic chambers even though phagocytosis proceeds at a normal rate.

Clinical evidence of the fundamental importance of oxygen-dependent microbicidal systems was the discovery that neutrophils and monocytes from patients with the clinical entity called chronic granulomatous disease do not respond to phagocytosis with a typical burst of oxidative metabolism. The circulating phagocytes from these patients phagocytize catalase producing bacteria and fungi normally, but cannot kill the intracellular organisms.

The oxidative metabolism during phagocytosis includes increased oxygen consumption, shift to hexose monophosphate shunt activity, and increased hydrogen peroxide production that occurs within a few seconds after there is attachment and beginning engulfment of microbes by neutrophils. The rapidity of the reaction suggests that the enzyme systems responsible for this response may be in the neutrophil plasma membrane. This location would also allow continued production of active oxygen radicals around the microbes encased in the inside out plasma membrane of the phagosomes.

Nitroblue tetrazolium dye (NBT) is used in a histochemical test to identify leukocytes with oxidase activity during phagocytosis. Oxidized NBT is colorless, but, when reduced, precipitates in the cytoplasm as blue formazan. Approximately 80–90% of normal leukocytes reduce NBT during phagocytosis. In contrast, leukocytes that do not respond to phagocytosis with increased oxidative metabolism do not reduce NBT.

One of the products of this metabolic burst, hydrogen peroxide, reacts with the granular enzyme myeloperoxidase which is discharged into phagosomes during degranulation, and this strong oxidizing complex in turn reacts with halides such as iodine and chloride. Iodination of bacteria has been demonstrated in phagocytic vacuoles, and chloride which is in high concentrations in neutrophils also participates in this bactericidal mechanism.

Other highly reactive oxygen molecules produced by neutrophils during phagocytosis include superoxide, singlet oxygen, and hydroxyl radicals. Superoxide is a reactive oxygen radical produced during phagocytosis by univalent reduction of oxygen. Evidence for the toxicity of this radical for bacteria is the fact that aerobic species of bacteria, i.e., species resistant to oxygen, have high levels of superoxide dismutase. This enzyme converts superoxide to hydrogen peroxide and oxygen. Bacterial species susceptible to oxygen (anaerobes) lack superoxide dismutase. Most mammalian cells contain superoxide dismutase. However, human neutrophils contain a very small amount of the enzyme located in the cytosol. Superoxide dismutase, therefore, does not interfere with the microbicidal action of superoxide within the phagosome but does protect the cytoplasm from this freely diffusible toxic oxygen radical.

Singlet oxygen is another electronically excitable oxygen molecule produced during phagocytosis by normal neutrophils. It emits light (chemiluminescence) which can be measured in a liquid scintillation counter. Singlet oxygen is formed during the spontaneous dismutation of superoxide and also during the reaction of myeloperoxidase, hypochlorite, and hydrogen peroxide, all of which are known to be present in phagosomes during phagocytosis. The high energy of singlet oxygen is believed to be capable of disrupting double carbon bonds in the membranes of microorganisms and therefore, this oxygen radical may be microbicidal.

Another product of the oxygen metabolism that occurs during phagocytosis is the hydroxyl radical formed by reaction of singlet oxygen with hydrogen peroxide. A role for hydroxyl radicals in microbial killing is suggested by the observation that bacterial killing is inhibited by hydroxyl scavengers, ethanol, manitol, and benzoate.

The measurable changes in metabolism of human neutrophils during phagocytosis are outlined in Table 18.1. Neutrophils from patients with chronic granulomatous disease and neutrophils without glucose-6-phosphate dehydrogenase do not have an oxidative metabolic response during phagocytosis, and the laboratory differences between these neutrophils and normal neutrophils are outlined in Table 18.2.

The rate limiting factors in the oxidative response of neutrophils during phagocytosis appears to be the puridine nucleotides NADH and NADPH which provide electrons for conversion to oxygen into hydrogen-peroxide and other oxygen radicals. Recently NADPH was shown to be the primary electron donor for superoxide production in homogenates of human neutrophils. The enzyme(s) (as yet unidentified but presumed in the cell membrane) which activate the puridine nucleotide oxidases are critical factors for a normal oxidative metabolic response during phagocytosis.

Bacteria such as *Staphylococcus epidermidis* and *Pseudomonas aeruginosa* are killed by neutrophils in the absence of oxygen and certain Candida species are killed normally by neutrophils without an oxidative

TABLE 18.1. *Metabolic Response of Human Neutrophils during Phagocytosis*

1. There is increased NADH/NADPH oxidase activity.
2. Oxygen is converted to superoxide.
3. A shift to hexose monophosphate shunt activity occurs.
4. Hydrogen peroxide is produced.
5. Singlet oxygen and hydroxyl radicals are produced.
6. Chemiluminescence is produced.
7. NBT dye is reduced.

TABLE 18.2. *Abnormalities in Neutrophils that Do Not Have an Oxidative Metabolic Response*

1. Oxygen is not converted to superoxide.
2. No increase in NADH/NADPH oxidase activity.
3. H_2O_2 is not produced.
4. NBT dye is not reduced.
5. No shift to hexose monophosphate shunt.
6. There is no chemiluminescence response.
7. Iodination of particles does not occur.
8. Catalase producing microbes are not killed.

response and by myeloperoxidase-deficient neutrophils. Therefore, in addition to the oxidative metabolic activity discussed above, neutrophils also have "back-up" systems which are effective in killing certain microorganisms.

The pH of phagosome contents during phagocytosis becomes increasingly acid because of lactic acid production and this alone may inhibit microbial replication. Pneumococci are highly sensitive to an acid pH, but most other bacteria survive.

Lysozyme is present in neutrophil granules and is discharged into phagosomes during degranulation. While most bacteria and fungi are resistant to the lytic action of lysozyme, several species become sensitive when acted upon by antibody and complement or hydrogen peroxide. Lysozyme, therefore, may act synergistically with other antimicrobial systems in the phagosome, but its primary role appears to be digestive rather than bactericidal.

Specific neutrophil granules contain lactoferrin, which inhibits microbial growth by binding iron, an essential nutrient for most microbes. Lactoferrin may also react with hydrogen peroxide in the oxygen-dependent bactericidal activity of neutrophils. Cationic proteins extracted from human neutrophil granules can be separated into fractions and each fraction demonstrates specificity of antibacterial activity. These cationic proteins are believed to be toxic for microbes by interfering with acidic groups on the microbial membranes. The cationic proteins in human neutrophils are greatly amplified by the addition of hydrogen peroxide and halide.

Summary

There is accumulating evidence that rapid directional locomotion of phagocytes is important for adequate host defense. The cellular factors required for locomotion and regulation of locomotion in response to chemotactic stimulation are better understood than before; however, the molecular trigger for activating this system remains a mystery.

The greatest advance in knowledge of phagocyte function has been in identification of factors in neutrophils which contribute to the microbicidal activity. This knowledge has come primarily from intense investigation of neutrophils without oxidative metabolism and with defective microbicidal function, i.e., neutrophils from patients with "chronic granulomatous disease". The primary antimicrobial systems of human neutrophils and presumably monocytes depends on oxygen metabolism and several reactive oxygen radicals contribute to the microbicidal armamentarium. The products of oxidative metabolism together with myeloperoxidase and halides kill a wide spectrum of microbes with amazing rapidity. Factors such as lysozyme and cationic proteins, which are also microbicidal, may be considered as cofactors in human neutrophils.

Several new methods for studying the metabolic response of neutrophils during phagocytosis are evolving which may reveal subtle defects of metabolic response in neutrophils from patients with increased susceptibility to infection. These methods allow studies of pharmacologic agents which may "stimulate the phagocytes".

SELECTED REFERENCES

Allen, R. C., Stjernholm, R. L., and Steele, R. H.: Evidence for the generation of an electronic excitation state in human polymorphonuclear leukocytes and its participation in bactericidal activity. Biochem. Biophys. Res. Comm., *47:* 679–684, 1974.

Babior, B. M., Curnutte, J. T., and Kipnes, R. S.: Pyridine nucleotide-dependent superoxide production by a cell-free system from human granulocytes. J. Clin. Invest., *56:* 1035, 1975.

Clark, R. A., and Kimball, H. R.: Defective granulocyte chemotaxis in the Chediak-Higashi syndrome. J. Clin. Invest., *50:* 2645, 1971.

Gregory, E. M., and Fridovich, I.: Oxygen metabolism in *Lactobacillus plantarium.* J. Bacteriol., *117:* 166, 1974.

Hill, H. R., Goldberg, N. D., Estenson, R. C., Hogan, N. A., and Quie, P. G.: Modulation of human neutrophil chemotactic responses by cyclic 3′5′ guanosine monophosphate and cyclic 3′5′ adenosine monophosphate. Metabolism *24:* 447–456, 1975.

Hill, H. R., and Quie, P. G.: Association of eczema, hyperimmunoglobulin E, defective neutrophil chemotaxis and recurrent bacterial infections. Lancet *1:* 183, 1974.

Holmes, B., Page, A. R., and Good, R. A.: Studies of the metabolic activity of leukocytes from patients with a genetic abnormality of phagocytic function. J. Clin. Invest., *46:* 1422, 1967.

Johnston, R. B., Jr., Keele, B., Webb, L., Kessler, D., and Rajogopalan, K. V.: Inhibition of phagocytic bactericidal activity by superoxide dismutase. A possible role of superoxide anion in killing of phagocytized bacteria. J. Clin. Invest., *52:* 44a, 1973.

Klebanoff, S. J.: Antimicrobial mechanisms in neutrophilic polymorphonuclear leukocytes. Semin. Hematol., *12:* 117, 1975.

Lehrer, R. I.: Functional aspects of a second mechanism of candidacidal activity by human neutrophils. J. Clin. Invest., *51:* 2566, 1972.

Mandell, G. L.: Bactericidal activity of aerobic and anaerobic polymorphonuclear neutrophils. Infect. Immun., *93:* 37, 1974.

Miles, A. A., Miles, E. M., and Burke, J.: The value and duration of defense reactions of the skin to primary lodgement of bacteria. Br. J. Exp. Pathol., *38:* 79, 1957.

Miller, M. E., Oski, F. A., and Harris, M. B.: Lazy leukocyte syndrome, a new disorder of neutrophil function. Lancet *1:* 665, 1971.

Odeberg, H., Olsson, I., and Venge, P.: Cationic proteins of human granulocytes. IV. Esterase activity. Lab. Invest., *32:* 86, 1975.

Olmstead, J. B., and Borisy, G. C.: Microtubules. Ann. Rev. Biochem., *42:* 507, 1967.

Quie, P. G., White, J. G., Holmes, B., and Good, R. A.: *In vitro* bactericidal capacity of human polymorphonuclear leukocytes: diminished activity in chronic granulomatous disease of childhood. J. Clin. Invest., *46:* 668, 1967.

Robinson, W. A., and Mangolik, A.: The kinetics and regulation of granulopoiesis. Semin. Hematol. *12:* 7, 1975.

Sbarra, A. J., Paul, B. B., Jacobs, A. A., Strauss, R. R., and Mitchell, G. W., Jr.: Biochemical aspects of phagocytic cells as related to bactericidal function. J. Reticuloendothel. Soc., *11:* 492, 1972.

Steerman, R. L., Snyderman, R., Leikin, S. L., and Colten, H. R.: Intrinsic defect of the polymorphonuclear leukocytes resulting in impaired chemotaxis and phagocytosis. Clin. Exp. Immunol., *9:* 939, 1971.

Stossel, T. P., and Pollard, T. D.: Myosin in polymorphonuclear leukocytes. J. Biol. Chem., *248:* 8288, 1973.

Chapter 19

THE NEUTROPHIL IN ABNORMAL HOST RESISTANCE: NEUTROPENIA AND ABNORMAL CHEMOTAXIS

Mark S. Klempner, M.D. and Sheldon M. Wolff, M.D.

Over a century has passed since Metchnikoff's profound discovery that the neutrophil had a host protective function. Prior dogma maintained that the neutrophil was a disseminator of microbes, rather than a means of containment. Subsequent investigations and recognition of multiple "experiments in nature" have provided a concept of the requirements for competent neutrophil participation in the acute inflammatory response. There must be an adequate number of phagocytic cells to limit the microbial invasion; these cells must be able to localize at the inflammatory site; and, finally, there must be a means of destroying the infecting organism. Any defect in these integrated components renders the host susceptible to infections. The following is a brief review of abnormalities in the first two requirements; namely, an inadequate neutrophil population (neutropenia) and inability to localize at the appropriate site (defective chemotaxis). Phagocytic and bactericidal malfunctions are covered elsewhere in this volume (see Chapter 18).

Neutropenia

Neutropenia denotes fewer circulating neutrophils than is considered normal. Normal values vary with age, race, and sex but the generally accepted range is 4–10,000/mm^3 total white blood cells with neutrophils constituting some 50%. The major determinant when neutropenia exposes the patient to excessive risk of infection is primarily a matter of degree. Individuals with total neutrophils below 2000 per mm^3 are uncommon in the general population. However, many healthy black Africans and

Yemenite Jews have neutrophil counts in the 1000 per mm^3 vicinity without apparent disease.

These reservations aside, neutropenia of 500–1000 per mm^3, increases, to some degree, the risk of infection and decreases the ability to localize at inflammatory sites. Counts below 500 expose the individual to morbidity and mortality from infection, especially if the drop in count is sudden and induced by drugs or toxins.

A classification of neutropenias is limited by our incomplete understanding of the relevant kinetics. The mechanisms of egress from the bone marrow, division into circulating and marginated pools and finally, neutrophil destruction are imperfectly defined. Nevertheless, for convenience we can divide the neutropenias according to simple dynamics of inadequate production and excessive destruction (Table 19.1).

Inadequate Production

Familial Benign Chronic Neutropenia

Familial benign chronic neutropenia is a rare syndrome most striking for the paucity of clinical manifestations. First reported by Gansslen, these individuals are often recognized serendipitously when a white blood count is obtained. By definition, repeated infections do not occur and a normal life span is anticipated; however, some patients have been described with extensive pyorrhea. Inheritance is non-sex-linked dominant with absolute penetrance. There seems to be an especially high incidence among Yemenite Jews where inbreeding has been extensive.

The total leukocyte count is usually 2–4000 per mm^3 with 5–20% representing neutrophils. A relative lymphocytosis and monocytosis are present and a low-grade absolute eosinophilia is seen in 50% of patients. There is no anemia or thrombocytopenia. No good kinetic studies are available; however, bone marrow examination suggests "maturation ar-

TABLE 19.1. *Categories of Neutropenia*

Inadequate production
Inherited
Familial benign chronic neutropenia
Infantile genetic agranulocytosis and related disorders
Cyclic neutropenia
Acquired
Nutritional deficiencies
Noncytotoxic drugs
Cytotoxic drugs
Bone marrow replacement (myelophthisis)
Excessive destruction
Drug-related immune
Autoimmune
Splenomegaly
Infections

rest" with granulocytes represented in normal numbers to the myelocyte stage. Metamyelocytes, bands, and polymorphonuclear leukocytes are deficient.

Recognition of this syndrome is important to avert unnecessary diagnostic and therapeutic maneuvers. It should be easily definable by history and sampling from family members.

Infantile Genetic Agranulocytosis and Related Disorders

This group of neutropenias share two outstanding characteristics: (1) they are inherited; and (2) repeated infections occur from infancy and often end with death in early childhood. In 1956 Kostmann described 14 children from nine inbred Swedish families with severe neutropenia, recurrent infections, death before 1 year and a failure of neutrophil maturation beyond the early myelocyte stage. Inheritance followed an autosomal recessive pattern. Subsequently, similar families have been reported.

A variety of morbid congenital neutropenias that differ from Kostmann's syndrome in inheritance and associated disorders have also been described. Abnormalities of γ globulins (both hyper-γ-globulinemia and hypo-γ-globulinemia), lymphoid genesis (reticular/dysgenesis), cartilage hair hypoplasia, and pancreatic insúfficiency with lipomatosis are all described in association with severe neutropenia. Current knowledge does not allow unification of this heterogenous group beyond their shared features of congenital neutropenia and associated severe infections.

Cyclic Neutropenia

Little has been added to the clinical description of this rare, infrequently inherited (autosomal dominant) syndrome since Rutledge, in 1930, wrote of a young boy: "These periodical 'attacks' recur usually at intervals of three weeks. A typical attack was described approximately as follows: He looks yellowish. There is little fever 99°–100°F (rectal); he feels listless and fatigued. The temperature gradually rises to 104° or 105° reaching its height on the fourth day, when it gradually falls; it is irregular, suggesting sepsis. The gums become red and swollen, and show more or less numerous, usually rather deep indurated sores which appear also on lips, tongue and buccal surfaces from which Vincent's organisms have been found on several occasions in abundance. The glands of the neck swell. With the fall of temperature the buccal manifestation disappears. The patient may sleep through most of the attack. At other times he is very irritable and fretful. Occasionally he vomits. There is anorexia. The bowels remain regular. It has been observed from time to time that the white blood cell count is low during the attack with a marked depression, chiefly of granular elements.

Spontaneous cyclic fluctuations in neutrophil counts have also been observed in gray collie dogs and patients with chronic myelogenous leukemia and lymphosarcoma. Cycling can be induced in an animal model by constant daily myelosuppression with cyclophosphamide. Recent studies demonstrated periodic fluctuations in all formed blood elements with cycling of monocytes, eosinophils, reticulocytes, platelets, and lymphocytes. Bone marrow examination at various times in the cycle reveals periodic hypoproliferation antedating peripheral findings by 3–4 days. Thus, a more appropriate term for this disorder is cyclic hematopoiesis.

King-Smith and Morley have proposed a computer model of granulocytopoiesis (Fig. 19.1). In this scheme cyclic neutropenia could represent an abnormal negative production feedback control, cycling of a stimulator, an abnormal stem cell, or abnormal release control. No inhibitors have been demonstrated and since the bone marrow population also cycles the defect is not in release mechanism. However, colony stimulating factor, a possible positive feedback control, has been shown to cycle in both the human and canine syndromes. That a defective stem cell may play a role is supported by reversal of neutrophil cycling in gray collie dogs by allogenic bone marrow transplantation.

Nutritional Deficiency

Neutropenia is included in the panorama of abnormal neutrophil functions seen in malnutrition. In kwashiorkor and marasmus, the leukocyte count is usually normal. However, multiple functional parameters are defective. Patients with anorexia nervosa may have hypoplasia of all marrow elements. Similarly, the neutropenia observed with pancreatic insufficiency may partially be a reflection of malabsorption.

Specific deficiences of folic acid and B_{12} may result in neutropenia. Interference with nucleic acid metabolism akin to the mechanism of anemia is suspected. Replacement therapy promptly reverses the neutropenia. Recently, neutropenia has been described in some patients treated with long-term parenteral hyperalimentation. At least some of these individuals have reversible copper deficiency.

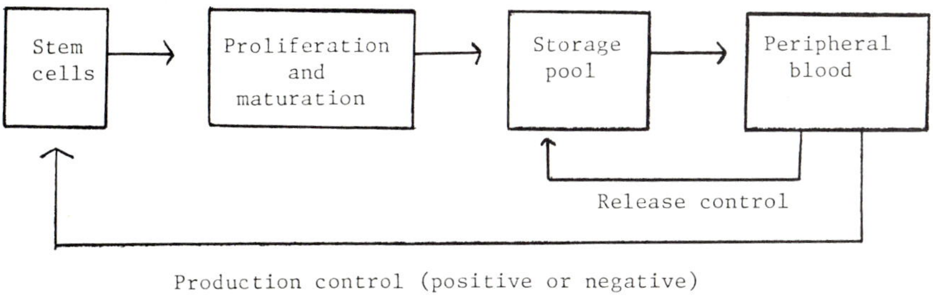

FIG 19.1. Model of granulocytopoiesis controls. (Adapted from King-Smith and Morley.)

Noncytotoxic Drugs

In the modern era of polypharmacy it is not surprising that many drugs have been implicated as causes of neutropenia. However, in the absence of precise definition of mechanisms, a note of reservation is appropriate. Association does not necessarily mean pathogenesis. Current knowledge permits the former but, except for a few drugs, the biologic basis for noncytotoxic drug-related neutropenias is conjecture. Nevertheless, it is clinically prudent to discontinue any drug suspect of causing neutropenia.

With the rapidly expanding pharmacologic armamentarium, any list of drugs associated with neutropenia is necessarily incomplete. Those agents where clinical experience has demonstrated repeated association are listed in Table 19.2. Some of the drugs in this list appear to directly inhibit bone marrow genesis and others seem to act via imprecisely defined immune mechanisms (see section on immune neutropenias). The phenothiazine group of drugs provide the best studied example of direct bone marrow toxicity.

The natural history of phenothiazine related neutropenia offers some mechanistic clues. Most examples have been observed after prolonged, high-dose administration (cumulative dose greater than 10 g). Patients who have developed severe neutropenia or agranulocytosis may be given smaller doses with recovery of a normal neutrophil population. Bone marrow examination during the neutropenic phase shows striking aplasia. However, when the drug is discontinued, the marrow becomes repopulated within 2 weeks. In vitro studies with phenothiazines confirm their broad spectrum of biochemical effects. DNA synthesis, protein synthesis, and certain enzyme reactivity are reduced by phenothiazines. With such protean biochemical interference, it has proved extremely difficult to pinpoint the mechanism of bone marrow suppression.

Cytotoxic Drugs

Because of the extensive use of cytotoxic drugs for immunosuppressive and cancer chemotherapy, this has become the most commonly encountered cause of severe neutropenia. The neutropenia is a result of direct

TABLE 19.2. *Noncytotoxic Drugs Associated with Neutropenia*

Phenothiazines (chlorpromazine, etc.)
Antibiotics (cephalothin, penicillin derivatives, chloramphenicol, sulfonamide derivatives, streptomycin, gentamicin, etc.)
Diuretics (thiazides, etc.)
Antithyroid (thiouracil derivatives)
Nonsteroidal antiinflammatory (indomethacin, phenylbutazone, gold salts)
Oral hypoglycemic (chlorpropramide, etc.)
Antiarrhythmic (quinidine, procainamide, propranolol)
Anticonvulsants
Miscellaneous (aminopyrine, penicillamine, hydroxychloroquine, allopurinol)

myelosuppression. In general, there is a direct relationship between cell turnover kinetics and sensitivity to these drugs. Because the granulocyte cell line is a rapidly dividing population, these cells rank high in their susceptibility to suppression by cytotoxic drugs. Moreover, the resultant neutropenia and its attendant risk of infection are often the limiting factors in continuing cytotoxic therapy.

Various authorities have questioned the reliance on the peripheral neutrophil count as an estimation of granulocyte reserve during myelosuppressive therapy. In addition, Godwin et al. showed that patients who had an impaired granulocyte reserve had a much greater risk for serious infectious complications following cytotoxic therapy. Measurements of marrow granulocyte reserve may improve our ability to predict which patients will benefit most from granulocyte replacement therapy (see section on therapy).

Bone Marrow Replacement (Myelophthisic Neutropenia)

When bone marrow is replaced by neoplastic cells, an infrequent and late manifestation may be neutropenia. More typically, a peripheral leukoerythroblastic anemia is seen characterized by many nucleated red blood cells and a few immature granulocytes. The malignancies most often associated with myelophthisic neutropenia are acute leukemia, multiple myeloma, lymphoma and, less commonly, breast and lung carcinoma.

Excessive Destruction

Immune Neutropenia

That immunologic mechanisms play a role in the development of neutropenia has been suspected for years. Nevertheless, convincing evidence has been difficult to obtain owing mainly to technical problems. Immune neutrophil destruction seems to occur in two settings: drug related and spontaneous. The mechanism of immune injury may be different in these categories.

Drug-Related Immune Neutropenia

Aminopyrine, a seldom used antipyretic/analgesic is the model for drug-induced immune neutropenia. Madison and Squier reported 14 patients who developed precipitous neutropenia after varying latent periods. Upon drug rechallenge, dramatic relapses occurred within 2 hours.

In another study, two normal individuals were given aminopyrine without ill effect. However, when blood from a patient with aminopyrine agranulocytosis was transfused, a prompt fall in neutrophil count resulted. Through further studies, a mechanism has been proposed whereby drug-antibody complexes are adsorbed to leukocytes and the cells are destroyed as carriers of antigen-antibody complexes. A similar hapten immune mechanism is thought to be operant with other drugs.

Non-Drug-related Immune Neutropenia

Validity of the most commonly used method of demonstrating antineutrophil antibodies, the leukoagglutinin reaction, has been questioned. More recently developed techniques seem to offer greater specificity. Nevertheless, caution is warranted in interpreting the presence of leukoagglutins as the cause, rather than the result, of associated neutropenia.

These reservations aside, the demonstration of specific antineutrophilic antibodies has awaited the recognition of unique neutrophil antigens. Standard histocompatibility testing has identified neutrophil antigens with NA1, NA2, and NB1 specificity. Other specific antigens have been proposed but convincing evidence is lacking.

The best characterized non-drug-related immune neutropenia is isoimmune neonatal neutropenia (INN). Fetal maternal incompatibility results in transient selective absence of neutrophils in the neonates peripheral blood and bone marrow. During the neutropenic period, infection, especially pyoderma, is common, although usually not fatal. Normal repopulation of bone marrow and blood occurs by three months, and there are no apparent sequellae. Maternal IgG isoantibodies with NA1, NA2, and NB1 specificity, and, specific absorption of this antibody with paternal and infant neutrophils have been demonstrated. No other cells are affected. The analogy to erythroblastosis fetalis is apparent.

Perhaps the most exciting recent advance in studies on neutropenia has been the demonstration of autoantibodies. Autoimmune neutropenia is an extension of previously reported autoantibodies with pathophysiologic significance. Too few cases have been adequately studied to warrant dogmatic statements on clinical syndromes. Nevertheless, certain themes are evident: (1) occurrence of antigen specific neutrophil autoantibodies in nulliparous, never transfused individuals; (2) appropriate target antigen present in these individuals; (3) development of neutropenia after a period of normal neutrophil counts (age range 3 months to 72 years); (4) normal to increased bone marrow granulocyte cellularity; (5) mild, recurrent infections concomitant with neutropenia; and (6) response to steroids and relapse when they are discontinued. It is not surprising that leukoagglutinins have been described in other "autoimmune" diseases (systemic lupus erythematosus, Felty's syndrome, polyarteritis nodosa) and certain infections (chronic active hepatitis, mononucleosis). What initiates and stimulates the production of these autoantibodies remains obscure.

Splenomegaly

A variety of diseases are associated with splenomegaly and in some, neutropenia is occasionally observed. This has led to the nebulous concept of splenic neutropenia. Kinetic studies with labeled neutrophils have revealed a large, sequestered population of granulocytes in certain patients with splenomegaly. Neutropenia may be the result of intrasplenic destruction or margination.

In systemic lupus erythematosus and Felty's syndrome (rheumatoid arthritis, splenomegaly, and neutropenia), the spleen may play several roles in depressing neutrophil counts. Leukoagglutinins are present in some patients with both syndromes. Whether the spleen is the primary source of these antibodies, analogous to some cases of autoimmune hemolytic anemia, is unknown. Splenic sequestration of labeled neutrophils has, however, been documented in both of these rheumatic diseases. In a long-term follow-up study of patients with Felty's syndrome who underwent splenectomy, 60% had reversal of neutropenia and concomitant decrease in infectious complications. Similar results have been reported with other "splenic sequestration syndromes".

Approach to the Patient

From the preceding discussion, there can be little doubt that the most powerful tool available to the clinician in assessing a patient with neutropenia is the history. Attention to details of family history, drug use, dietary habits and weight, pattern of infectious episodes, and associated diseases are all essential. Recurrent infections is the hallmark of clinically significant neutropenia. It should be remembered that a low neutrophil count, in and of itself, is not a disease.

A few laboratory studies are helpful. Serial total white cell and differential counts exclude spurious laboratory results and document the pattern of neutropenia. Folic acid, B_{12}, antinuclear antibodies, rheumatoid factor, and immunoglobulin levels may point to an associated disease. Bone marrow examination may suggest a defect in granulopoiesis and clarify the mechanism. Although currently limited by availability, leukocyte antibody testing may become more widespread as further investigation clarifies their significance. More specialized studies of leukokinetics with measurement of pool size and determination of colony stimulating factor remain appropriate research tools yielding limited clinical information.

Therapy

Therapeutic decisions rest on a balance between morbidity of the disease and morbidity of the treatment. Clearly, certain of the neutropenias are transient benign phenomena that require no intervention. In others, treatment may be life saving.

The kinetic division of neutropenias provides a convenient approach to therapy.

Hypoproliferative; Specific Therapy

When a specific etiology for the failure of granulopoiesis is discovered, therapy should be appropriately tailored. In the case of noncytotoxic, drug-induced neutropenia, elimination of the offending drug usually suffices. Similarly, nutritional deficiencies respond to replacement therapy albeit at variable rates. The neutropenia of certain infectious diseases usually resolves with treatment of the specific organism. When no treatment is available (i.e., measles), concomitant spontaneous resolution of both is the rule.

Several agents have been used in an attempt to stimulate the hypoproliferative marrow. Brodsky et al. reported a patient with cyclic neutropenia responding to testosterone. Periodicity was unaltered but the granulocyte nadir was increased to > 500. Symptomatic improvement was also reported as was an increase in the granulocyte reserve pool. Despite the encouraging results in this patient, many others have been refractory to androgens. Steroid therapy has also been tried in cyclic neutropenia, but with no consistent benefit has been noted.

Although currently an experimental approach, the report by Dale et al. of reversing the canine syndrome with isologous bone marrow transfusion may become clinically applicable.

Hypoproliferative; Supportive Therapy

While specific therapy for many of the neutropenic syndromes remains unavailable, the most common cause (cytotoxic drugs) is a self-limited process providing the patient survives the initial insult. Major effort should be directed at defining specific infectious agents and antibiotic therapy tailored according to sensitivity testing. At the outset of suspected sepsis in these patients, empirical antibiotic therapy may be warranted. A five-drug regimen reported by Tattersall resulted in a 30% increase in survival.

A natural extension of the specific blood product replacement for anemia and thrombocytopenia has been the increasing use of granulocyte transfusions for temporary neutropenic states. The idea is far from new. In 1934 Strumia gave intramuscular injections of "leukocytic cream" to neutropenic patients. Over the last 40 years experimentation has demonstrated that (1) infused granulocytes circulate; (2) enter inflammatory exudates; (3) are capable of phagocytosis; and (4) bacterial killing. More recent methods in collection and donor/recipient matching have facilitated clinical studies. In studies using the canine model, after irradiation-induced neutropenia, Pseudomonas pneumonia was experimentally produced in 18 animals treated with antibiotics alone (no white blood cell transfusions). The median survival was four days, and there was only one long-term survivor. In the experimental group treated with antibiotics and white blood cell transfusions, the median survival was 20 days and there were six of 11 long-term survivors. In infected neutropenic humans, several investigators have shown a significant increase in survival among patients receiving granulocyte transfusions. Patients who fail to achieve a remission from their underlying malignancy seem to benefit to an even greater extent.

Excessive Destruction

Analogous to autoimmune hemolytic anemia, three basic approaches to therapy of excessive destructive neutropenias have been used: (1) removal of the site of destruction; (2) suppression of antineutrophil antibody production; and (3) elimination of the offending antigen or antigen/antibody complex. When the inciting antigen is borne on the neutrophil as a genetic surface marker, it is clear that elimination of the antigen would require the extreme measure of ablative chemotherapy and repopulation. However, when the neutrophil is a carrier of antigen/antibody complexes, removal of the antigen is often feasible. This usually means discontinuation of a drug. As previously mentioned, when leukoagglutinins are associated with specific infections, treatment of the microbial disease usually corrects the neutropenia. Pharmacologic suppression of antineutrophil antibody production has been attempted with corticosteroids. Patients with autoimmune neutropenia are generally responsive to such chemotherapy and often relapse when steroids are withdrawn. During the period of steroid therapy, leukoagglutinin titers fall as the neutrophil count returns toward normal. Whether steroids may also act by eluting antibody from the neutrophil surface, analogous to certain hemolytic anemias, is unknown. Cytotoxic drugs (e.g., of cyclophosphamide) have also been noted to decrease leukoagglutinin titers. This, however, is often in the setting of an associated disease requiring such therapy, i.e., systemic lupus erythematosus. The reduction in leukoagglutinins may be a nonspecific manifestation of better control of the underlying disease.

Finally, limited kinetic studies have shown the spleen to be the primary locale of neutrophil over-destruction. Splenectomy may reverse the neutropenia in Felty's syndrome and "splenic neutropenia". Unfortunately, there are no established guidelines for splenectomy under these conditions, and such a decision must be made according to individual circumstances.

Chemotaxis

An adequate number of neutrophils does not, in and of itself, protect the host from infection. There must be a means of localizing phagocytes at the inflammatory site. This requires that neutrophils leave the intravascular space through a series of integrated processes including adherence to the endothelial surface, emigration between endothelial cells, and migration to the appropriate site. The capacity of leukocytes to move in a directed fashion toward a gradient of chemical stimulus (chemoattractant) is chemotaxis. In the clinical setting there are two commonly used techniques for assessing chemotaxis. The first, an in vivo method described by Rebuck et al., requires making a standardized skin abrasion and evaluating the sequential influx and adherence to glass slides of phagocytes into the wound. In the normal individual, polymorphonuclear leukocytes are seen within 2 hours and peak at 4–6 hours. Monocytes and lymphocytes follow over the next 12–24 hours. The in vivo nature of this test makes it difficult to state with certainty that chemotaxis is being measured. A second technique, described by Boyden et al., is an in vitro method whereby cells and chemoattractant are separated by a filter and migration of cells into the filter is measured.

Recent investigations have led to the concept of normal, directed cell migration requiring: (1) adequate generation of chemotactic stimulus; (2) cell responsiveness to the stimulus; and (3) the absence of inhibitors that interfere with either genesis or response. Defects in each part of this system have been described resulting in abnormal chemotaxis and often in recurrent infections. The following is a brief discussion of recognized defects of chemotaxis in each category. No attempt has been made to be all-inclusive.

Chemoattractants

Agents which promote directed cell migration are designated chemoattractants. In general, these molecules are derived from six sources: (1) complement component cleavage fragments; (2) enzymes involved in the coagulation/fibrinolytic pathway (kallikrein and plasminogen activator); (3) products from bacteria and viruses which both activate complement components and release chemoattractants during replication; (4) products of tissue breakdown (collagen and fibrin fragments); (5) proteins derived from activated lymphocytes (lymphokines) and phagocytes; and (6) lipids from mammalian and microbial cells.

Some of the chemotactic factors exhibit specificity for different leukocyte populations. Eosinophilic chemotactic factor of anaphylaxis and histamine are found in basophils and mast cells and have preferential attraction for eosinophils. Kallikrein, on the other hand, is much more active on neutrophils.

Defects in Chemoattractant Generation (Table 19.3)

The best characterized defects in chemoattractant generation involve complement components. This is a heterogeneous group of disorders, only some of which are clearly associated with pathology. As is the case of many disorders involving proteins, inadequate synthesis and synthesis of functionally inactive components are described.

C1r deficiency has been described in two families. Endotoxin activation of serum chemotactic factors is delayed about 45 min; however, total activity is normal. This agrees with the kinetics of alternate pathway

TABLE 19.3. *Chemotactic Defects Associated With Abnormal Generation of Chemoattractant*

1. Complement components
   a. C1r
      C2
      C3
      C5
   b. Immunoglobulin deficiencies
2. Coagulation/fibrinolytic pathway
   a. Prekallikrein
   b. Hageman factor
3. Cell-derived
   a. Mucocutaneous candidiasis
   b. Wiskott-Aldrich syndrome

generation of C5a being slower than in the classical pathway. These patients do not suffer from severe infections, although necrotizing vasculitis and dermatitis are associated findings.

As in C1r deficiency, patients with C2 deficiency have a delay in generation of chemoattractants but total activity after one hour is normal. The incidence of infections in these patients is difficult to assess since there is a high incidence of lupus-like syndromes often requiring steroid therapy.

Alper et al. have reviewed the role of C3 in defense against bacterial infections. Three mechanisms resulting in C3 deficiency have been elucidated: (1) deficient or absent synthesis; (2) C3 inactivator deficiency resulting in consumption of C3 by unchecked activation of the alternate pathway; and (3) hypercatabolism of C3 by excessive activity of C3ase activity. Although all of these patients suffer from recurrent infections, it is unclear whether deficient chemotaxis plays any role. Recent studies indicate that C3a may not be a chemotactic factor.

C5 deficiency results in recurrent, severe infections and marked subnormal generation of serum chemotactic activity. Normal chemotactic factor production is restored by the addition of pure C5. Two biochemical types of C5 deficiency have been described. In one, an immunologically present but functionally abnormal protein (Leiner's syndrome) is observed; and in the other, failure of synthesis occurs. C6 deficiency has also been described. Generation of chemotactic factors is normal and there is no increased incidence of infection. This has led to speculation on the biologic importance of C$\overline{567}$ trimolecular complex as a chemoattractant.

In addition to complement component deficiencies, abnormal genesis of chemotactic factors has been recognized in patients with immunoglobulin deficiencies. Serum from patients with hypo- or a-γ-globulinemia fails to generate normal chemotactic activity when stimulated with endotoxin. This is thought to result from insufficient antigen-antibody complexes to activate complement components via the alternate pathway. The contribution of deficient chemoattractant activity to the increased incidence of infection seen in these patients is difficult to evaluate. Failure of opsonization and ingestion also occurs and certainly contributes to the recurrent pyogenic infections. Finally, several defects of cell-derived chemotactic factor generation have been described. A patient with mucocutaneous candidiasis failed to produce lymphocyte-derived chemotactic activity when exposed to Candida antigen. Children with Wiskott-Aldrich syndrome also have an abnormal monocyte chemotactic response, but this is in the presence of excessive lymphocyte-derived chemotactic factor production. The high level of lymphocyte-derived chemotactic factor may inhibit directed migration by interference with the development of a stimulus gradient. Further studies on these and other patients with abnormal lymphocyte function should provide new insights into the interaction of different cellular participants at the inflammatory site.

Cellular Defects of Chemotaxis (Table 19.4)

Although certain morphologic and biochemical events are known to accompany the interaction of leukocytes with chemoattractants, the pathophysiologic basis for the various cellular defects of chemotaxis is unclear. Classification of these defects remains descriptive of clinical features common to the particular patient population. What follows is a brief description of the clinical settings in which cellular defects of chemotaxis have been recognized.

In 1971, Miller et al. described two children with mild, recurrent infections, neutropenia, abnormal directed and random migration, failure of either epinephrine or hydrocortisone to stimulate release of the granulocyte reserve pool, and virtually no influx of polymorphonuclear leukocytes into a Rebuck skin window. Serum chemotactic factor generation and bactericidal capacity were normal. These investigators picturesquely dubbed this the "lazy leukocyte syndrome". In 1974, Boxer et al. described

TABLE 19.4. *Cellular Defects of Chemotaxis*

1. Lazy leukocyte syndrome
2. Actin dysfunction
3. Hyperimmunoglobulin E
4. CHS
5. Diabetes mellitus
6. Drugs
7. Bone marrow transplantation
8. Burn injury
9. α-Mannosidase deficiency
10. Hypophosphatemia
11. Neonates
12. Congenital ichthyosis

an intriguing patient with recurrent, severe infections, deficient adherence to glass, and abnormal random and directed migration. Particle ingestion was also abnormal, thus differing from Miller's patient. Studies of the contractile protein actin revealed marked decrease in polymerization. Whether actin-myosin polymerization and coupling play a role in phagocyte movement analogous to muscle remains speculation.

Several investigators have reported children with recurrent pyogenic infections, extreme hyperimmunoglobulin E, and abnormal chemotaxis. The first report in 1966 described two females with red hair, hyperextensible joints, atopic dermatitis, and recurrent "cold" staphylococcal abscesses (Job's syndrome). Subsequent reports have included patients with associated mucocutaneous candidiasis, eczema, urticaria, asthma, and allergic rhinitis. The mechanism of abnormal chemotaxis in this constellation of disorders remains obscure. Histamine inhibition, phagocytosis of antigen-antibody complexes and binding of IgE to the neutrophil membrane have all been suggested without convincing evidence.

The Chediak-Higashi syndrome (CHS) is a rare, inherited disease characterized by partial oculocutaneous albinism, recurrent pyogenic infections, and neutropenia. Morphologically, granulocytes contain giant, lysosomal granules, and defects in polymorphonuclear leukocyte and monocyte chemotaxis have been described.

These in vitro defects are enhanced by using progressively smaller filter pore sizes in the Boyden chamber assay. This has led to the suggestion that cellular deformability is abnormal. More recently, abnormal microtubule assembly has been proposed as an alternative mechanism of deficient leukocyte function. Several manifestations of abnormal microtubule function can be corrected by increasing intracellular cyclic guanosine monophosphate (cGMP). In a recent report, the in vitro addition of ascorbic acid (which raises intracellular cGMP) to CHS neutrophils and a clinical trial of ascorbate in a patient with CHS reversed the usual chemotactic and bactericidal defects.

Although epidemiologic studies have provided conflicting results, clinicians have long suspected that diabetics suffer from more frequent infections. Defects of phagocytosis, bactericidal activity, and Rebuck skin window responses have inconsistently been described, as well as the demonstration of a chemotactic defect, not correlated with blood sugar, blood urea nitrogen, or serum insulin. Perhaps more interesting is the reversal of the defect by incubation of polymorphonuclear leukocytes with insulin and glucose. This may be related to intracellular ion fluxes analogous to the reversal by potassium of oubain-induced abnormal chemotaxis.

As is the case with neutropenia, a variety of drugs are associated with depressed in vitro chemotaxis. These include corticosteroids, colchicine, griseofulvin, and vinblastine. The observation that prednisone, but not dexamethasone, interferes with leukocyte mobilization in vivo may have clinical significance.

After bone marrow transplantation, neutrophil chemotaxis is abnormal. This is directly associated with graft-versus-host disease or treatment with anti-thymocyte globulin. Clinically, those patients with deficient chemotaxis have more frequent infections. Finally, a number of case reports of patients with abnormal chemotaxis in various clinical settings have been described. Some patients with severe burns have abnormal chemotaxis. The appearance of this defect seems to correlate with a poor prognosis. A child with α-mannosidase deficiency, recurrent infections, and abnormal chemotaxis but normal random migration has been recently reported. Abnormal neutrophil chemotaxis has also been described in hypophosphatemia, neonates, and congenital ichthyosis.

Chemotactic Defects Associated with Inhibitors (Table 19.5)

Several investigators have described circulating inhibitors that interfere with either cell responsiveness to chemoattractants or the activity of the chemotactic factor. A 4-year-old boy with recurrent pyogenic infections, abnormal chemotaxis, defective bactericidal activity against *Escherichia coli* and Klebsiella (normal against *Staphylococcus aureus*) and decreased reduction of nitroblue tetrazolium consistent with chronic granulomatous disease was the first patient described with a cell-directed inhibitor. However, several chronic granulomatous disease patients have had normal chemotaxis with no inhibitors. Another patient with a cellular inhibitor showed partial resolution of clinical and in vitro abnormalities by transfusion with normal plasma.

A serum inhibitor in patients with rheumatoid arthritis, although poorly characterized, seems to irreversibly attach to the neutrophil membrane and be heat stable. There is no correlation between presence of this inhibitor and seropositivity, age, drug treatment, sex, or disease activity.

In addition to these inhibitors, at least two leukocyte-derived cellular inhibitors have been described. The first, neutrophil immobilizing factor, is produced by neutrophils and exhibits specificity for the neutrophil and eosinophil (i.e., monocyte chemotaxis is unaffected). No other neutrophil

TABLE 19.5 *Chemotactic Defects Associated with Inhibitors*

1. Rheumatoid arthritis
2. Systemic lypus erythematosus
3. Hodgkin's disease
4. Lepromatous leprosy
5. Sarcoidosis
6. Alcoholic liver disease
7. Uremia
8. IgA myeloma

function is affected. The second, leukocyte inhibitory factor, is a protein with a molecular weight of 68,000 and is liberated from stimulated lymphocytes after antigen or concanavalin A challenge. In a physiologic scheme it would seem logical to have a substance liberated at the inflammatory site to inhibit further migration once the neutrophil reached the target site. Neutrophil immobilizing factor or leukocyte inhibitory factor may be active in this modulating role.

A chemotactic factor inactivator (CFI) present in low concentration in normal serum inhibits both complement-derived and complement-independent chemotactic factor activity. It has no direct effect on the neutrophil's ability to migrate. Studies suggest that CFI is more likely a heterogeneous group of serum proteins. Excessive CFI has now been reported in a variety of diseases associated with frequent infections and abnormal chemotaxis. The initial report was among patients with cirrhosis. Nineteen of 22 patients had at least 50% reduction in chemotaxis. Recent studies of patients with sarcoidosis, lepromatous leprosy, Hodgkin's disease, and systemic lupus erythematosus have confirmed the association of elevated serum CFI, abnormal chemotaxis, and recurrent infections.

Therapeutic Perspective

The array of clinical disorders associated with abnormal chemotaxis and frequent infections has dramatically expanded over the last 10 years. However, the current state of the art is more descriptive than mechanistic. As a result, specific therapy is not available for chemotactic disorders. Nevertheless, several observations have provided some exciting insights. Disorders of chemotactic factor generation should be amenable to replacement therapy. Owing to the physicochemical properties of complement components, replacement of specific fractions is not available. However, in the setting of life-threatening infection, plasma infusions may be of benefit. Miller et al. have given plasma transfusions to C5-deficient infected patients with encouraging results. Since the cellular events underlying chemotaxis are poorly understood, it is difficult to comment on specific therapy for these abnormalities. Snyderman has reported a patient with defective monocyte chemotaxis and mucocutaneous candidiasis whose chemotactic abnormality resolved with transfer factor. Similarly, BCG therapy has been reported to restore normal chemotaxis in certain patients with cancer. The antihelminthic agent, levamisol, increases intracellular cGMP and promotes in vitro chemotaxis. Several patients with the hyper-IgE syndrome are currently part of a clinical study with this drug. As previously noted, ascorbic acid also raises cGMP levels and has had an encouraging trial in a patient with the Chediak-Higashi syndrome. Results of these and similar trials with new agents may provide exciting additions to our ability to effectively treat infections in these compromised hosts.

SELECTED REFERENCES

Agnello, V., de Bracco, M. M. E., and Kunkel, H. G.: Hereditary C2 deficiency with some manifestations of systemic lupus erythamatosus. J. Immunol., *108:* 837, 1972.

Alper, C. A., Stossel, T. P., and Rosen, F. S.: Genetic defects affecting complement and host resistance to infection. In *The Phagocytic Cells,* edited by J. Bellanti and D. Dayton. New York: Raven Press.

Altman, L. C., Snyderman, R., and Blaese, R. M.: Abnormalities of chemotactic lymphokine synthesis and mononuclear leukocyte chemotaxis in Wiskott-Aldrich syndrome. J. Clin. Invest., *54:* 486, 1974.

Boxer, L. A., Greenberg, M. S., Boxer, G. J., and Stossel T. P.: Autoimmune neutropenia. N. Engl. J. Med., *293:* 748, 1975.

Boxer, L. A., Hedley-Whyte, E. T., and Stossel, T. P.: Neutrophil action dysfunction and abnormal neutrophil behavior. N. Engl. J. Med., *291:* 1093, 1974.

Boxer, L. A., and Stossel, T. P.: Effects of anti-human neutrophil antibodies *in vitro:* quantitative studies. J. Clin. Invest., *53:* 1534, 1974.

Boxer, L. A., Watanabe, A. M., Rister, M., Besch, H. R., Jr., Allen, J., and Baehner, R. L.: Correction of leukocyte function in Chediak-Higashi syndrome by ascorbate. N. Engl. J. Med., *295:* 1041, 1976.

Boyden, S.: The chemotactic effect of mixtures of antibody and antigen on polymorphonuclear leukocytes. J. Exp. Med., *115:* 453, 1962.

Brodsky, I., Reimann, H. A., and Dennis, L. H.: Treatment of cyclic neutropenia with testosterone. Am. J. Med., *38:* 802, 1965.

Clark, R. A., Johnson, F. L., Klebanoff, S. J., and Thomas, E. D.: Defective neutrophil chemotaxis in bone marrow transplant patients. J. Clin. Invest., *58:* 22, 1976.

Clark, R. A., Root, R. K. Kimball, H. R., and Kirkpatrick, C. H.: Defective neutrophil chemotaxis and cellular immunity in a child with recurrent infections. Ann. Intern. Med., *78:* 515, 1973.

Craddock, P. R., Yawata, Y., Van Santen, L., Gilberstadt, S., Silvis, S., and Jacob, H. S.: Acquired phagocyte dysfunction. A complication of the hypophosphatemia of parenteral hyperalimentation. N. Engl. J. Med., *290:* 1403, 1974.

Dale, D. C., Brown, C. H., Carbone, P., and Wolff, S. M.: Cyclic urinary leukopoietic activity in grey collie dogs. Science, *173:* 152, 1971.

Dale, D. C., and Graw, R. G.: Transplantation of allogeneic bone marrow in canine cyclic neutropenia. Science, *183:* 83, 1974.

Dale, D. C., Reynolds, H. Y., Pennington, J. E., Elin, R. J., Pitts, T. W., and Graw, R. G. Jr.: Granulocyte transfusion therapy of experimental *Pseudomonas* penumonia. J. Clin. Invest., *54:* 664, 1974.

Deinard, A. S., Fortuny, I. E., Theologides, A., Anderson, G. L., Boen, J., and Kennedy, B. J.: Studies on the neutropenia of cancer chemotherapy. Cancer, *33:* 1210, 1974.

Dunlap, W. M., James, G. W. III, and Hume, D. M.: Anemia and neutropenia caused by copper deficiency. Ann. Intern. Med., *80:* 470, 1974.

Gallin, J. I., Clark, R. A., and Frank, M. M.: Kinetic analysis of chemotactic factor generation in human serum via activation of the classical and alternate complement pathway. Clin. Immunol. Immunopathol., *3:* 334, 1975.

Gallin, J. I., Klimerman, J. A., Padgett, G. A., and Wolff, S. M.: Defective mononuclear leukocyte chemotaxis in the Chediak-Higashi syndrome of humans, mink, and cattle. Blood, *45:* 863, 1975.

Gallin, J. I., and Wolff, S. M.: Leukocyte chemotaxis: Physiological considerations and abnormalities. Clin. Haematol. *4:* 567, 1975.

Gänsslen, M.: Konstitutionelle familiäre leukopenia (neutropenie). Klin Wochenschr., *20:* 922, 1941.

Godwin, H. A., Zimmerman, T. S., Kimball, H. R. Wolff, S. M., and Perry, S.: Correlation of granulocyte mobilization with etiocholanolone and the subsequent development of myelosuppression in patients with acute leukemia receiving therapy. Blood, *31:* 580, 1968.

Graw, R. G., Jr., Herzig, G., Perry, S., and Henderson, E. S.: Normal granulocyte transfusion therapy: treatment of septicemia due to gram-negative bacteria. N. Engl. J. Med., *287:* 367, 1972.

Guerry, D., Adamson, J. W., Dale, D. C., and Wolff, S. M.: Human cyclic neutropenia: urinary colony-stimulating factor and erythropoietin levels. Blood, *44:* 257, 1974.

Guerry, D., Dale, D. C., Omine, M., Perry, S., and Wolff, S. M.: Periodic hematopoiesis in human cyclic neutropenia. J. Clin. Invest., *52:* 3220, 1973.

King-Smith, E. A., and Morley, A. A.: A computer model for the mammalian (human) leukocyte system. In *Proceedings of the Twentieth Annual Conference on Engineering in Medicine and Biology,* Boston, Mass., 1976. New York: Institute of Electrical and Electronics Engineers, 1967, Vol. 9, Sect. 19, Abstr. 9.

Kostmann, R.: Infantile genetic agranulocytosis (agranulocytosis infantalis hereditaria). Acta Paediatr., *105:* 1, 1956.

Leddy, J. P., Frank, M., Gaither, T., Baum, J., and Klempner, M. R.: Hereditary deficiency of the sixth component of complement in man. I. Immunochemical, biologic and family studies. J. Clin. Invest., *53:* 544, 1974.

Lux, S. E., Johnston, R. B., Jr., August, C. S., Say, B., Penchaszadeh, V. B., Rosen, F. S., and McKusick, V. A.: Chronic neutropenia and abnormal cellular immunity in cartilage-hair hypoplasia. N. Engl. J. Med., *282:* 231, 1970.

Maderazo, E. G., Ward, P. A., Woronick, C. L., Kubik, J., and DeGraff, A. C., Jr.: Leukotactic dysfunction in sarcoidosis. Ann Intern. Med., *84:* 414, 1976.

Miller, M. E., and Nilsson, U. R.: A familial deficiency of the phagocytosis-enhancing activity of serum related to a dyfunction of the fifth component of complement (C5). N. Engl. J. Med., *282:* 354, 1970.

Miller, M. E., Oski, F. A., and Harris, M. B.: Lazy-leukocyte syndrome: a new disorder of neutrophil function. Lancet, *1:* 665, 1971.

Moeschlin, S., and Wagner, K.: Agranulocytosis due to the occurrence of leukocyte agglutinins. Acta Haematol., *8:* 29, 1952.

Moore, R. A., Brunner, C. M., Sandusky, W. R., and Leavell, B. S.: Felty's syndrome: Long-term follow-up after splenectomy. Ann. Intern. Med., *75:* 381, 1971.

Oliver, J. M., and Zurier, R. B.: Correction of characteristic abnormalities of microtubule function and granule morphology in Chediak-Higashi syndrome with cholinergic agonists. J. Clin. Invest., *57:* 1239, 1976.

Pachman, L. M., Schwartz, A. D., Barron, R., and Golde, D. W.: Chronic neutropenia: response to plasma with high colony-stimulating activity. J. Pediatr., *87:* 713, 1975.

Rebuck, J. W., and Crowley, J. H.: A method of studying leukocytic functions *in vivo.* Ann. N. Y. Acad. Sci., *59:* 757, 1955.

Rosenfeld, S. I., Baum, J., Steigbigel, R. T., and Leddy, J. P.: Hereditary deficiency of 5th component of complement of man. II. Biological properties of C5-deficient human serum. J. Clin. Invest., *57:* 1635, 1976.

Rutledge, B. H., Hansen-Prüss, O. C., and Thayer, W. S.: Recurrent agranulocytosis. Bull. Johns Hop. Hosp., *46:* 369, 1930.

Schiffman, E., Corcoran, B. A., and Wahl, S. M.: N-formylmethionyl peptides as chemoattractants for leukocytes. Proc. Natl. Acad. Sci. USA, *72:* 1059, 1975.

Snyderman, R., Altman, L. C., Frankel, A., and Blaese, R. M.: Defective mononuclear leukocyte chemotaxis: a previously unrecognized immune dysfunction; studies in a patient with chronic mucocutaneous candidiasis. Ann. Intern. Med., *78:* 509, 1973.

Soriano, R. B., South, M. A., Goldman, A. S., and Smith, C. W.: Defect of neutrophil motility in a child with recurrent bacterial infections and disseminated cytomegalovirus infection. J. Pediatr., *83:* 951, 1973.

Squier, T. L., and Madison, F. W.: Drug sensitivity as a cause of acute primary granulocytopenia. Wis. Med. J., *34:* 175, 1935.

Strumia, M.: The effect of leukocyte cream injections in the treatment of the neutropenias. Am. J. Med. Sci., *187:* 527, 1934.

Tattersall, M. H., Spiers, A. S., and Darrell, J. H.: Initial therapy with combination of five antibiotics in febrile patients with leukemia and neutropenia. Lancet, *1:* 162, 1972.

Van Epps, D. E., Palmer, D. L., and Williams, R. C.: Characterization of serum inhibitors of neutrophil chemotaxis associated with energy. J. Immunol., *113:* 189, 1974.

Vogel, J. M., Kimball, H. R., Wolff, S. M. and Perry, S.: Etiocholanolone in the evaluation of marrow reserves in patients receiving cytotoxic agents Ann. Intern. Med., *67:* 1226, 1967.

Ward, P. A. and Berenberg, J. L.: Defective regulation of inflammatory mediators in Hodgkin's disease: supernormal levels of chemotactic-factor inactivator. N. Engl. J. Med., *290:* 76, 1974.

Ward, P. A., Goralnick, S., and Bullock, W. E.: Defective leukotaxis in patients with lepromatous leprosy. J. Lab. Clin. Med., *87:* 1025, 1976.

Warden, G. D., Mason, A. D., and Pruitt, B. A.: Evaluation of leukocyte chemotaxis *in vitro* in thermally injury patients. J. Clin. Invest., *54:* 1001, 1974.

Wolfsdorf, J., and Nolan, R.: Leukocyte function in protein deficiency states. S. Afr. Med., *48:* 528, 1974.

Chapter 20

IMMUNOLOGIC ASPECTS OF THE SPLEEN

Craig S. Kitchens, M.D.

The spleen consists of an intricate spongework of reticular cells arranged in a lattice supporting a dense population of lymphocytes and macrophages. Through this sieve-like arrangement runs an elaborate vascular system consisting of arterioles, sinuses, and veins. While other tissues of the "reticuloendothelial system" contain similar cells, the spleen is unique in its compactness and seemingly singular mission of filtering and perusing the blood's contents.

The functions of the spleen are best understood if one appreciates the structure of the organ. Blood is received from the general circulation via the splenic artery. After branching into trabecular arteries, the vessels are surrounded by either white or red pulp. The white pulp is circumferentially arranged around the more proximal part of the artery and consists primarily of macrophages and small unstimulated lymphocytes, the majority of which are T cells. Small arterioles branch off at right angles from the central artery and "skim" relatively more plasma than cells from the whole blood of the central artery. This low hematocrit blood is released into the white pulp. The remaining high hematocrit blood is released directly into the red pulp by the open ends of the central artery and its more distal branches. The red pulp consists primarily of macrophages, red blood cells, B lymphocytes, and plasma cells. It is chiefly involved in filtration of the formed elements of the blood. Blood cells must survive sluggish flow and physiologic extremes while percolating through an obstacle course of reticular cells and macrophages. After reaching the sinuses, the blood returns to the general circulation. Defective and effete cells are cleared. Approximately 30% of the total mass of platelets is passively sequestered in the red pulp. Monocytes readily transform into macrophages under appropriate stimulation.

The white pulp serves the immunologic function of primary antibody formation. Plasma borne particles and proteins enter the white pulp and are antigenically scrutinized. If deemed "foreign", the material is phagocytized by the macrophage and "processed" into an antigenic message to which the adjacent lymphocytes react by producing antibody. By this synergistic action between macrophages and lymphocytes, primary antibody formation is rapidly initiated against a new antigen. The newly stimulated lymphocytes move from the white pulp, enter the bloodstream and circulate back to the red pulp of the spleen or to the lymph nodes, evolve into plasma cells, and produce and secrete antibody against the stimulating antigen. The white pulp functions appear to be blocked by corticosteroids while the filtration function of the red pulp does not.

Other tissues of the reticuloendothelial system (liver, bone marrow, lymph nodes) can filter blood and phagocytize foreign material; however, in the absence of antibody coating, clearance is limited. The spleen is singular in its ability to phagocytize antigenic material without prior existing antibody. Once antibody production has been initiated by the spleen, other reticuloendothelial tissues can readily phagocytize antibody-coated antigen.

Several experimental models and clinical observations have demonstrated the role of the spleen in immunity. Splenectomized animals and humans seem normal in their ability to produce antibodies to antigen administered subcutaneously or intraperitoneally. Thus, antibody titers after innoculation of normal and splenectomized patients with diphtheria toxoid rise at equal rates. Splenectomized and control rats given sheep red blood cells intraperitoneally developed anti-sheep red blood cell antibodies to the same degree. However, if the sheep red blood cells are administered intravenously, the splenectomized model fails to produce antibody. Ellis and Smith demonstrated that rapid production of type-specific, antipneumococcal antibody is dependent on the spleen. If normal rabbits are given heat-killed type II pneumococci intravenously, rapid antibody production permits survival when the animal is challenged 8 hours later with a bolus of live type II pneumococci. Splenectomized rabbits fail to produce the protective antibody and succumb to the subsequent challenge of the live bacteria.

The human counterpart of these experiments has been observed. A small percentage of splenectomized patients may become victims of fulminant bacterial sepsis complicated by the Waterhouse-Friderichsen syndrome, disseminated intravascular coagulation, and usually death. This syndrome is rare except in the splenectomized or hyposplenic patient. Typically the offending organism is a virulent organism having a phagocytic-resistant capsule. The most common bacteria involved are *Diplococcus pneumoniae, Hemophilus influenzae,* or Klebsiella sp. Presumably, the host has not previously encountered the antigenic species and the lack of a functioning spleen delays primary antibody production and, hence, antibody-dependent phagocytosis by the remaining reticuloendothelial system is impeded to the point that rapid bacterial proliferation may prove fatal. A recent report of a survivor of this syndrome, exemplifies those points. Low acute phase serum antibodies were found against the offending organism (type VI pneumococcus) but convalescent sera drawn 1 month later demonstrated antibody production. The patient likewise was found to produce antibody to a polyvalent pneumococcal vaccine, and was, therefore, able to show an antibody response to a "new" antigen over a 1 month period. Presumably, the significant delay in antibody production is within the first hours to days of the illness. Other immunologic tests (quantitative immunoglobulin levels, B and T lymphocytes, serum opsonins, Staphylococcal killing ability of white cells, and antibody production in response to diphtheria and tetanus toxoid inoculation) were found to be normal.

SELECTED REFERENCES

Ellis, E. F., and Smith, R. T.: The role of the spleen in immunity with special reference to the post-splenectomy problem in infants. Pediatrics, *37:* 111, 1966.

Kitchens, C. S.: The syndrome of post-splenectomy fulminant sepsis. Case report and review of the literature. Am. J. Med. Sci., *274:* 303, 1977.

Krivit, W.: Overwhelming post-splenectomy infection. Am. J. Hematol., *2:* 193, 1977.

Weiss, L.: *The Cells and Tissues of the Immune System: Structure, Functions, Interactions.* Englewood Cliffs, N.J.: Prentice-Hall, 1972.

Weiss, L.: A scanning electron microscopic study of the spleen. Blood, *43:* 665, 1974.

Whitaker, A. N.: Infection and the spleen: association between hyposplenism, pneumococcal sepsis, and disseminated intravascular coagulation. Med. J. Aust., *1:* 1213, 1969.

Chapter 21

IMMUNOHEMATOLOGY

Neil Abramson, M.D.

Few fields of medicine have bridged the gap between the basic and clinical sciences as effectively as hematology. Immunohematology has provided basic science with knowledge and skill for the clinical immunologist and hematologist and these disciplines have returned understanding and considerable insight into basic immunology.

The major emphasis of this chapter is the review of immunology as it affects red cells. Rather than using the classic terminology of immunohematology, the specific immunoglobulins, or the specific complement components will be interrelated.

Historical Background

Formed in the bone marrow and presumably destroyed in the reticuloendothelial system, red cells live approximately 120 days, moving repeatedly from arterial to venous system through small capillaries. They travel between 175–200 miles. Since some capillaries are half the diameter of the cells, the cells' shapes must be altered and deformed. Immunoglobulins impair irreversible shape alterations and complement causes premature detection by the reticuloendothelial system or frank lysis, thus shortening the life-span.

The history of immune hemolytic anemia began recently. Vanlair and Masius described a form of jaundice distinct from liver disease caused by liberation of "coloring material" from red cells in 1871. Donath and Landsteiner detected immune factors in the serum of a patient with clinical hemolytic anemia. In 1913 Banti's experiments identified an antibody later referred to as "incomplete". An antibody he produced by injecting rabbits with dog red cells caused spherocytosis, splenomegaly, and hemolytic anemia when reinjected into dogs. The antibody, however, caused no hemolysis or spherocytosis in vitro. The "incomplete" antibody eluded further description until Coombs reported the antiglobulin test

(Coombs' test) which characterized the antibody as IgG. In 1958 Jandl demonstrated the relationship between antibody coated red cells and white cells which led eventually to the pathogenesis of spherocytosis.

Confusion has occurred because of the terms "warm" and "cold" antibodies, hemolysins and agglutinins, complete and incomplete antibodies. It is simpler to review pathophysiologic mechanisms as IgG, IgM, and components of complement.

IgG Antibodies

IgG antibodies are maximally active at 37°C, hence the classification warm. They are "incomplete" in that they are not as potent in causing agglutination or complement fixation as IgM antibodies and do not result in morphologic or metabolic aberration in vitro. Agglutination may fail to occur because IgG is insufficient in length to bridge the natural gap between red cells created by electrical forces. Most IgG antibodies found in disease have specificity for the Rh antigen. Despite the lack of activity in vitro, this antibody produces spherocytosis, splenomegaly, and hemolytic anemia in vivo.

The work of Jandl and coworkers help explain the pathophysiologic mechanisms of IgG red cell antibodies. Studies using anti-D, an IgG antibody directed against the Rh antigen, show that these antibodies when placed on red cells in vitro or in vivo cause the cells to disappear from the plasma within an hour, with little or no hemolysis, and sequester in the spleen. When the cells were coated with anti-D or other IgG antibodies and mixed with normal white blood cells in vitro, they were observed bound circumferentially about the central white cell into a "rosette." The attached red cells appeared spherocytic whereas the unattached red cells did not. The white cell responsible for rosette formation is the monocyte or tissue macrophage by light and electron microscopic criteria. Polymorphonuclear leukocytes do not participate in rosette formation unless complement is present on red cells. Examination of points of attachment between the monocyte and red cells often reveal multiple, short finger-like projections from the monocyte which interdigitate with the red cell. In some areas pieces of the red cell membrane appear fragmented. In other areas long, finger-like projections appear to envelop the red cell; in the center of the cup-like monocyte projection, the red cell appears to be siphoned into the monocyte. The attachment of red cells to monocytes is firm and they can be dislodged only with proteolytic enzymes, such as papain, which cleave the gamma globulin molecule binding them. Measurements of cells after attachment indicated that they have lost some membrane and become spherocytic.

IgG is responsible for attaching red cells to monocytes. On the basis of in vitro experiments such as those with papain it can be assumed that the Fc end of the molecule attaches to the monocyte and the antigen-binding end to the red cell. Most IgG antibodies, such as those induced by drugs, blood group antibodies, and those in idiopathic acquired autoimmune hemolytic anemia, mediate rosette formation. The selectivity of IgG for rosette formation is more restricted within the subclasses. IgG_1 and IgG_3 have specific monocyte receptors, IgG_3 binding being the most avid. These subclasses are those of anti-Rh antibody.

The relationship between antibodies and red cells not only must include class of antibody but also subclass specificity, reticuloendothelial blood flow, and monocyte function. Well known are examples of hemolysis with little, if any, detectable antibody as well as examples of excess antibody with no hemolysis. In the majority of cases in which IgG_3 is present on red cells, rosette formation can be shown in vitro and hemolysis in vivo. Rosette formation and hemolysis are less likely with a mixture of subclasses or when red cells contain only a sublcass without monocyte receptor activity, such as IgG_4. The elution of antibody from red cells, blood flow to the reticuloendothelial system and monocyte function are all affected by corticosteroid therapy; hence, these drugs may terminate hemolysis in Coombs' positive hemolytic anemia.

The incomplete IgG antibody is ineffective on red cells until met by the monocyte or macrophage of the spleen. Once detained by or attached to a monocyte or macrophage, red cell membrane is lost and destruction occurs in the adverse conditions of the spleen. If the cells exit the spleen before destruction they are observed as the spherocytes of IgG-related hemolytic anemia.

IgM Antibodies

IgM antibodies are "complete" in that they are high molecular weight proteins large enough to bridge the gap between red cells and cause agglutination. In addition they fix complement very strongly and are capable of producing lysis. Since their activity in vitro is optimum at temperatures less than 37°C, they are referred to as cold agglutinins.

A pathophysiologic mechanism of red cell destruction is exemplified by infusion of ABO incompatible red cells. Anti-A or anti-B antibodies are usually IgM. Within moments the incompatible cells disappear from peripheral blood. Simultaneously hemoglobin appears in the plasma, indicating hemolysis. In contrast to the situation with anti-D (IgG), red cell sequestration is localized in the liver. A distinct monocyte receptor for IgM has not been found; however, IgM fixes complement which may be important since the Kupffer cells have a receptor for the third component of complement.

Complement

Complement's effects upon red cells begin with activation of C3. The classical pathway may be initiated by IgM, IgG_1, IgG_2 or IgG_3. Endotoxin and other immunoglobulins may trigger the alternate (properdin) pathway. In either, when enzymatic activity occurs, C3 is cleaved into two components, C3a which has anaphylotoxic and chemotactic properties and C3b which attaches to red cell membranes. The C3 inactivator acting upon cell-bound C3b produces a fragment referred to as C3c which elutes or washes free of the cell and C3d which remains on the cell but is functionally inactive. Alternatively when C5 through C9 are sequentially activated, lysis occurs and electron microscopy shows defects on the red cell membrane.

Complement-mediated red cell destruction may occur when cells coated with immunoglobulin and C3b are removed by monocytes or macrophages and polymorphonuclear leukocytes. Despite these postulated mechanisms, however, complement-coated red cells often are resistant to lysis in vitro and have a normal life-span in vivo. Recent studies show that C3b-coated cells, when injected in vivo, rapidly sequester in the liver where they are converted to C3d-coated cells presumably by the C3 inactivator. C3d cells are tolerant to lysis which possibly explains the normal survival of complement coated cells.

Clinical Features

The hemolytic anemias often are divided into primary and secondary forms. The latter is associated with an underlying disorder or drug-induced mechanism and the relative frequency varies in great part with the vigor with which one seeks an underlying mechanism. The drug-induced condition provides a good example of the pathophysiologic mechanisms previously reviewed.

The complement fixing type of drug-induced immune hemolysis was the first example of a secondary form to be clearly recorded. Stibophen, an antimonial compound used in the treatment of schistosomiasis, induces hemolysis on an immunologic basis. Serum from certain patients treated with this drug contained an antibody which did not react with red cells until the offending drug was added. In vitro tests confirmed the presence of complement on red cells or complement-mediated hemolysis. Antibody activity and complement activation were not directed against the red cells but the drug; the red cells were "innocent bystanders." Other drugs responsible for this type of hemolysis include quinine, quinidine, aminopyrine, phenacetin, paraaminosalicylic acid, and chlorpropamide. Treatment of this disorder is discontinuation of the drug. Hemolysis abates as soon as the drug or its metabolites disappear.

The second type of drug-induced hemolytic anemia is referred to as the hapten form, best shown by penicillin or its analogs. Penicillin is an incomplete antigen (hapten), hence unable to induce production of antibody unless bound to a macromolecular substance or tissue protein. When bound to red cells it may induce an IgG antibody which is responsible for Coombs' positive red cells and hemolysis. This antibody does not bind to normal red cells but only to those coated with penicillin. The pathophysiologic mechanism of red cell destruction is identical to the situation with anti-D IgG antibodies including the lack of significant complement activation. Antipenicillin antibodies cross-react with penicillin analogs or with drugs sharing the β lactam configuration such as cephalothin. Clinically the antipenicillin IgG red cell antibody does not appear unless large doses of penicillin are administered, allowing for the coating of red cells. Treatment requires discontinuation of the drug, if hemolysis occurs. Hemolysis abates as soon as the drug elutes from the cells or as soon as the drug-coated cells are removed. The presence of the antibody without hemolysis is no indication for discontinuation of the drug.

The third example of drug-induced hemolytic anemia is referred to as "autoimmune" and is associated with α-methyldopa, L-dopa, and mefenamic acid. Coombs' positive red cells may be detected in approximately 10% of hypertensive patients taking α-methyldopa. It is produced for unknown reasons and closely resembles that of idiopathic autoimmune hemolytic anemia. It is a warm noncomplement fixing IgG globulin with specificity directed against the Rh antigen and may induce spherocytosis, splenomegaly, and hemolytic anemia. In these patients the drug is associated with antibody production. The antibody may appear after 3–4 months of drug administration and remain 3–4 months after discontinuation. Differentiation of this anemia from idiopathic immune hemolytic anemia is exceedingly important in terms of prognosis and therapy. Corticosteroids, immunosuppressive therapies, and splenectomy often used in idiopathic anemia are not needed; rather, the most appropriate therapy is discontinuation of the drug.

The last type of drug-induced mechanism is referred to as aggregation, best illustrated by cephalothin. Like penicillin, cephalothin avidly binds to red cells, however, normal serum proteins are aggregated with it which results in the binding of IgG or C3. This nonspecific deposition of serum protein onto red cells may not be associated with hemolysis. In man and subhuman primates experimentally given cephalothin daily Coombs' positivity occurred without hemolysis. Coombs' positivity also may occur among patients with impaired renal function who are being given cephalothin. High drug levels may be related to impaired catabolism, however, when hemolysis appears it may not be immunologic but associated with underlying disease. Anticephalothin and antipenicillin antibodies do cross-react which adds to the confusion.

The common secondary forms of immune hemolytic anemia other than those caused by drugs are associated with lymphoproliferative and connective tissue diseases. In addition hemolytic anemia may be seen with myeloproliferative diseases, benign and malignant tumors, infections, granulomatous diseases, and chronic diseases such as ulcerative colitis and liver disease. When underlying disease cannot be found, the term primary, idiopathic, or autoimmune is frequently used.

Clinical features of IgG induced immunohemolytic anemia are those of hemolysis plus the signs and symptoms of the secondary disease. Laboratory features include spherocytic hemolytic anemia and a positive Coombs' test. Treatment must be directed to the associated or secondary disease. If no disease is present corticosteroids are frequently employed in high doses, which benefit 50 to 75% of these patients. Once a response is apparent, the dosage is decreased to the lowest effective dose. The mechanism of the corticosteroids' action is not precisely known, but there may be effects upon reticuloendothelial flow, binding of antibody to cells, and function of monocytes. When corticosteroid therapy is not successful, splenectomy or "immunosuppressive" therapy (cyclophosphamide or azathioprine) are often considered. Demonstration of an excess accumulation of radiolabeled red cells in the spleen may predict beneficial results from splenectomy. Transfusions should be avoided where possible because of additional antibody formation to red cells, white cells, or platelets.

A much different disease is IgG induced immune hemolytic anemia associated with a cold hemolysin (Donath-Landsteiner antibody) and referred to as paroxysmal cold hemoglobinuria. It may occur without underlying cause, associated with viral infections, congenital or acquired syphilis. This IgG antibody is active at temperatures less than 37°C (cold), fixes complement more strongly and is directed against the P-antigen of red cells. A striking syndrome is presented with severe hemolysis and hemoglobinuria occurring within hours after exposure to cold. Symptoms include shaking chills, fever, flank pain, urticaria, prostration, weakness, dyspnea, and pallor. Laboratory evaluation confirms an acute hemolytic anemia but the definitive procedure is demonstration of a cold active antibody in the patient's serum by the cold hemolysin (Donath-Landsteiner) test. The peripheral blood smear may show spherocytosis and red cell fragmentation. Leukopenia may occur early and may be followed by leukocytosis and occasionally erythrophagocytosis. The Coombs' test may detect IgG (IgG_3 in one case) or C3 on red cells which may explain spherocytosis and phagocytosis respectively. The prognosis is good. Except for penicillin therapy in patients with coexistent syphilis, drug treatment is not necessary.

IgM-induced immune hemolytic anemia is exemplified best with the cold agglutinin syndrome. Often this entity may be idiopathic or secondary to an underlying disease. The idiopathic form occurs mainly among older patients and may be a chronic disorder. The secondary form has been noted in association with a variety of infections such as influenza, infectious mononucleosis, infectious hepatitis, mycoplasma pneumonia, or the lymphoproliferative diseases. The relationship between the infectious diseases and the production of cold agglutinin is not clear. In most, the cold agglutinin is directed against the I-antigen but in infectious mononucleosis it may be directed against the i-antigen. This antibody may cause only minimal hemolysis, perhaps because the i-antigen is present in minute quantities on adult red cells. Normal quantities of cold agglutinins exist but their titers are less than 1:50 and they result in no hemolysis. When cold agglutinins follow infection, titers may be in hundreds or thousands. They are polyclonal and do not usually result in hemolysis; however, when hemolysis occurs it may be severe.

In the cold agglutinin syndrome associated with the lymphoproliferative diseases or in the idiopathic types, high titers of cold agglutinins may occur. They are often monoclonal and can appear on electrophoresis as an M component. Despite these high titers the anemia is often mild. Clinically, patients may have venous sludging in peripheral vessels, acrocyanosis, Raynaud's phenomena and, at times, frostbite or gangrene. Agglutination may be demonstrated by routine tests and the Coombs' test detects C3 or C4 on red cells deposited by the action of the IgM antibody.

Treatment for these disorders is environmental control. When an underlying lymphoma is present, treatment of it often corrects the cold agglutinin problem. The results of splenectomy are predictably poor in view of the pathophysiologic mechanisms of IgM and complement-mediated hemolysis. In the acute cold agglutinin syndrome associated with infections such as mycoplasma, treatment with appropriate antibiotics has been associated with diminution of the cold agglutinin titer.

Finally, clinical examples of complement-mediated hemolysis are seen in association with transfusions and drug-induced reactions, and the bizarre paroxysmal nocturnal hemoglobinuria. In paroxysmal nocturnal hemoglobinuria the membranes of red and white cells and platelets are exquisitely sensitive to complement, however, there is no known antibody present that activates the complement system. Activation of the alternate or classical pathway may cause hemolysis. Test procedures include the sugar water, Ham test, or inulin test. Complement activation is produced by an acid medium in the Ham test, low ionic strength solutions in the sugar water, or the alternate pathway in the inulin test.

Summary

Several features of hemolytic anemia and specific features of immune hemolytic anemia have been reviewed. These are examples of research begun at the bedside which have resulted in a great deal of basic science information. These findings have allowed the investigator and clinician to understand the pathogenesis of immune hemolytic anemia and have provided new tools for treatment of this disease. Hopefully the concepts will continue to assure better patient care and return additional stimulation and information for the basic scientists.

SELECTED REFERENCES

Abramson, N., Alper, C. A., Lachmann, P. J., Rosen, F. S., and Jandl, J. H.: Deficiency of C3 inactivator in man. J. Immunol., *107:* 19, 1971.

Abramson, N., LoBuglio, A. F., Jandl, J. H., and Cotran, R. S.: Interaction between human monocytes and red cells. Binding characteristics. J. Exp. Med., *132:* 1191, 1970.

Aster, R. H., and Enright, S. E.: Platelet and granulocyte defect in paroxysmal nocturnal hemoglobinuria; usefulness for detecting platelet antibodies. J. Clin. Invest., *48:* 1199, 1969.

Banti, G.: Splénomégalia hémolytique and hémopoietique: le role de la rate dans l'hémolyse. Semaine Med., *33:* 313, 1913.

Brown, D. L., and Nelson, D. A.: Surface fragmentation of red cells as a mechanism for complement-mediated immune spherocytosis. Br. J. Haematol., *24:* 301, 1973.

Donath, J., and Landsteiner, K.: Über Paroxysmale Hemaglobinuria. Munch Med. Wochenschr., *51:* 1590, 1904.

Gelfand, E. W., Abramson, N., Segel, G. S., and Nathan, D. G.: Buffy coat observations and red cell antibodies in acquired hemolytic anemia. N. Engl. J. Med., *284:* 1250, 1971.

Götze, O., and Müller-Eberhard, H. J.: Paroxysmal nocturnal hemoglobinuria. Hemolysis initiated by the C3 activator system. N. Engl. J. Med., *286:* 180, 1972.

Harris, J. W.: Studies on mechanism of drug-induced hemolytic anemia. J. Lab. Clin. Med., *44:* 809, 1954.

Jandl, J. H., Jones, A. R., and Castle, W. B.: Destruction of red cells by antibodies in man. I. Observation on sequestration and lysis of red cells altered by immune mechanisms. J. Clin. Invest., *36:* 1428, 1957.

Jandl, J. H., and Kaplan, M. E.: Destruction of red cells by antibodies in man. III. Quantitative factors influencing the patterns of hemolysis in vivo. J. Clin. Invest., *39:* 1145, 1960.

Jandl, J. H., and Tomlinson, A. S.: Destruction of red cells by antibodies in man. II. Pyrogenic, leukocytic and dermal responses to immune hemolysis. J. Clin. Invest., *37:* 1202, 1958.

LoBuglio, A. C., Cotran, R. S., and Jandl, J. H.: Red cells coated with immunoglobulin G.: binding and sphering by mononuclear cells in man. Science, *158:* 1582, 1967.

LoBuglio, A. F., and Jandl, J. H.: Nature of alpha-methyl DOPA antibody. N. Engl. J. Med., *276:* 658, 1967.

Rosse, W. F.: Quantitative immunology of immune hemolytic anemia. II. Relationship of cell-bound antibody to hemolysis and effect of treatment. J. Clin. Invest., *50:* 734, 1971.

Chapter 22

NONSPECIFIC IMMUNITY

Rama Ganguly, Ph.D.

The major divisions of host defenses are specific and nonspecific immunity. Most of this book has dealt with the former. Nonspecific or native immunity refers to the ability of the normal host to stay unaffected by most infectious agents arising within and present in the environment. Native immunity or innate host resistance factors constitute an original grant for survival which provides a baseline of defense against foreign agents. Sometimes native immunity is absolute, i.e., all members of a species are entirely unsusceptible to an agent; in other cases, the resistance is relative. In the latter, racial and individual differences become apparent within the same species.

Native defenses are of much greater importance than is usually appreciated. Animal tissues have all the makings of an excellent culture medium, but most microbes cannot or do not grow in them. In the case of those that can, actual invasion is rather infrequent compared to the ubiquity of microbes in our environment. This indicates the vital importance of natural defenses by which the normal animal stays unharmed in its hostile surroundings.

Native defenses function as a barrier to the penetration of organisms through the integument; to inhibit or destroy microorganisms in tissues, or to eliminate toxic substances liberated by living or dead microbes.

These mechanisms of native defenses are indicated by various factors, some of which are listed in Table 22.1. This list is not all-inclusive, but includes the more important factors.

Skin and Epithelial Membranes

The unbroken skin presents a more or less impassable barrier to penetration of microorganisms. Epithelial tissues are composed of cells held firmly together by a viscous intercellular substance containing hyaluronic acid. Bacteria are found normally on the skin between the

TABLE 22.1 *Classification of Natural Defense Mechanism*

1. Physical: epithelial membrane, skin, ciliary movement, peristalsis
2. Biochemical: lysozyme, basic peptides, natural antibodies, β lysins, plakins, and leukins
3. Cellular: phagocytes, inflammation, reticuloendothelial system
4. Others: body temperature, oxygen tension in tissues, indifference of tissues to toxins, antagonism of indigenous flora.

superficial horny cells but ordinarily are not able to penetrate deep into the tissues unless favored by some cutaneous injury. In diseases like leptospirosis and syphilis, penetration through small breaches of the skin is the mechanism of infection. Staphylococcal and streptococcal infections have been demonstrated to occur via the ducts of the sweat glands and hair follicles. The skin has bactericidal properties due to fatty acids in the sweat and sebaceous secretions. This property is inhibited by serum albumin.

The moist surface of the respiratory tract catches many passing particles. The mucous film with the trapped objects is continuously swept outward by ciliary movement. By this mechanism, plus structural barriers like the nasal turbinates, the inhaled air is kept free of floating objects. Small particles of 1.5μ diameter or less, which penetrate into the lungs, are phagocytosed by macrophages.

The bacterial flora of the mouth is subject to constant depletion because of the flushing action of the saliva. The microorganisms flushed to the back of the mouth combine with those from the nose and are swallowed. Bacteria reaching the stomach are subjected to high acidity and the majority is destroyed. Bacteria are bountiful in the intestine; however, the intestinal mucosa possess antimicrobial properties so that invasion usually does not occur. Mucus forms a meshwork coating and the mucus, with the embedded microbes, is rolled into small masses and moved outward by peristalsis. Therefore, bacteria, which enter the mouth or nasopharyngeal tract, are eventually eliminated in the feces.

The moisty mucous film of the respiratory and genital passages, as well as other bathing fluids such as tears and saliva, possess antimicrobial properties due to presence of various enzymes. The urethra in both males and females is remarkably free of bacteria, probably as a result of the flushing action of the slightly acid urine. Normal vaginal secretions are markedly bactericidal toward most bacterial species.

Antimicrobial Factors of Tissues and Body Fluids

Blood and various tissue extracts have antimicrobial properties. This has been ascribed to factors like β-lysins, leukins, and plakins. β-Lysins are thermostable serum factors, whereas leukins and plakins are present in extracts of leukocytes and platelets respectively. These are basic substances and act by combining with the acidic substances of the bacterial cell wall. They are most active against spore-forming aerobes. They also enhance antibody-mediated bacteriolysis. Phagocytin, on the other hand, is active against gram-negative bacteria. This is present in the granulocytes and is discharged into the cytoplasm along with a host of other hydrolytic enzymes after phagocytosis.

Lysozyme

Many tissue extracts and secretions inactivate bacteria and even viruses, this activity being due to hydrolytic enzymes, the main one being lysozyme. It lyses gram-positive bacteria and enhances antibody-complement mediated action against gram-negative bacteria. It breaks the bond between N-acetylglucosamine and N-acetyl muramic acid of the mucopeptide complexes of the bacterial cell wall. Lysozyme may also be involved in antibacterial action of secretory IgA and complement. Lysozyme is widely distributed in various body fluids, tissue extracts, and secretions. Since most microorganisms enter the body via mucosal surfaces, the presence of such antimicrobial factors in mucosal secretions contributes significantly to natural body defenses.

A very important and distinct mode of natural immunity is the production of interferon. Interferon and its mechanism of action will be discussed in detail in Chapter 23. In short, interferon is produced promptly into the circulation of experimental animals by a variety of inducers, classically virus infection, but also bacterial products and other chemicals. It acts by limiting intracellular viral synthesis and may be involved importantly in antiviral resistance. Since it is non or weakly immunogenic, exogenous interferon application for clinical purposes is of great interest and potential.

Natural Antibodies

Natural antibodies are important mediators of native resistance. These antibodies are absent at birth but develop against a wide range of exotic microbes during the first few years of life. They are usually of the IgM immunoglobulin class and are active against gram-negative microbes in the presence of complement. These antibodies are widely distributed in nature, present in low titers, and persist for prolonged time periods. They may develop after exposure to heterologous microbes sharing common antigens or arise from subclinical infection. Whatever the cause of these antibodies, they act in the same way as do "immune" antibodies against microbes. Limited experimental evidence suggests that these antibodies may be related to protection.

The presence of cross-reacting antigens between microbes has been utilized for vaccine development. Robbins and coworkers fed adults 10^7 *Escherichia coli,* strain Easter. All subjects showed heavy growth of the organism 24–48 hours following feeding and colonization persisted for 5–6 weeks. All responded with a 2- to 10-fold increase in serum antibody titer against *Haemophilus influenza* type b. No untoward effect was observed. These observations suggest that it may be possible to utilize nonpathogenic cross-reacting organisms to develop effective vaccines against pathogenic microbes. Normal endogenous flora like other *E. coli* strains and *Bacillus pamilis,* have also been shown to possess cross reactive antigens against *Neisseria meningitidis* and *Streptococcus pneumoniae.*

Phagocytosis and Inflammatory Process

Phagocytosis is important in defense of the body against invading organisms, processing of antigens, ridding the body of worn out and alien (malignant) cells, as well as in inducing delayed hypersensitivity. The process of phagocytosis is influenced by the nature of the microbial agent, types of phagocytic cells involved and the presence of antibodies, calcium ions, and complement. A lower pH and deviation from isotonicity depress phagocytic function.

The process of inflammation develops in four stages: (1) In response to infection or noxious stimuli, vascular permeability increases due to the influence of histamine and histamine-like substances released locally by mast cells. (2) Emigration of neutrophils to the infected area occurs due to chemotactic stimuli accumulated in the area. These neutrophils actively ingest and digest the foreign substances, furnishing an important first line host defense. They also release substances that maintain the inflammatory response by increasing permeability and attracting more neutrophils. (3) Emigration of mononuclear cells from the circulation follows synthesis of messenger RNA and proteins by these cells triggered by some unknown substances liberated from the inflammed site. (4) Resolution and repair are the final stages, mediated by proliferation of fibroblasts and synthesis of mucopolysaccharides and collagen fibers. Phagocytosis is discussed in more detail in Chapter 18.

Phagocytes are scavenger cells which take up microbial pathogens, foreign materials, and worn out host tissue components, and include polymorphonuclear leukocytes and various mononuclear phagocytes such as blood monocytes, tissue histiocytes or macrophages. The latter group of cells are part of the reticuloendothelial system. Phagocytic cells of the reticuloendothelial system are scattered throughout the connective tissues in the body. The lung is an example of a rich source of tissue macrophages. These cells constantly remove dust or carbon particles inhaled in air. Both the neutrophils (polymorphonuclear leukocytes) and macrophages are involved in the ingestion and killing of bacteria. Neutrophils constitute the first line of resistance of the host and are produced in large numbers in the bone marrow and are short-lived. Macrophages, in contrast, are long-lived and persist in tissues for weeks and months. Macrophages of the alveoli and peritoneum are wandering cells whereas those present in liver (Kupffer cells), spleen, and lymph nodes are fixed type. When the polymorphonuclear leukocytes cannot kill certain intracellular parasites such as *Mycobacterium tuberculosis,* they are ultimately taken up by the macrophages along with their ingested pathogen. The process of phagocytosis and killing by either polymorphonuclear leukocytes or macrophages is enhanced if opsonizing antibodies are present and when the macrophage is activated by lymphokine production from sensitized lymphocytes, the digestion of intracellular parasites also is accelerated.

In nonimmune animals, some bacteria survive and proliferate within macrophages, the examples being *M. tuberculosis, Brucella abortus, Salmonella typhimurium,* and *Listeria monocytogenes.* Influenza virus is phagocytosed by leukocytes but remain viable for a long time and in general, virulent bacteria such as streptococci tend to persist and might destroy the phagocyte. For viruses like vaccinia, the viral envelope interacts with the vacuolar membrane of the phagocytic cell, resulting in dissolution of the membrane, and viral DNA is thereafter released into the cytoplasm in nonimmune animals. If antibody is present, the virus-antibody complex similarly enters the phagocytic vacuole, but cannot escape from the vacuole. The phagocytic vacuole fuses with lysosome, the released acid hydrolases degrade the viral nucleic acids to acid soluble fragments. Viral proteins are probably broken down in a similar fashion.

Other Factors

The degree of availability of oxygen in various tissues may deter microorganisms which would otherwise be parasitic, e.g., anaerobic spore-bearing bacilli (*Clostridium tetani*) can proliferate to produce lethal neurotoxin only in devitalized tissues. As a reverse example tubercle bacilli are inhibited in areas where oxygen supply is limited.

Indifference of tissues to a microbial toxin constitutes another natural host resistance mechanism. Rats can resist about 1000 times the minimal lethal dose of diphtheria toxin for the guinea pig. Cold blooded animals such as the toad and frog appear to be entirely unsusceptible to this as well as tetanus toxin.

The presence of endogenous flora in some locations in the body exert a very significant influence upon the outcome of infection by exogenous pathogens. An example of the deleterious effect of disturbing the normal flora is seen in patients treated with antibiotics who occasionally develop rapidly progressive staphylococcal enterocolitis. Normal resident viridans streptococci in saliva inhibit the growth of diphtheria bacilli in certain media. The mechanisms of antagonism by endogenous flora is not clearly delineated, however, competition for nutrients or production of toxic substances may be involved.

Pasteur demonstrated that chickens, normally resistant to anthrax bacilli, become susceptible when immersed in cold water. Fever as a native resistance mechanism has been demonstrated with the type III pneumococcus in rabbits. It was observed that in response to pneumococcal infection, the rabbits developed fever (102–104°F). At this higher temperature growth of the organism was inhibited and degeneration of the capsule occurred. This loss of capsule finally helped in phagocytosis and killing of the bacteria. Recent evidence from human studies also suggests that administration of antipyretic drugs like aspirin prolongs the period of virus shedding in rhinovirus infection. In a recent report, Bernheim and Kluger studied the effects of drug-induced antipyresis on survival. They determined whether the prevention of fever affects the survival of an animal infected with pathogenic bacteria. The body temperature of an ectotherm (or behavioral thermoregulator) can be easily controlled at either the normothermic or febrile level by simply adjusting the ambient temperature; so the lizard was used in this study as a suitable animal model for study of the role of fever in disease. Lizards were infected with live *Aeromonas hydrophila* and received varying doses of sodium salicylate. The animals which increased their mean body temperature at least 0.6°C, survived the week, whereas those which did not develop a fever died within 3 days. These data indicate that the prevention of fever by use of an antipyretic drug increases the rate of mortality from a bacterial infection. Thus, it would seem that judicious application of antipyretic drugs in fever is warranted.

SELECTED REFERENCES

Bernheim, H. A., and Kluger, M. J.: Effect of drug-induced antipyresis on survival. Science, *193:* 237, 1976.

Cohen, A. B., and Gold, W. M.: Defense mechanisms of the lungs. Ann. Rev. Physiol., *37:* 325, 1975.

Daniele, R. P., Altose, M. D., and Rowlands, D. T., Jr.: Immunocompetent cells from the lower respiratory tract of normal human lungs. J. Clin. Invest., *56:* 986, 1975.

Donaldson, D. M. Beta-lysin. In *Microbiology,* edited by D. Schlessinger. Washington, D.C.: Am. Soc. Microbiology, 1974, pp. 223–226.

Gottschalk, A. Correlation between composition, structure, shape and function of a salivary mucoprotein. Nature, *186:* 949, 1960.

Kluger, M. J., Ringler, D. H., and Anver, M. R.: Fever and survival. Science, *188:* 166, 1975.

Robbins, J. B., Schneerson, R., Liu, T. Y., Schiffer, M. S., Schiffman, G., Myerowitz, R. L., McCracken, Jr., G. H., Ørskov, I., and Ørskov, F.: Cross-reacting bacterial antigens and immunity to disease caused by encapsulated bacteria. In *The Immune and Infectious Diseases.* Buffalo, N.Y.: Fourth Int. Convoc. Immunol., 1974, pp. 218–241.

Stanley, E. D., Jackson, G. G., Panusarn, C., Rubenis, M., and Dirda, V.: Increased virus shedding with aspirin treatment of rhinovirus infection. J.A.M.A., *231:* 1248, 1976.

Stossel, T. P. Phagocytosis. N. Engl. J. Med., *290:* 717, 1974.

Veres, J. Natural antibodies in healthy adults. Acta Microbial Acad. Sci. Hung., *22:* 65, 1975.

Chapter 23

INTERFERON AND THE IMMUNE SYSTEM

George E. Gifford, Ph.D.

Interferon

The interferon system was first recognized as a normal defense phenomenon of animal cells to viral infection. In recent years, it has become increasingly recognized as a defense mechanism against all intracellular parasites and, indeed, its role may be even more inclusive and may play an important role in the elimination or inhibition of cells modified in a variety of ways and including tumor cells. It also has dramatic effects on the immune system.

Role in Viral Infection

The first known effect of interferon was an inhibitory effect on virus replication. When cells are exposed to a virus, the cells are induced to briefly synthesize and secrete a glycoprotein called interferon. When noninfected cells come in contact with interferon, they become resistant for a period of time to subsequent virus infection. This sequence of events is schematically represented in Figure 23.1. Interferon synthesis in the initially infected cell usually occurs too late to prevent virus replication in that cell and a normal cycle of virus replication results. However, since interferon secretion usually precedes virus release, interferon may interact with surrounding cells and protect them before they are infected. This newly synthesized interferon may also be disseminated in the blood and protect cells at distant sites.

The actual induction event for interferon synthesis remains elusive. The inducing virus may be inactivated but still induce interferon synthesis; the only prerequisite seems to be that the virus must still be able to recognize cellular receptors and react with the cell membrane. Indeed, the original discovery of the interferon system was made with an inacti-

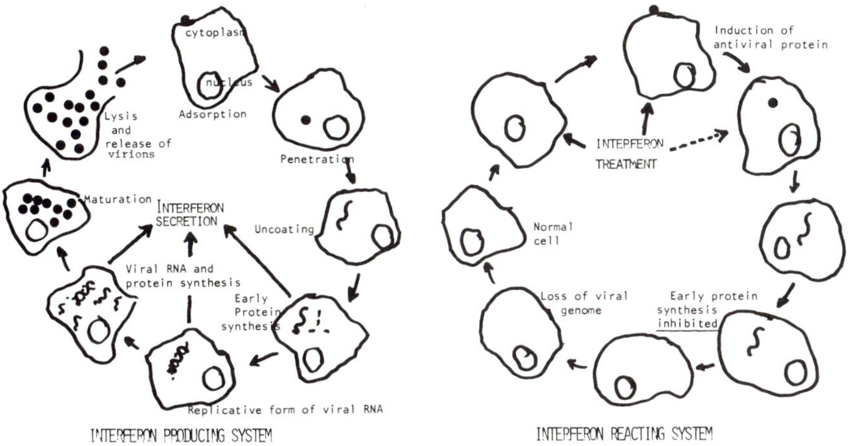

FIG. 23.1. Schematic diagram of the interferon producing and reacting systems. Interferon synthesis in the initially infected cell usually occurs too late to prevent virus replication in that cell and a normal cycle of virus replication results. Interferon treatment of cells prior to infection, or shortly afterwards, will prevent virus replication in that cell. Note that adsorption, penetration, and uncoating of the virion are not inhibited in the interferon treated cell but that early protein synthesis and subsequent viral nucleic acid synthesis are inhibited; presumably with the eventual destruction of the viral genome and restoration of the cell to normalcy.

vated influenza virus. In some cases, as with influenza, the inactivated virus is a better inducer than the active virus. An important observation is that double-stranded polyribonucleotides, both natural and synthetic, may be inducers of interferon, even in submicrogram quantities. It is important in this regard that double-stranded polyribonucleotides are found in cells infected by RNA viruses (except for the Oncornaviruses) and are either an intermediate in viral replication or a product thereof. Double-stranded RNA molecules also appear in cells infected with DNA viruses although their function in DNA virus replication is not known.

Thus, these double-stranded RNA molecules seem to be a common denominator in cells permissively infected with almost any virus. Double stranded RNA does not seem to be the only natural inducer in virus infected cells since double-stranded RNA is not found in cells exposed to inactivated viruses which induce interferon.

In addition to the induction of interferon, these double-stranded RNA molecules have other effects which are probably very important in the pathogenesis of viral disease and may be responsible for some of the symptoms of the disease. These effects include pyrogenicity and the ability to inhibit host cell protein synthesis.

The mode of action of interferon is also somewhat elusive. It is known that for maximal effectiveness, the interferon molecule must interact with the cell *before* infection. Interferon induces another protein, called the viral inhibitory protein, which is actually responsible for the antiviral effect. Interferon apparently does not have to enter the cell to induce the antiviral protein. In this respect interferon is like a peptide hormone in its action. The induction event takes time and the full expression is usually found about 8 hours after interferon has initially reacted with the cell. Virus adsorption, penetration, and uncoating is quite similar regardless of whether or not the cell has been treated with interferon. However, virus replication does not occur in interferon-treated cells. The block in virus replication seems to occur at the level of viral transcription and/or translation.

Characteristics of the Antiviral Action of Interferon

An important characteristic of interferon is that it is not specific for a particular virus. All animal viruses induce interferon synthesis to a variable extent and the replication of all viruses in interferon-treated cells is inhibited to a variable extent. This spectrum of inducibility and response is shown in Table 23.1. There is, however, some variation in the spectrum, this being dependent on the animal and virus which are interacting. Usually, RNA viruses seem to be the better inducers and responders.

Another important characteristic of interferon is its species specificity. Interferon acts only in the animal species in which it is produced although there are some important exceptions. This is important in the clinical use of exogenous interferon in that it must be prepared in human tissues to be useful in the therapy or prophylaxis of human disease. It is difficult to obtain and purify sufficient quantities of interferon to be useful. In limited studies, however, exogenously supplied interferon has been shown to be effective in modifying viral disease. The difficulty of purifying and preparing large amounts of interferon for clinical trials has led many workers to consider the use of interferon inducers for the prevention and treatment of viral disease. The high toxicity of the inducers, such as the synthetic polyribonucleotide, poly I:C, has precluded their general use. A

TABLE 23.1. Spectrum of Activity of Various Viruses in their Ability to Induce and Respond to Interferon (viruses are listed in decreasing order)

Togaviruses	RNA
Myxoviruses	RNA
Reoviruses	RNA
Rhabdoviruses	RNA
Picornaviruses	RNA
Poxviruses	DNA
Herpesviruses	DNA
Papovaviruses	DNA
Oncornaviruses	RNA[a]
Adenoviruses	DNA

[a] Oncornaviruses have a DNA replicative form.

notable exception is the surface application of poly I:C in eye or nose drops which has shown some protective effects.

The sequence of events shown in Figure 23.2 depicts what may happen in an experimental animal exposed to a sublethal dose of virus. Virus replication and interferon synthesis occur and the synthesis of both seem to be terminated before the appearance of a significant immune response. Of course, when massive amounts of virus are used, the interferon system can be overwhelmed, as can most defense systems, virus synthesis continues, and the animal dies. This, however, is not the usual situation in naturally acquired viral disease.

When exposed to the same virus again at a later time, the immune system plays the most important role and little interferon is induced. A very important aspect of the interferon system is the hyporesponsive period which follows the initial production. The reason for the hyporesponsive period is unknown but interferon synthesis is transiently inhibited. The hyporeactive period is variable in length and may last for several days. It is probable a second virus infection during the hyporeactive period may result in a more serious disease since the interferon response is repressed.

Another important attribute of interferon is that it is not generally considered to be toxic to noninfected cells, although it may temporarily prevent DNA synthesis and cell division. Since interferon has not yet been highly purified, it is possible that the cellular inhibitory effects may be due to other molecules present in the interferon preparation. In any

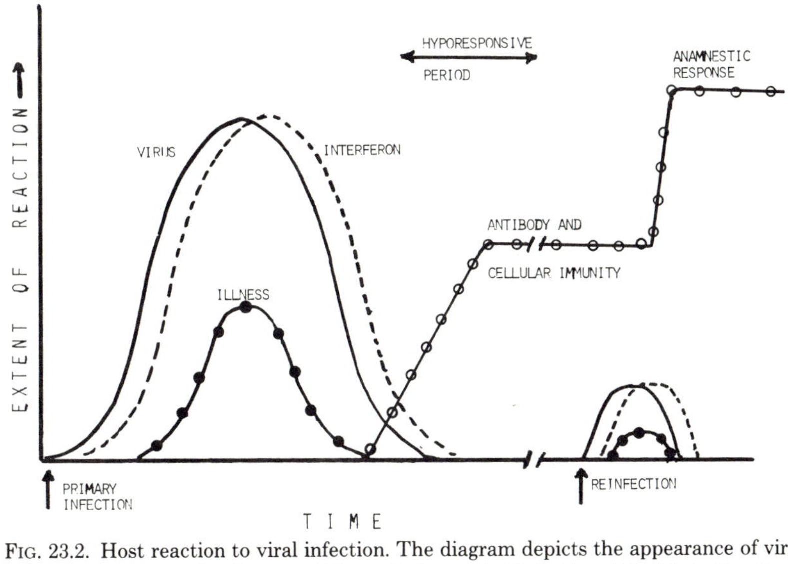

FIG. 23.2. Host reaction to viral infection. The diagram depicts the appearance of virus, interferon, immune mechanisms, and illness during a viral infection. (Modified after Baron, S., J. Gen. Physiol. *56:* 196, 1970 (Suppl.)).

case, the inhibitory effects of interferon preparations on DNA synthesis seem to play an important role in immune phenomena.

Role in the Immune Systems

During the course of many viral diseases, immunity to other nonrelated antigens may be suppressed. Antibody synthesis and the induction and expression of delayed type hypersensitivity may all be inhibited.

Indeed, certain immune reactions which do not involve viruses may result in interferon production. Thus, for example, white cells from individuals previously immunized with diphtheria toxoid will respond to diphtheria toxoid by the production of interferon whereas cells from nonimmunized individuals will not so respond. The mixed lymphocyte reaction, which is an in vitro correlate of a primary immune response will also induce the production of interferon (Fig. 23.3). In fact, all substances which induce lymphocytes to undergo blastogenesis seem to induce interferon as well as lymphokines (Fig. 23.4). Thus, there seems to be another kind of interferon induction system which involves the cells of the immune system and this kind of interferon, sometimes called "immune interferon" or "type II interferon," seems to be a lymphokine.

Either kind of interferon can suppress the mitogenic activity of various mitogens, both specific and nonspecific. Figure 23.5 shows the effect of interferon on phytohemagglutinin (a T cell mitogen) and endotoxin (a B cell mitogen) stimulation of lymphocyte proliferation as measured by the

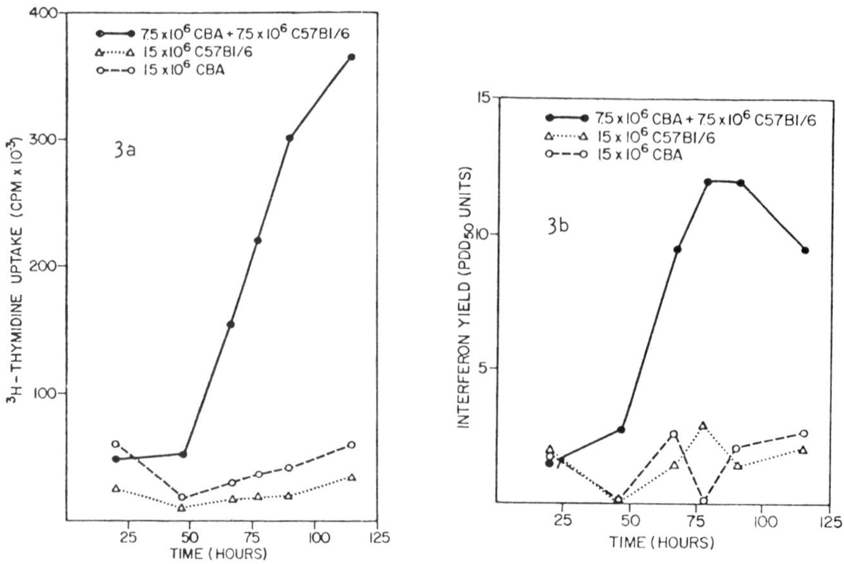

FIG. 23.3. Induction of interferon in the mixed lymphocyte reaction. (a) shows the stimulation of DNA synthesis and (b) the time course of interferon synthesis. (Reprinted from Gifford, et al., Infect. Immun. *3:* 164, 1971.)

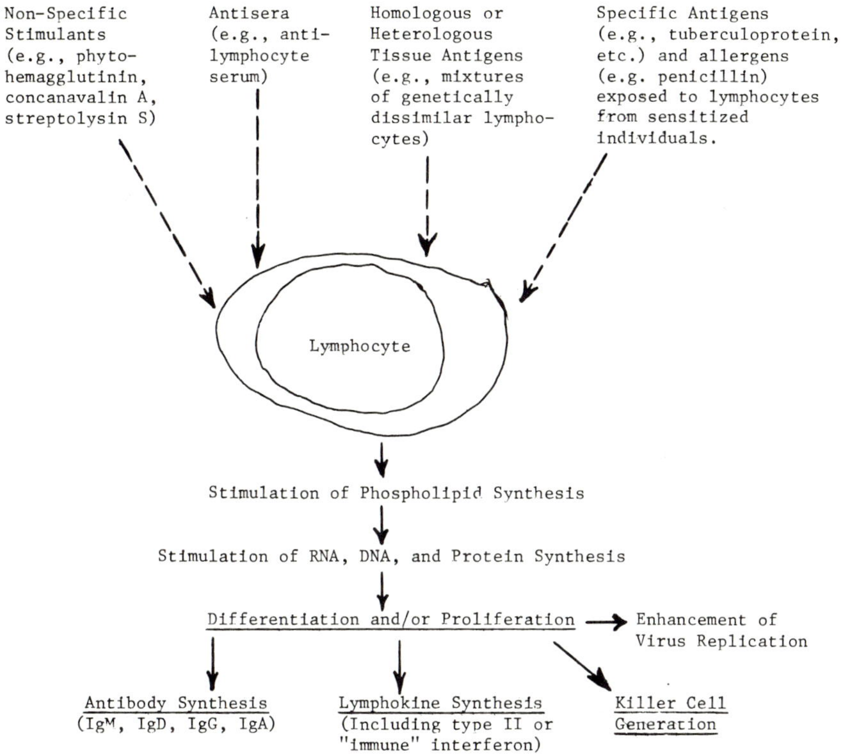

FIG. 23.4. Factors involved in blastogenesis and the subsequent or concomitant production and secretion of antibody, lymphokines, and interferon.

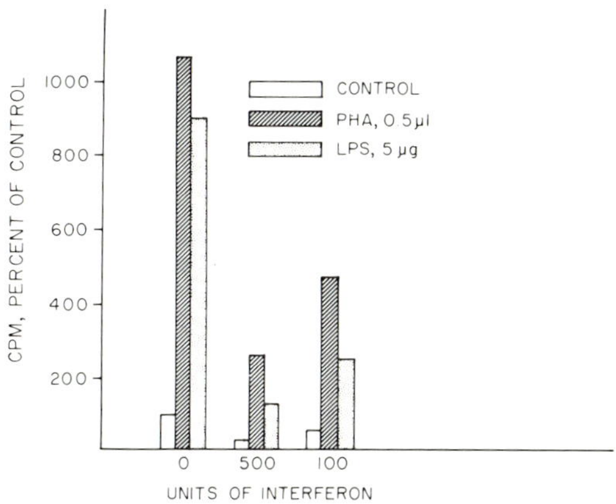

FIG. 23.5. Effect of interferon on the mitogenic effects of a T cell mitogen (phytohemagglutinin, PHA) or a B cell mitogen (lipopolysaccharide, LPS).

incorporation of tritiated thymidine. Interferon suppresses the effect of both mitogens to a similar extent. Using spleen cells from influenza immunized mice, with virus used as a specific mitogen, the immune response is markedly inhibited by interferon (Fig. 23.6). Similarly, the mixed lymphocyte reaction is inhibited by interferon (Fig. 23.7). Recently, others, using a massive amount of interferon or interferon inducers, have shown an inhibition of the primary and secondary immune responses in vivo as well as inhibition of the induction and expression of delayed-type hypersensitivity. Thus, much of the suppression of the

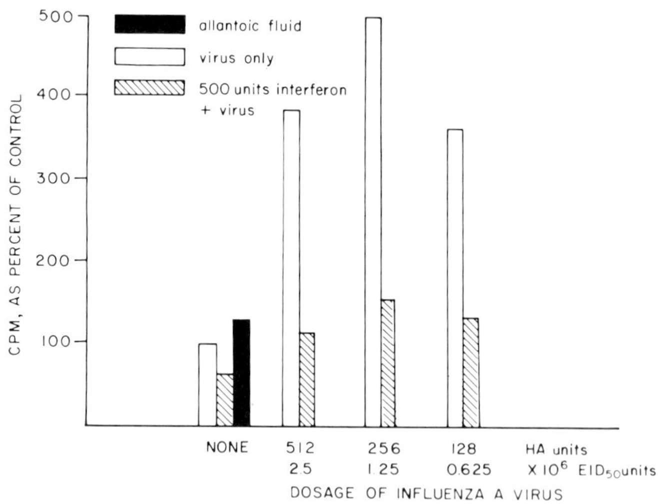

FIG. 23.6. Effect of interferon on the mitogenic effect of a specific mitogen (influenza virus). Mice were immunized with influenza virus two weeks prior to removal of the spleen which was then minced and cultivated in the presence of the indicated amounts of virus.

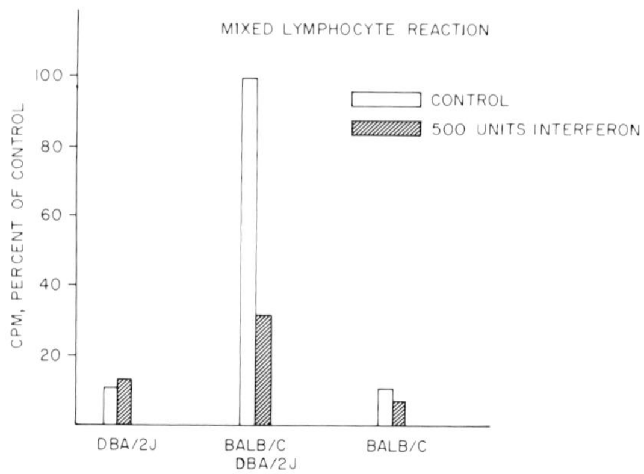

FIG. 23.7. Effect of interferon on the mixed lymphocyte reaction. Mice used were the inbred strains DBA/2J and BALB/C.

immune response seen during viral disease can be attributable to interferon. It is not clear, however, why an important natural defense mechanism should have an adverse effect on another important defense mechanism. It is possible that interferon may have a modulating role in many of the interrelationships that occur among the components of the immune system; Figure 23.8 is a schematic model of some of these possible roles.

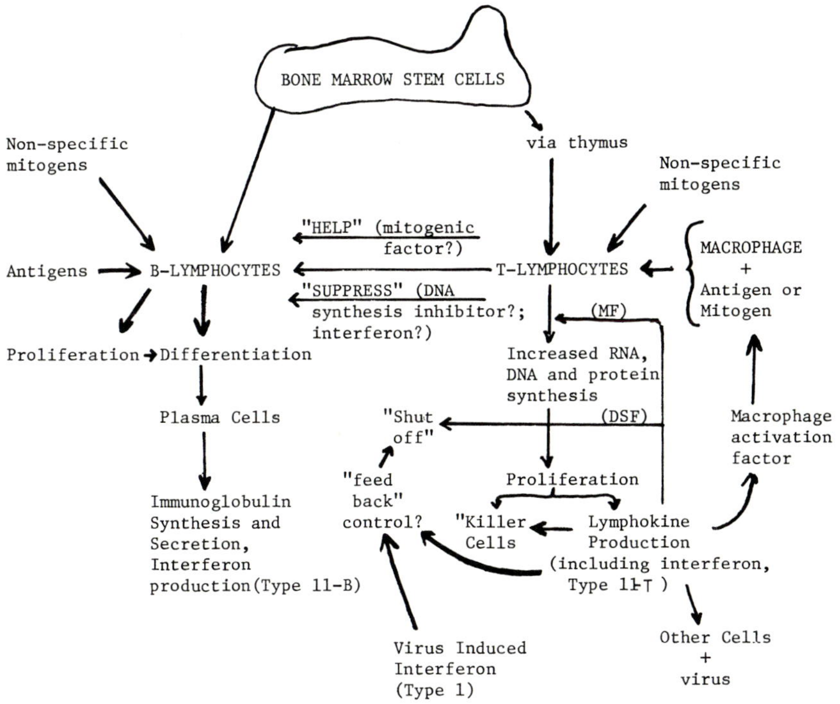

LYMPHOKINES

Positive Control (turn on a function)	Negative Control (turn off a function)
CHEMOTACTIC FACTOR (CF)	MIGRATION INHIBITORY FACTOR (MIF)
MITOGENIC (BLASTOGENIC) FACTOR(MF)	DNA SYNTHESIS INHIBITOR (DSI)
	CYTOTOXIN OR LYMPHOTOXIN (LT)
MACROPHAGE ACTIVATION FACTOR (MAF)	COLONAL INHIBITORY FACTOR (CIF)
MACROPHAGE AGGREGATION FACTOR (MAF)	PROLIFERATION INHIBITORY FACTOR
SKIN REACTIVE FACTOR	
TRANSFER FACTOR	INTERFERON (Type 1, 11-T and (11-B)

FIG. 23.8. Schematic model of the function and possible interrelationships of interferon and other factors in the immunologic system. Included is a list of some of the lymphokines. Note that lymphokines have either a "positive" or "negative" control function and that interferon is a lymphokine with negative control function.

Other Roles of Interferon

Interferon also seems to play an important role in inhibiting other intracellular parasites such as rickettsia, chlamydia, protozoa (toxoplasma and plasmodia) and even bacteria, and also in inhibiting tumor cell growth. The mechanisms underlying these effects are not known but indicate that interferon plays an important role in *all* cellular immune phenomena.

SELECTED REFERENCES

Braun, W., and Levy, H. B.: Interferon preparations as modifiers of immune responses. Proc. Soc. Exp. Biol. Med., *141:* 769, 1972.

Brodeur, B. R., and Merigan, T. C.: Mechanism of the suppressive effect of interferon on antibody synthesis in vivo. J. Immunol., *114:* 1323, 1975.

Gifford, G. E., Tibor, A., and Peavy, D. L.: Interferon production in mixed lymphocyte cell cultures. Infect. Immun. *3:* 164, 1971.

Glasgow, L. A.: Cellular immunity in host resistance to viral infection. Arch. Intern. Med., *126:* 125, 1970.

Green, J. A., Cooperband, S. R., and Kibrick, S.: Immune specific induction of interferon production in cultures of human blood lymphocytes. Science, *164:* 1415, 1969.

Ho, M., and Armstrong, J. A.: Interferon. Ann. Rev. Microbiol., *29:* 131, 1975.

Johnson, H. M., Smith, B. G., and Baron, S.: Inhibition of the primary *in vitro* antibody response by interferon preparations. J. Immunol., *114:* 403, 1975.

Lindahl, P., Leary, P., and Gresser, I.: Enhancement by interferon of the specific cytotoxicity of sensitized lymphocytes. Proc. Natl. Acad. Sci. (USA), *69:* 721, 1972

Lindahl-Magnussen, P., Leary, P., and Gresser, I.: Interferon inhibits DNA synthesis induced in mouse lymphocyte suspensions by phytohemagglutinin or by allogeneic cells. Nature (New Biol.), *237:* 120, 1972.

Machara, N., Ho, M., and Armstrong, J. A.: Differences in mouse interferons according to cell source and mode of induction. Infect. Immun., *17:* 572, 1977.

Younger, J. S., and Salvin, S. B.: Production and properties of migration inhibitory factor and interferon in the circulation of mice with delayed hypersensitivity. J. Immunol., *111:* 1914, 1973.

Chapter 24

EVALUATION OF PATIENTS WITH IMMUNOLOGIC DISEASES

Eric P. Brestel, M.D., Jeffrey C. Delafuente, M.S., Selden Longley, M.D., and Richard S. Panush, M.D.

A number of techniques is useful for investigating patients with immunologic diseases. Many of these methods are now available to the practicing clinician. It is important to understand the manner in which immunologic tests are performed so that they can be meaningfully ordered and interpreted. This chapter will (1) review general principles of evaluating (a) humoral immune function, (b) cellular immune function, and (c) immediate hypersensitivity; (2) indicate information imparted by various tests; and (3) discuss the relevance of immunologic abnormalities to (a) diagnostic, (b) prognostic and (c) therapeutic aspects of certain disease states.

Humoral Immune Function

Detection of Antigens and Antibodies

Electrophoresis. Serum proteins may be separated on the basis of net charge by zone electrophoresis. The sample is applied to a supporting medium, usually cellulose acetate. An electropotential is placed across the medium, and serum proteins migrate toward respective electrodes. The cellulose acetate strip is then stained, and the separated proteins appear visually as dense bands (Fig. 24.1). Five gross bands may be determined by this method and include albumin and the globulins α-1, α-2, β, and γ. Albumin migrates closest to the anode.

Scanning the strip permits quantitation of the amount of protein in each region. Some disease states give characteristic patterns. During acute illness, there may be increases in the α-1 and α-2 fractions and decreases in the levels of prealbumin, albumin, and transferrin proteins.

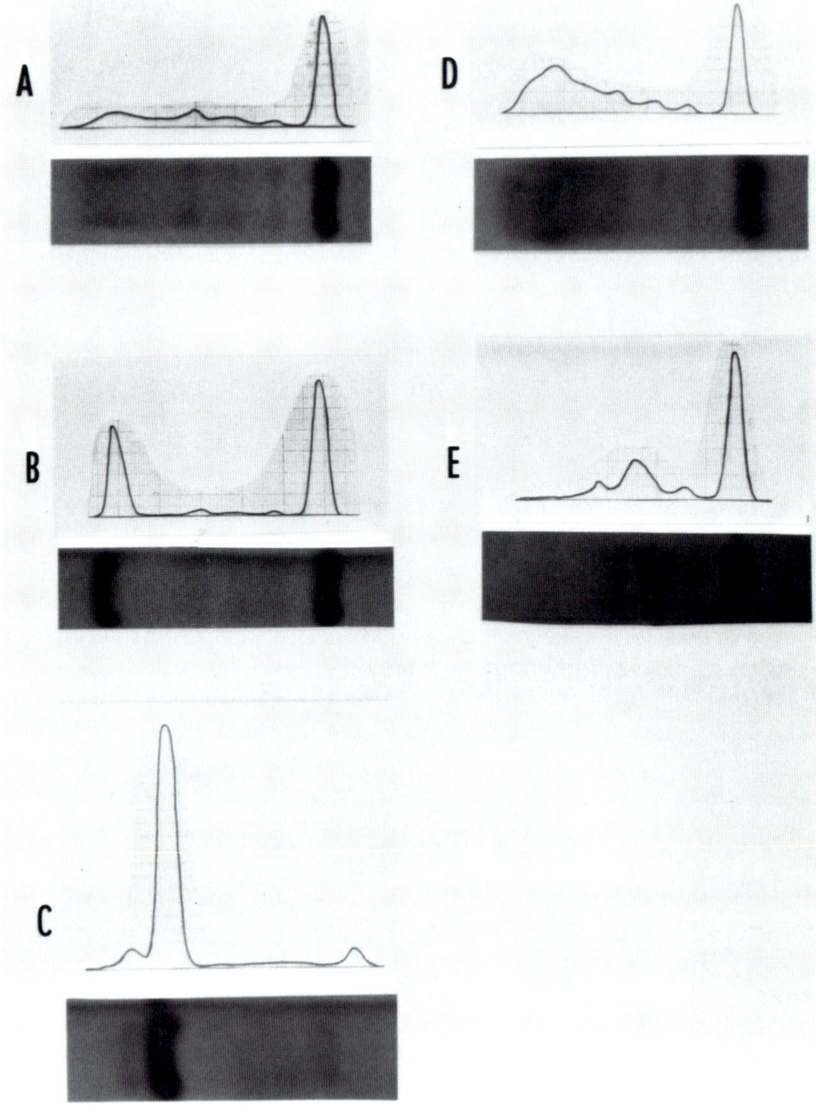

FIG. 24.1. Zone electrophoresis of serum in cellulose acetate. Anode is toward right. A, normal human serum; B, multiple myeloma serum; C, urine with Bence Jones protein; D, diffuse hyper-γ-globulinemia; and E, hypo-γ-globulinemia.

Occasionally, C-reactive protein is markedly increased in acute inflammatory states. This migrates in the gamma region and may be confused with monoclonal spikes of multiple myeloma. In chronic diseases diffuse elevations of the gamma globulins may be noted. These may be marked in chronic liver disease, systemic lupus erythematosus, rheumatoid arthritis, sarcoidosis, and Sjögren's syndrome. Hypo-γ-globulinemia, multiple myeloma, Waldenstrom's macroglobulinemia, and α-1-antitrypsin deficiency may be suggested by abnormalities on serum electrophoresis. In patients suspected of having multiple myeloma, the urine may be concentrated, electrophoresed, and examined for light chains of γ mobility. Cerebrospinal fluid may also be concentrated and examined for increased levels of γ globulins, which is helpful in the diagnosis of multiple sclerosis.

Serum electrophoresis is a useful screening technique for evaluating serum proteins. Patients with abnormalities of gammaglobulins (hypo-γ-globulinemia, polyclonal, or monoclonal increases) can be detected. Further studies of such patients to more carefully define the abnormalities would include radial immunodiffusion or immunoelectrophoresis. Unless the serum protein electrophoresis is abnormal, further laboratory studies (i.e., quantitative or qualitative Ig) are not usually informative.

Immunodiffusion in Gel. The double-diffusion technique of Ouchterloney involves placing antigens and antibodies in wells cut into an inert supporting gel. A visible line of precipitation forms where the reagents are in equivalence. By this method antigens may be compared for identity, partial identity (cross-reactivity) or nonidentity against a given antibody(Fig. 24.2). Simple gel diffusion is clinically helpful in determining the qualitative presence of precipitating antibodies seen in hypersensitivity pneumonitis, and in detecting low molecular weight (7S) IgM observed in some vasculitides and in lymphosarcoma-associated angioedema.

Radial Immunodiffusion. Antigens may be quantitated by allowing them to diffuse into gels containing dilute, specific antibody. Wells are cut into the gel, and the antigen sample or dilutions of a standard are applied to the wells. As the antigen diffuses into the gel, a visible precipitate forms, the area of which is proportional to the amount of antigen present (Fig. 24.3). This method is sensitive to about 10 μg/ml

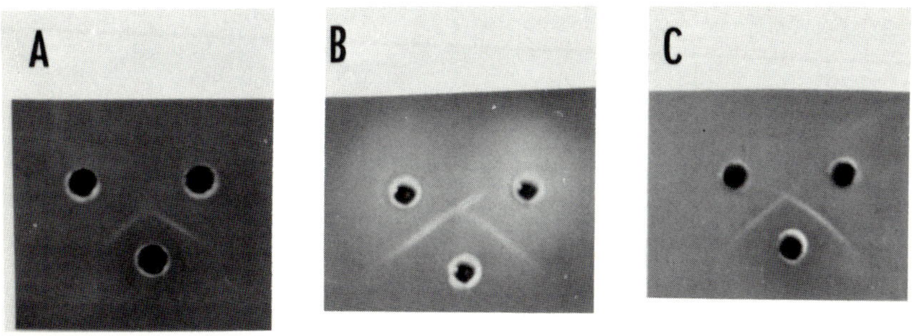

FIG. 24.2. Ouchterlony immunodiffusion in gel. A, lines of identity; B, lines of partial identity; and C, lines of nonidentity.

and is commonly used to quantitate IgG, IgA, IgM, IgD, C3, C4, the C1 esterase inhibitor, and other proteins.

Quantitation of complement levels may be helpful in following and managing patients with systemic lupus erythematosus, glomerulonephritis, and certain others with complement-mediated diseases and in whom disease and complement changes correlate. Immunoglobulin levels are altered in many diseases, with little specificity of patterns in individual patients. They are, therefore, usually quantitated in patients with hypo-γ-globulinemia or monoclonal protein "spikes" by electrophoresis (Table 24.1).

Immunoelectrophoresis. This is a qualitative tool and at best is semiquantitative. It is carried out by dissolving gel in a special buffer. A well is cut to receive the sample. An electropotential applied across the gel allows the proteins in the sample to migrate toward respective electrodes. At the completion of the procedure, a trough is cut parallel to

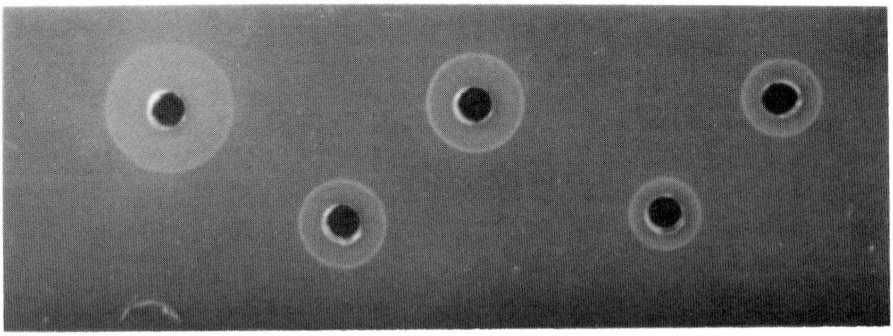

FIG. 24.3. Radial immunodiffusion. Quantitation of antigen (in wells) by antibody-containing gel. Area of precipitate is proportional to antigen concentration. The agarose gel contains anti-human C4. The top wells contain (left to right) normal human serum diluted 1:1, 1:2, and 1:4. The bottom wells contain, at the left, active SLE serum 1:1, and at the right, acute hereditary angioedema serum 1:1.

TABLE 24.1. *Measurement of Serum Immunoglobulins*

Methods of Detection
Quantitative
Radial immunodiffusion
Radioimmunoassay
Single electroimmunodiffusion ("rockets")
Nephelometry
Qualitative
Immunoelectrophoresis
Crossed immunoelectrophoresis
Diagnostic value
Immunodeficiency diseases
Monoclonal gammopathies
Polyclonal gammopathies

the direction of the protein migration and is filled with an antiserum (Fig. 24.4). The size of the arcs and their closeness to the trough depend on the concentration and molecular weight of the particular protein. This method is commonly used for screening protein preparations for purity. It may be applied clinically to further study patients with hypo-γ-globulinemia and monoclonal gammopathies found on protein electrophoresis.

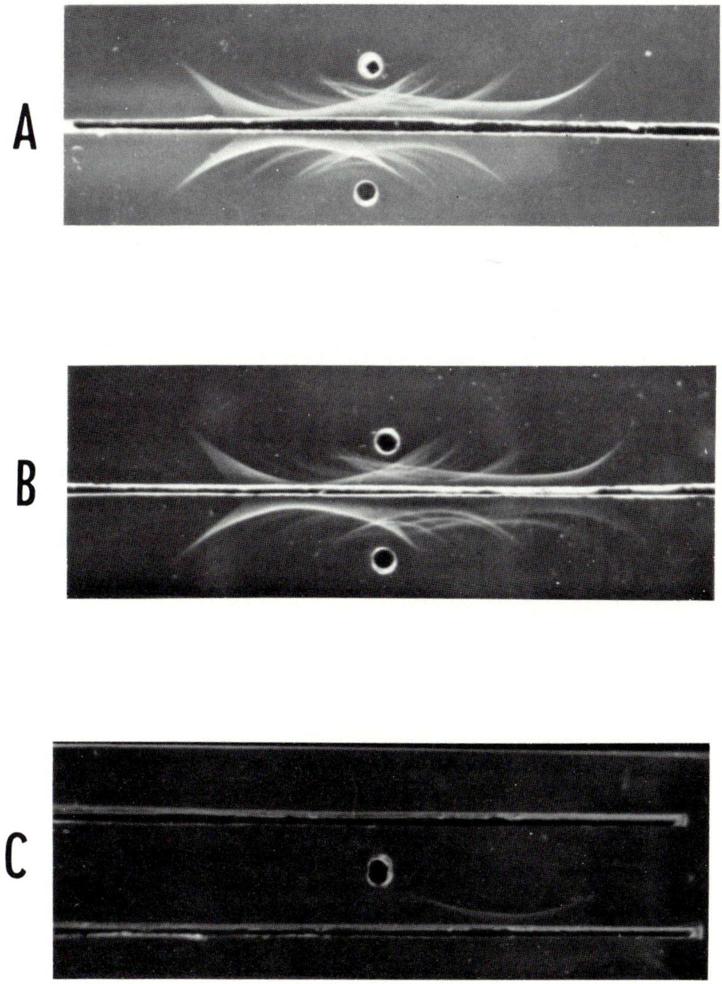

FIG. 24.4. Immunoelectrophoresis. Anode is toward the left. A, top well, normal human serum; bottom well, hypogammaglobulinemic serum; trough, anti-normal human serum. Notice the absence of the gamma globulin arc in hypogammaglobulinemic serum (toward the right). B, top well, normal human serum; bottom well, IgG myeloma serum; trough, anti-normal human serum. Notice the broad arc in the gamma region in the myeloma serum (toward the right). C, well, urine with Bence Jones protein; top trough, anti-κ chain; bottom trough, anti-λ chain. This indicates light chains of the λ type only.

Urine may be tested for light chains but may need to be concentrated before they can be detected.

Electroimmunodiffusion. The sensitivity of immunodiffusion in agar may be increased by the technique of electroimmunodiffusion. The method of single electroimmunodiffusion (rocket electrophoresis) is performed by electrophoresing antigen of relatively negative charge into an agarose gel containing monospecific antiserum. A rocket-shaped precipitin is formed in the gel. Its length is used to quantitate antigen concentration (Fig. 24.5). With double electroimmunodiffusion (counter-immunoelectrophoresis), antigens with a relatively negative net charge migrate toward specific antibody in an adjacent well. Its clinical value is that results can be rapidly obtained (i.e., during the course of a clinic) and used promptly for clinical decisions (e.g., antinuclear antibody levels in lupus patients). This method is somewhat less sensitive than others (such as DNA binding assays).

Electrofocusing. A slight variation of gel electrophoresis involves gel electrofocusing in which proteins migrate to their isoelectric points in specially prepared medium. This allows greater resolution and definition of mixtures of proteins and is largely used in the investigative laboratory for purification and analysis of proteins.

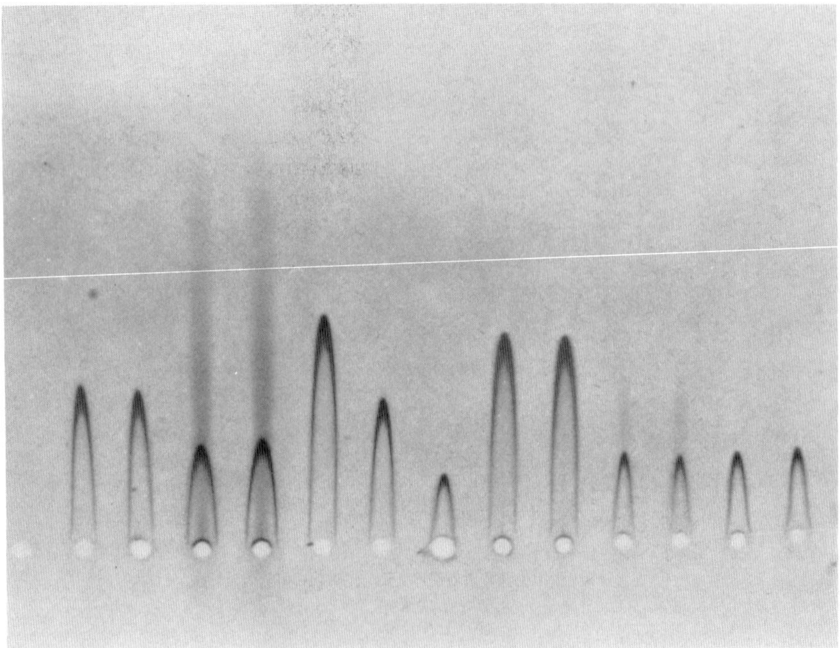

FIG. 24.5. Single immunoelectrodiffusion (rocket electrophoresis). The gel contains antiserum to α-1-antitrypsin. The fifth, sixth, and seventh wells (left to right) contain 1:1, 1:2, and 1:4 dilutions of standard human serum whereas the others contain unknown samples.

Radioimmunoassay. The greatest technical advance for measuring antigens or antibodies at concentrations $< 1\ \mu g/ml$ is the radioimmunoassay. Commonly, a purified antigen is radioisotope labeled and is used to compete with unlabeled standard or unknown samples for a specific antibody. The degree of competition (and thus, concentration of unknown antigen) may be quantitated by radioactive emission. Separation of bound and unbound antibody may be achieved by ammonium sulfate precipitation of the antigen-antibody complex (the Farr assay), precipitation of high molecular weight complexes by polyethylene glycol, convalently linking specific antigen or antibody to an insoluble matrix (as cellulose paper disks or Sepharose beads) and washing away unbound radiolabeled material, and by precipitation by the double-antibody method. The radioimmunoassay has been used to measure hormones, drugs, Australia antigen, IgE, antibodies to DNA, and other substances present in low concentration.

Agglutination and Agglutination Inhibition. Agglutination reactions may be direct or indirect. Direct agglutination is used to measure antibodies to some erythrocyte, bacterial, and fungal surface antigens. For indirect agglutination reactions, antigens may be adsorbed or covalently linked to insoluble matrices as erythrocytes, bacteria, or polystyrene-latex particles. When serum containing antibodies to these antigens is added, the cells agglutinate and form a visible clump. Quantitation is usually determined by titration. Agglutination and hemagglutination reactions may be used to detect antibodies to a variety of antigens. These include antinuclear antibodies, anti-γ-globulins (rheumatoid factors), anti-red blood cell antibodies, antithyroglobulin, antimicrobial antibodies, and others. Hemagglutination inhibition detects soluble antigens by their ability to inhibit a standard antibody concentration from agglutinating the sensitized erythrocytes. It has been used to detect Australia antigen and factor VIII antigen.

Detection of Immune Complexes

Immune complexes have a pathogenic role in such diseases as rheumatoid arthritis, systemic lupus erythematosus, hypersensitivity pneumonitis, the Arthus reaction, some forms of glomerulonephritis, and vasculitis. Although a number of methods have been developed to quantify complexes, their detection has proved difficult. Most measurements have been based on complexes' high sedimentation velocity or on their interactions with rheumatoid factors, the complement system, platelets, or lymphocyte surface receptors (Table 24.2).

Ultracentrifugal analysis may reveal "intermediate" or macromolecular complex of antigens and antibodies. In rheumatoid arthritis 7S IgG (antigen) may complex with 7S IgG or 19S IgM anti-γ-globulins producing either 11-14S or 22S complexes. This method is not widely available and

TABLE 24.2. *Immune Complexes*

Methods of detection
Clq precipitation
Monoclonal rheumatoid factor (M RF) precipitation
Ultracentrifugation
Radioimmunoassays (rheumatoid factor, aggregated IgG, Clq)
Anticomplementarity
Tissue immunofluorescence
Tissue elution
Cryoprecipitation
Binding to cells with C receptors
Platelet aggregation test
DNAase digestion and anti-DNA titers
Diagnostic value
Documentation of immune-complex-mediated disease
Identification of immunoreactants
M RF (+) 26–57% rheumatoid arthritis (RA), 7–8% systemic lupus erythematosus (SLE) patients
Clq (+) 23–91% SLE, 0–80% RA patients
Prognostic value
Correlates with disease severity and exacerbations (RA and SLE)

is relatively insensitive. Immune complexes have also been identified by coupling monoclonal rheumatoid factor to cellulose particles. Immune complexes in test serum compete for the rheumatoid factor with ^{125}I-aggregated IgG complexes. This method has been used to detect immune complexes in the serum and synovial fluid of patients with rheumatoid arthritis and correlates directly with the severity of the disease and inversely with the serum C4 level. This method was not sensitive for detecting immune complexes in systemic lupus erythematosus and other vasculitides.

Various methods used the ability of C1q to bind to immune complexes. The method of precipitating C1q with aggregated γ globulin or immune complexes in agarose gel was used to detect immune complexes in patients with systemic lupus erythematosus and in joint fluids of patients with rheumatoid arthritis. Immune complexes may also be detected by mixing ^{125}I-C1q with test serum plus disodium ethylenediamine tetra-acetate (EDTA) and precipitating the immune complex-^{125}I-C1q with polyethylene glycol. This method was used to find immune complexes in more than 70% of patients with rheumatoid arthritis, regardless of seropositivity for rheumatoid factor. The presence of complexes correlated inversely with the serum C4 level. Additionally, immune complexes may compete with antibody-sensitized erythrocytes for ^{125}I-C1q. The degree of inhibition is measured by separating the soluble immune complex-^{125}I-C1q by centrifugation. Immune complexes have also been measured by their ability to compete with radiolabeled aggregated IgG for C1q bound to polystyrene tubes. These radioimmunoassays are currently under development and may prove useful clinically. They are presently restricted to investigative laboratories.

Another recently developed method for detecting immune complexes uses the Raji cell. This is a human lymphoblastoid cell with B cell characteristics but without surface immunoglobulin. Raji cells have receptors for the immunoglobulin Fc region and C3b. Immune complexes may be quantitated by reacting patient serum with the Raji cells and then measuring the ability of these cells to take up ^{125}I-antihuman IgG. Results are evaluated by comparison with the ability of Raji cells mixed with aggregated human gammaglobulin to take up ^{125}I-antihuman IgG. This method was used to detect immune complexes in serum hepatitis, systemic lupus erythematosus, and malignancies.

Cryoproteins

Blood to be examined for cryoproteins is drawn into warm syringes at 37°C. For cryofibrinogens the sample is anticoagulated with disodium EDTA or citrate. The serum or plasma is separated by centrifugation at 37°C and is then stored at 4°C for at least 72 hours. A precipitate or gel should be redissolved at 37°C before confirming the presence of the cryoprotein. Immunochemical analyses may be performed on the precipitates. Cryofibrinogens have been observed in association with malignancies and rheumatic disorders, especially scleroderma.

Cryoglobulins are found in many infectious, rheumatic, and malignant diseases (Table 24.3). They are thought to consist of immune complexes and may contain a variety of immunoreactants (Ig, complement, antinuclear antibodies, antigammaglobulins, and others). Cryoglobulins have been classified into three types. Type I contains monoclonal Ig. Type II consists of a monoclonal component with antibody activity to a polyclonal

TABLE 24.3. *Cryoproteins*

Methods of measurement
Serum/plasma incubation at 4°C
Cryocrit
Quantitative cryoprotein determination
Diagnostic value
Immune-complex-mediated diseases
Dysproteinemias
Malignancy
Infection
Prognostic value
May be associated with vasculitis

component (i.e., IgG or IgM anti-γ-globulin (monoclonal) – IgG (polyclonal)). Type III is mixed polyclonal, usually Ig with or without non-Ig.

Methods of Serum Protein Separation

Although the separation and purification of serum proteins are seldom of concern to the practicing clinician, he/she will encounter such methods in reading reports relating to clinical immunology. The methods used include "salting-out" procedures and ion-exchange, gel-filtration, and affinity chromatography.

Salting out neutralizes protein charges, thus insolubilizing proteins. Ion-exchange chromatography allows proteins to bind to a charged matrix with differing affinities. Proteins can then be differentially eluted by adding gradients of salt solutions. Gel filtration uses polysaccharide beads that admit low molecular sized molecules but allow molecules to pass around the beads. Thus, the compounds of high molecular weight elute from the column first and compounds of lower molecular weight are retained. Affinity chromatography is helpful in isolating pure proteins. With this procedure antigens or antibodies are covalently linked to polysaccharide beads. A protein sample will bind to this immunoadsorbent and can subsequently be eluted off.

Detection of Complement

The details of activation of human complement are discussed in Chapter 10. A brief description of the methods of measurement is included here.

CH50 Assay. This is used to measure the entire complement system. This is far less sensitive than hemolytic methods for the individual complement components. Sheep erythrocytes (E) are washed and coated with antibody(A) specific for the cell. Dilutions of the serum to be tested are added to a standard number of sensitized cells (EA). A standard serum of known complement content is used as a control. Lysis of the erythrocyte is accomplished by complement activation through the classical pathway. Once C9 is activated, the erythrocytes lyse and release hemoglobin into the supernatant fluid. The degree of lysis is measured by the amount of hemoglobin released and depends on the concentration of complement in the original serum sample. The serum titration that lyses 50% of the sensitized erythrocytes is taken as the CH50 value.

Measurement of Individual Components. Individual complement components may be titrated by diluting the sample to be tested and adding all other components in excess. For example, to measure C4, purified C1 is added to sensitized sheep erythrocytes (EAC1). Dilutions of the C4 source are incubated with EAC1 cells. After this, C2 and then C3-9 are added in excess and the mixture incubated for a standard time interval. The degree of hemolysis is measured by the spectrophotometric detection of hemoglobin in the supernatant.These methods require considerable time and expense in maintaining fresh reagents and are not generally available to the clinician.

Some complement components are more easily measured by radial immunodiffusion in gel, but this method is far less sensitive than the more laborious hemolytic assay. C3, C4, and C1 esterase inhibitor may be measured by radial immunodiffusion.

Extensive consideration of complement abnormalities in disease is beyond the scope of this discussion. Complement levels are generally determined by radial immunodiffusion, since the assay is readily available and relatively easy to perform. Hemolytic measurements are technically more difficult and require resources not generally available (Table 24.4).

Complement levels may be elevated in many diseases, particularly acute infectious or inflammatory states. Certain uncommon congenital deficiencies of complement components might be detected by low values of CH50 or individual complement proteins. Hereditary angioneurotic edema is such an entity. It is characterized by functional absence of the C1 inhibitor. Patients usually have low C4 and C2 levels as well as deficient C1 inhibitor. Acquired serum hypocomplementemia occurs in many immunologic diseases, such as lupus erythematosus glomerulonephritis, cryoglobulinemia, and other immune-complex-mediated processes. Classical complement activation leads to depressions of C1, C4, and C2, as well as C3. Alternative pathway utilization produces low values for properdin, C3 and later-acting components. Acquired hypocomplementemia also occurs in effusions (synovial, pericardial, and pleural) from patients with rheumatoid arthritis and lupus.

Hypocomplementemia is occasionally helpful diagnostically since it supports a presumption of immune-complex-mediated disease. It may also lead to diagnosis of a congenital complement deficiency syndrome.

TABLE 24.4. *Complement*

Methods of Detection
Hemolytic (functional) assays
Immunochemical (protein) assays
Diagnostic Value
Inherited C component deficiencies
Hereditary angioedema (C1 inhibitor deficiency)
Decreased (C4, C3) in rheumatoid arthritis synovial fluid, systemic lupus erythematosus, glomerulonephritis, cryoglobulinemias, immune-complex diseases
Prognostic value
↓ C associated with active immune-complex disease
↓ C associated with active severe rheumatoid arthritis, systemic lupus erythematosus (SLE)
↑ or ↓ C may respectively antedate clinical remission or exacerbation of SLE

Patterns of abnormalities are sufficiently nonspecific so that they are not often useful in trying to establish a specific diagnosis. Once it is clear that a patient has an immune-complex-mediated disease, and when complement abnormalities correlate with clinical abnormalities, it is useful to follow complement levels serially. This information is helpful to many clinicians in caring for certain patients with lupus nephritis and vasculitis.

Complement Fixation. When fluid-phase antigens and antibodies are allowed to react in the presence of complement (standard fresh serum with a known content of complement), complement components are fixed and activated. After a standard time of incubation the mixture is diluted, and its ability to lyse sensitized sheep erythrocytes (EA) is determined. If large quantities of antibody are present in the patient's serum, a greater quantity of complement will be used in the original incubation. This will leave less complement to lyse the sensitized sheep cells. Sometimes the result of complement fixation will be reported as "anticomplementary". A number of factors are known to be responsible for this phenomenon, including contamination of the serum sample or test reagents with microorganisms, agents that bind calcium and magnesium ions, immune complexes, aggregated immunoglobulin, and prolonged storage of serum. Complement fixation tests are useful for detection of antigens and antibodies to microbial organisms, nuclear constituents, and others.

Immunofluorescence

Fluorescein and rhodamine are organic compounds that fluoresce brilliant yellow-green and red, respectively, upon absorption of ultraviolet light. These compounds can be covalently linked to macromolecules, such as proteins, for histochemical studies. With direct immunofluorescence the antibody specific to a given antigen is conjugated with a fluorescent compound and applied directly to the tissue or source of antigen to be examined. After a thorough rinsing the material is examined with a special fluorescent microscope using an untraviolet lamp. Localization of the antigen in the tissue is detected by fluorescence. With indirect immunofluorescence the tissue or source of antigen to be examined is first incubated with untagged specific antibody. Fluorescein-labeled heterologous antibody specific for the untagged immunoglobulin is then applied and the sample examined for immunofluorescence. This has also been called the "sandwich technique". Immunofluorescence is useful clinically in examining biopsy specimens for the presence of immunoglobulin, complement, and localization of specific antigens. Additionally, serum may be examined for specific antibodies by the indirect immunofluorescence method, as in the fluorescent treponemal antibody absorption and antinuclear antibody tests. These are discussed more fully in Chapter 15.

Erythrocyte sedimentation rate

Determination of the erythrocyte sedimentation rate (ESR) has been used to monitor patients with inflammatory diseases. It is usually performed by the method of Wintrobe or Westergren, but the Westergren method is preferred. Blood anticoagulated with disodium EDTA or citrate is drawn into a 200-mm column, which is allowed to stand vertically for 60 min. Normal values are usually 0–10 mm per hour for men and 0–15 mm per hour for women. Pregnancy, liver disease, and certain hematologic disorders (characterized by abnormally shaped erythrocytes that rouleaux poorly) will affect the ESR. Inflammatory states frequently have an elevated ESR. The ESR has its greatest applicability in following the course of patients with rheumatoid arthritis. It is of less value in managing patients with other inflammatory or rheumatic diseases (Table 24.5).

Cellular Immune Function

Lymphocytes

As has been covered in previous chapters, lymphocytes comprise heterogeneous populations of cells, which may be categorized by their distinctive surface characteristics and functions. The two major classes of lymphocytes are T and B cells. Lymphocytes that cannot be classified as typical T or B cells are known as "null" cells.

T cells are derived from the thymus and appear in peripheral lymphoid tissues. They are concentrated mostly in the paracortical regions of the lymph nodes, in the periarteriolar portion of the white pulp of the spleen, and in the blood. T cells constitute 50–70% of the circulating peripheral blood lymphocytes. B cells may be derived from bone marrow, spleen, or fetal liver and are located in the thymic-independent cortical regions of lymph nodes and in the blood.

Purification. Assays of lymphocyte populations or functions require a purified suspension of mononuclear cells from whole blood. Commonly, the suspension is obtained by certrifuging whole blood over a mixture of

TABLE 24.5. *Erythrocyte Sedimentation Rate*

Methods of Evaluation
Westergren
Wintrobe
Zeta sedimentation rates, others
Diagnostic value
Nonspecifically elevated with inflammation
Prognostic value
Reflects activity in chronic inflammatory diseases, particularly rheumatoid arthritis

Ficoll-Hypaque. This separates formed elements in the blood according to cell density and yields a highly purified population of mononuclear cells at the interface, consisting of 70–90% of lymphocytes, suitable for the studies to be described. (Erythrocytes and neutrophils fall to the cell pellet.)

T and B Cell Enumeration. Many in vitro methods are available for determining percentages of T and B lymphocytes in blood or pathologic specimens (Tables 24.6 and 24.7).

SURFACE IMMUNOGLOBULIN. Surface immunoglobulin serves as a marker for B cells. Human T cells have little, if any, immunoglobulin on their surface. Immunofluorescent staining with anti-human immunoglobulin will detect B cells. When living B cells react with the fluorescein-labeled antisera, the cell surface becomes uniformly stained (Fig. 24.6).

FC RECEPTORS. Another marker on B cells is the Fc receptor. These receptors bind the Fc portion of an immunoglobulin in the form of an immune complex or as aggregated immunoglobulin. The Fc receptor will not bind native immunoglobulin. The assay for Fc receptors usually consists of radioisotope labeling or fluorescein labeling antigen-antibody complexes or heat-aggregated immunoglobulin. These complexes are then allowed to react with cell suspension and are detected by scintillation counting or fluorescent microscopy. Other cells, such as macrophages, T cells, and some null cells also have Fc receptors; corrections for these cells must be made when enumerating B cells by this method.

TABLE 24.6. *Enumeration of Human T and B Lymphocytes*

Assay	Specificity	
	T cell	B cell
Surface Ig	±	+
Fc receptors	±	+
EAC rosettes	−	+
C1q receptor	+	+
C3b receptor	−	+
C3d receptor	−	+
C4b receptor	−	+
Anti-B cell antisera	−	+
E rosettes	+	−
Anti-T cell antisera	+	−
EA rosettes	+	+

TABLE 24.7. *Quantitation of Lymphocyte Subclasses*

Methods of detection
- B cells: surface Ig, C3b (EAC rosettes)
- T cells: sheep red blood cell rosettes

Diagnostic value
- Lymphoproliferative disorders
- Immunodeficiency diseases

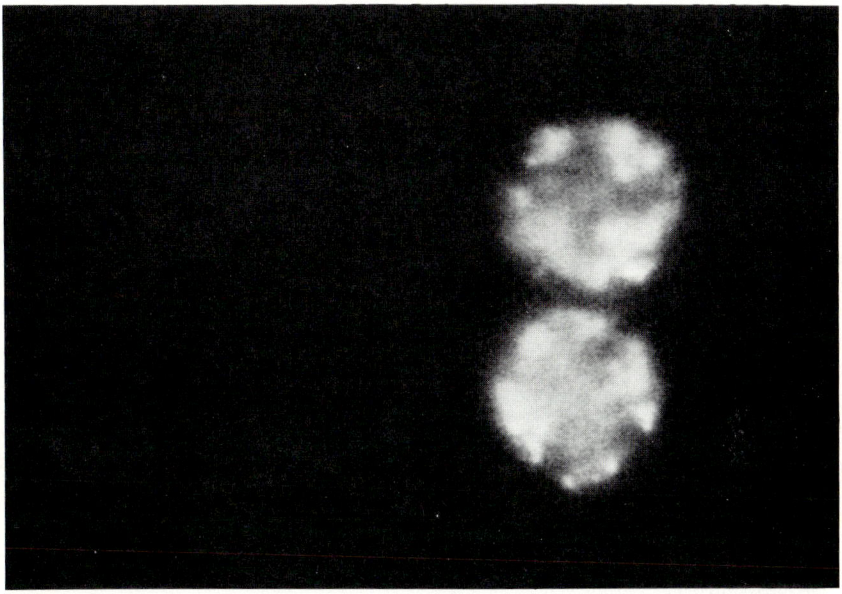

FIG. 24.6. Membrane immunofluorescence of human B lymphocytes stained with fluoresceinated goat anti-human Ig (original magnification ×810; kindly provided by Dr. Perry O. Teague).

COATED SHEEP CELL ROSETTES. B cells have also been shown to have surface receptors for C3b, C3d, and C4b. The method most used for detecting this receptor is coating sheep erythrocytes with antibody and complement (C3b, C3d, or C4b). Under appropriate conditions, these coated sheep cells (EAC) will form rosettes with B cells. Since neutrophils and monocytes can also form EAC rosettes, they need to be identified by other procedures.

ANTI-B CELL ANTIBODY. Purified B cells can be used to immunize animals to produce anti-B cell antibodies. These antibodies can be fluorescein-labeled and will bind living B cells and cells in frozen tissue sections. This, however, is not a commonly used technique for B cell enumeration, since good antiserum is not widely available.

E ROSETTES. Unlike the B cell, most T cells are devoid of Fc receptors and C3b receptors. The T cell is most commonly identified by its ability to form rosettes with normal sheep erythrocytes (Fig. 24.7). This is carried out by methods similar to the EAC rosette assay, except that the sheep erythrocytes have not been reacted with antibody and complement components. Thus the E rosette provides a good marker for human T cells.

ANTI-T CELL ANTIBODY. Antisera to human T cells can be produced by immunization of animals with T cells. The antibodies produced can be fluorescein labeled, and immunofluorescence studies can be done as described for B cells.

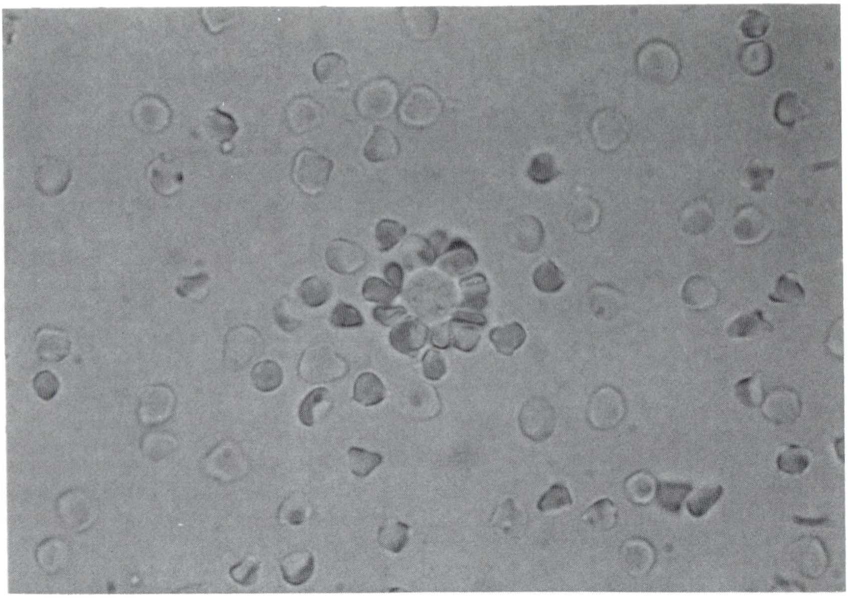

FIG. 24.7. Rosette formed by human T lymphocyte with sheep erythrocytes (original magnification ×388).

Quantitation of lymphocyte subclasses has been carried out on patients with many diverse diseases. Results have helped characterize immunologic abnormalities for patients with certain diseases (i.e., rheumatic, infectious, neoplastic) but have not yet generally proved helpful diagnostically for individual patients. T and B cell enumeration is most useful for identifying patients with T or B cell malignancies or immunodeficiency syndromes (Table 24.6).

In Vivo Assays of Lymphocyte Function. In vivo skin testing can be performed to assess delayed hypersensitivity responses of patients. When certain antigens are injected intradermally, a delayed type of hypersensitivity reaction will occur. Antigens often used include mumps, streptokinase-streptodornase, purified protein derivative, trichophyton, and *Candida albicans.* Erythema and induration are measured after 48 hours. Contact sensitization to dinitrochlorobenzene can also be tested. More than 90% of normal persons will react to two or more antigens (Table 24.8). Cutaneous reactivity is often depressed in the congenital and acquired defects that are listed in Table 24.9. Cutaneous delayed type hypersensitivity remains a clinically useful way of evaluating host cell-mediated immunity (Tables 24.8 and 24.9).

In Vitro Lymphocyte Activation. The integrity of cell-mediated immune function in vitro can be assessed by testing lymphocyte activation or lymphokine production (Table 24.10). Immunologic activation of

TABLE 24.8. *Delayed-Type Hypersensitivity Skin-Testing*

Methods of evaluation
- Intracutaneous skin-testing (purified protein derivative, Candida, streptokinase-streptodornase, trichophyton, mumps)
- Dinitrochlorobenzene sensitization
- Phytomitogens

Diagnostic value
- Congenital or acquired anergy (malnutrition, infectious, rheumatic, inflammatory, malignant diseases)
- Tuberculosis screening

Prognostic value
- Acquired anergy usually associated with severe disease

TABLE 24.9. *Clinical Disorders with an Impaired, Delayed Type of Hypersensitivity to Skin Tests*

Congenital
- Combined immunodeficiencies
- Wiskott-Aldrich syndrome
- Nezelof syndrome
- DiGeorge syndrome
- Ataxia-telangiectasia
- Candidiasis

Acquired
- Chronic lymphocytic leukemia
- Lymphomas
- Carcinoma
- Anemia
- Rheumatic disease
- Cirrhosis
- Pregnancy
- Aging
- Sardoidosis
- Immunosuppressive agents
- Surgery

Infectious
- Influenza
- Mumps
- Rubeola
- Rubella
- Vaccines
- Typhus
- Tuberculosis
- Fungal infections
- Scarlet fever

lymphocytes in vitro by plant lectins (phytomitogens), antigens, chemicals, or cell surface alloantigens in the mixed-lymphocyte culture leads to the proliferation of lymphocytes. Stimulation of blast transformation involves the induction or enhancement of RNA, protein, and DNA synthesis. It is the increase in DNA synthesis that results in cell division and is the basis for most of the activation assays. A radioisotope-labeled nucleoside precursor is added to the cells near the end of a culture period and then can be quantitated by liquid scintillation counting. Stimulated lymphocytes incorporate more nucleoside precursor than do unstimulated cells. A list of activators of blast transformation and their probable specificities for human T or B cells is shown in Table 24.11.

Abnormalities in lymphocyte activation have been seen in many disease states, including malignancies, rheumatic diseases, and infectious diseases. These types of abnormalities have been nonspecific and not uniquely characteristic for any given disease state. These assays thus

TABLE 24.10. *Functional in Vitro Lymphocyte Responses*

Methods of evaluation
Proliferation (antigens, mitogens)
Lymphokine production
Diagnostic value
Congenital or acquired cellular immunodeficiencies
Transplantation
Prognostic value
Acquired hyporesponsiveness associated with severe disease

TABLE 24.11. *Functional Activity in Vitro of Human T and B Lymphocytes*

Response	T cells	B cells
Proliferative response to:		
Phytohemagglutinin, pokeweed mitogen, concanavalin A	+	+
Sodium periodate	+	−
Anti-Ig	−	+
Lipopolysaccharide	−	±
Antigen	+	−
Mixed lymphocyte culture	+	+
Lymphokine production:		
Migration inhibitory factor	+	+
Blastogenic factor	+	−
Lymphotoxin	+	+
Chemotactic factor	+	+
Interferon	+	+
Cytotoxicity:		
Cell-mediated	+	+

remain largely investigative and are used to elucidate immunologic abnormalities in diseases. They do not usually provide important information to the clinician regarding individual patients.

Lymphokines. As discussed in detail in Chapter 2, when sensitized lymphocytes interact with antigens, a number of soluble substances are generated. These nonimmunoglobulin products of the activated lymphocyte possess in vitro biologic activities that appear to mediate cellular immune responses. These substances have been termed lymphokines. Many of these lymphokines have been shown to be glycoproteins that range in molecular weight from 30,000–100,000. In the laboratory, lymphokines are present in the supernatant fluids from sensitized lymphocytes cultured with an antigen. They may also be produced by nonspecific mitogenic stimulation. Biologic assays for the detection of lymphokines are numerous and difficult to perform.

Neutrophils

As discussed in Chapter 18, the primary functions of polymorphonuclear neutrophils (PMN) are phagocytosis and killing of particulate materials, such as bacteria. The PMN's gain access to the areas of inflammation and invading pathogens by attraction by chemotactic factors derived from serum complement, lymphocytes, and other sources. Neutrophil phagocytosis, motility, and bacterial killing can be assayed.

Nitroblue Tetrazolium Test. A clinically useful assay for phagocytosis is the nitroblue tetrazolium (NBT) dye reduction test. Nitroblue tetrazolium is a water soluble yellow compound. Reduction of dye in the phagocytic vacuole can be measured photometrically. This is a useful test for determining the metabolic integrity of phagocytes and is a diagnostically important test in chronic granulomatous disease.

Intracellular Killing Assay. Another useful assay of phagocytosis is the microbial killing technique in which the ability of the phagocytes to kill ingested bacteria is determined. Phagocytes are incubated with bacteria and numbers of viable ingested organisms determined from colony counts. This method provides information about the rate of intracellular killing, as well as the ability of the phagocyte to kill (Table 24.12). Clinical disorders of phagocytosis are discussed elsewhere (Chapter 19).

Chemotaxis. The ability of neutrophils and macrophages to undergo directional migration, known as chemotaxis, can be assessed in vitro. Chemotaxis is usually measured using a Boyden chamber. This consists of two compartments separated by a filter membrane. The leukocytes are placed in the upper chamber and the chemotactic factors (complement, bacteria, and lymphocyte derived) in the lower chamber. After incubation, the filter membrane is removed, rinsed with saline, and stained. The number of cells on the underside of the filter are quantitated microscopically. Defective chemotactic responses of mononuclear and PMN leukocytes have been described in congenital disorders, such as Wiskott-Aldrich syndrome and chronic mucocutaneous candidiasis, and in acute influenzal infections, rheumatic diseases, cirrhosis, renal disease, and others (Table 24.13).

Other Tests. Other methods to test PMN functions include phagocytosis of lipopolysaccharide emulsified in oil red 0, phagocytosis of insoluble particles with microscopic visualization, or assays for lysosomal enzymes.

Macrophages

Macrophages are mononuclear cells present in various tissues, such as the spleen, lungs, and lymph nodes, and in the blood. Circulating macrophages are known as monocytes. Macrophages phagocytize bacteria, viruses, damaged cells, and neoplastic cells. They also affect induction of the immune response through interaction with T and B lymphcoytes.

Human macrophages are usually obtained from surgical specimens of tonsils, thymus, spleen, lymph nodes, and synovium. Tests have not yet been standardized for evaluating macrophage functions and their relevance to human disease. The nitroblue tetrazolium test, intracellular killing assay, and chemotaxis assays described for PMN's can be applied to macrophages and blood monocytes.

TABLE 24.12. *Phagocytosis*

Methods of evaluation
Nitroblue tetrazolium test
Intracellular killing assays
Particle ingestion and enumeration
Lysosomal enzyme release
Diagnostic value
Congenital disorders (Job's syndrome, Chediak-Higashi, chronic granulomatous disease, complement deficiency, others)
Acquired disorders (malignant, infectious, rheumatic diseases, drugs, sickle cell disease, others)

TABLE 24.13. *Chemotaxis*

Methods of evaluation
Boyden chambers
Agarose gels
Skin window
Guinea pig peritoneal cavity
Diagnostic value
Congenital disorders (Wiskott-Aldrich, mucocutaneous Candidiasis, complement deficiencies, agammaglobulinemia)
Acquired disorders (infections, malignancy, rheumatic disease, liver disease, renal disease, diabetes, drugs)

Immediate Hypersensitivity

Prausnitz-Kustner Reaction

Passive anaphylaxis was described by Prausnitz and Kustner in 1921. This phenomenon involved passive transfer of immediate-type cutaneous sensitivity by serum to a previously insensitive individual. Clinical application of the Prausnitz-Kustner test is limited by its potential for transmission of infection. It can be used investigatively to assay for skin sensitizing antibody and measure blocking antibody.

Passive Cutaneous Anaphylaxis

Passive cutaneous anaphylaxis is performed like the P-K reaction. When carried out in animals the reaction may be partially quantitated by means other than wheal size. It may be produced as follows. A subject is sensitized passively by treatment with serum from a previously sensitized subject. Antigen is injected intracutaneously and dye intravenously. Prompt leakage of dye at the injection site indicates increased capillary permeability. This reaction is now recognized to be mediated by homocytotropic antibody which becomes fixed with increasing affinity to tissue mast cells in the 24–72 hours after passive transfer. The IgE antibodies may remain fixed for as long as 3–6 weeks. IgG antibodies may also attach to mast cells but usually dissociate within 24 hours. It is a highly sensitive means of detecting antibody and it is used experimentally to investigate mediators and roles of medication in the immediate hypersensitivity reactions.

Schultz-Dale Reaction

This reaction is named for the investigators who described smooth muscle contractility in immediate hypersensitivity reactions. Responses of isolated guinea pig ileum, actively or passively sensitized, is a valuable investigative tool for quantitating mediator release (as histamine and slow-reacting substance of anaphylaxis) in the immediate hypersensitivity reaction.

Histamine Release Studies

Histamine release in response to antigen challenge occurs with isolated organs (lung) and leukocytes (basophils). Basophils bind the immunoglobulins (IgE) and can release mediators of immediate hypersensitivity. Cellular responsiveness to antigens is measured by quantitating histamine release. Serial dilutions of antigen are incubated with atopic or passively sensitized leukocytes. Sensitivity reflects dose-response characteristics of antigen concentration and amount of histamine released. The concentration of reaginic antibody in atopic sera can also be assayed by this method. Leukocytes from a nonatopic donor are incubated with serial dilutions of atopic sera and then challenged by standard concentrations of antigen.

Leukocyte histamine release correlates well with the severity of clinical symptoms. These techniques are applicable to patients with allergic diseases and probably allow a more physiological evaluation of antigen-antibody relationship and mediator release than other in vitro assays. In addition to measuring reaginic antibody, the rise in blocking antibody during the course of hyposensitization can be quantitated. Also, effects of antigen can be evaluated in vitro without unnecessary hazard to patients. Although the manual histamine-release assay is cumbersome and requires large amounts of blood, automated methods have partially overcome these barriers. However, technical complexities remain limiting factors in the clinical application of this technique.

IgE Quantitation

Precise identification of IgE as reaginic antibody was the result of the investigations of the 1960's. Since concentrations of IgE in normal serum are below the sensitivity of radial diffusion in gels, it is usually measured by radioimmunoassays (Table 24.14). In the radioimmunosorbent test (Fig. 24.8), standard and unknown sera are incubated with antibody to IgE (A-IgE), insolubilized by attachment to the walls of polystyrene test tubes, paper disks, cellulose, or Sephadex microspheres. A second incubation is then performed with ^{125}I-antibody to IgE. The amount of bound radioisotope-labeled antibody is directly related to the IgE content of the original sera. In the radioimmuno-precipitation (double antibody) technique, rabbit antibody to IgE is incubated with standard or unknown serum and radiolabeled IgE myeloma protein. The bound antibody is precipitated with goat anti-rabbit Ig and separated from free antibody.

Concentrations of serum IgE are often increased in patients with parasitic infections, atopic disorders, bronchopulmonary aspergillosis, Wiskott-Aldrich syndrome with eczema, and "hyper-γ-globulinemia-E" syndrome. When eosinophilia occurs with normal IgE levels parasitism or bronchopulmonary aspergillosis are improbable diagnoses. Eosinophilia with normal IgE concentration often occurs in nonatopic (intrinsic) asthma.

Specific IgE Antibodies

Antigen-specific IgE is measured by the radioallergosorbent test (RAST) (Fig. 24.8). Allergen is coupled to an insoluble matrix and is incubated with unknown and reference sera. A second incubation is performed with ^{125}I-antibody to IgE. Bound radioactivity reflects antigen-specific IgE in the test serum. The direct radioimmunosorbent test and RAST require similar technical skills and resources.

The utility of RAST is limited by expense and the requirement of sufficiently pure antigen. RAST results are scored by comparison with known strongly positive reaginic sera and correlate with clinical skin

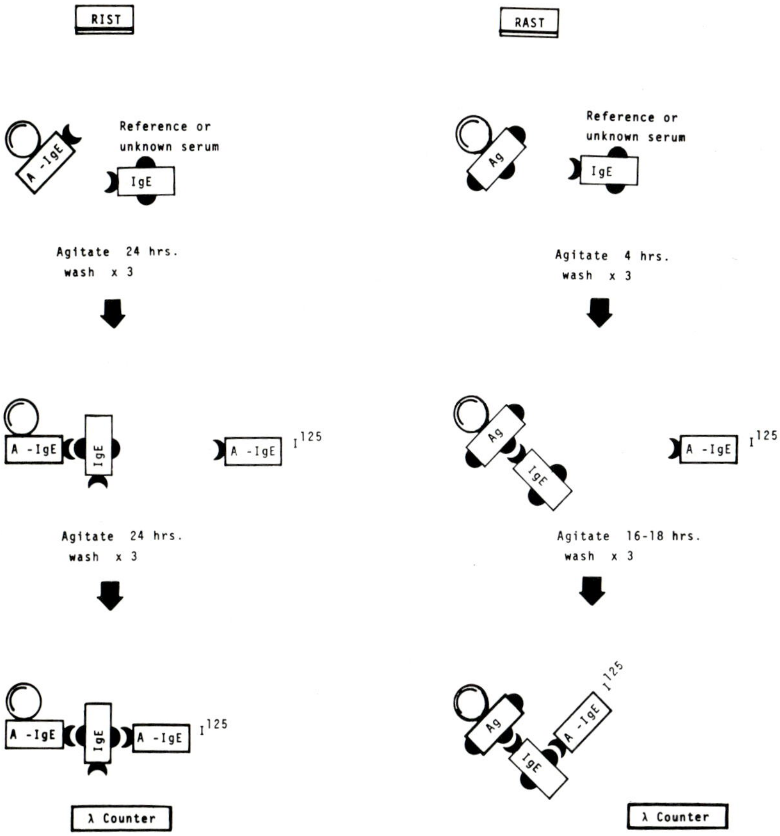

FIG. 24.8. Schematic diagram of radioimmunosorbent test (RIST) and the radioallergosorbent test (RAST). See text for explanation.

TABLE 24.14. *IgE*

Methods of detection
- Qualitative
  - Investigational
    - Prauskitz-Kustner reaction (P-K)
    - Passive cutaneous anaphylaxis (PCA)
    - Schutz-Dale reaction (S-D)
  - Clinical
    - Leukocyte histamine release
    - Skin testing
- Quantitative
    - Radioimmunoassays: radioimmuno-precipitation (RIP), radioimmunosorbent test (RIST), RAST

Diagnostic value
- Documentation of atopy (P-K, PCA, S-D, histamine release, RIP, RIST)
- Quantitation of specific allergen sensitivity (RAST, skin tests)

testing. The RAST has been useful in demonstrating antibodies to such diverse agents as pollens, foods, hymenoptera extracts, insulin, and the penicilloyl derivative of penicillin. False-positive results are rare with this technique except in the case of house dust. Clinically, the RAST may provide an alternative to skin tests in persons with dermographism, severe dermatitis, in apprehensive adults, or in small children.

Immediate Hypersensitivity Skin Testing

Cutaneous (scratch) or intracutaneous tests are used to evaluate immediate hypersensitivity in atopic patients. Allergen promptly induces IgE-mediated histamine release with the wheal and flare response. Antihistamines will reduce responses and should be stopped 48–72 hours prior to evaluation. When a high degree of sensitivity is suspected cutaneous (scratch) tests are performed first. Weakly positive or questionable results are repeated by more sensitive intracutaneous testing. Allergens tested are selected by the history and geographical considerations. Allergy skin testing correlates well with clinical allergy and is used to help document contributory factors in certain clinical syndromes (i.e., rhinitis, conjunctivitis, asthma, food allergy) that have an atopic component. Together with historical information, skin test results also help in selection of allergens for patients undergoing hyposensitization.

Conclusion

This chapter has summarized methods used to evaluate immunologic features of diseases and reviewed their underlying principles. Specific immunologic abnormalities in certain conditions and their importance in the pathogenesis, manifestations, course, and treatment of diseases were briefly discussed.

SELECTED REFERENCES

Boyden, S.: The chemotactic effect of mixtures of antibodies and antigens on polymorphonuclear leukocytes. J. Exp. Med., *115:* 453, 1962.

Chess, L., MacDermott, R. P., Sondel, P. M., and Schlossman, S. F.: Isolation and characterization of cells involved in human cellular hypersensitivity. In *Progress in Immunology.* edited by L. Brent and J. Holborow. New York: American Elsevier Publishing Co., Inc., 1974, Vol. 3, pp. 125–132.

Evans, R.: *Advances in the Diagnosis of Allergy: RAST.* Miami: Symposia Specialist, 1975.

Fudenberg, H. H., Stites, D. P., Caldwell, J. L., and Wells, J. V.: *Basic and Clinical Immunology.* Los Altos, Calif.: Lange Medical Publications, 1976.

Greaves, M. D., Owen, J. J. T., and Raff, M. C.: *T and B Lymphocytes, Origins, Properties and Roles in Immune Responses.* New York: American Elsevier Publishing Co., Inc., 1974.

Ishizaka, K.: Structure and biologic significance of IgE. Hosp. Pract., *12:* 57, 1977.

Johansson, S. G. O., Bennich, H. H., and Berg, T.: The clinical significance of IgE. Prog. Clin. Immunol., *2:* 157, 1972.

Kabat, E. A., and Mayer, M. M.: *Experimental Immunochemistry.* Springfield, Ill.: Charles C Thomas, 1961, pp. 22–96.

Laurell, C. B.: Electroimmunoassay. Scand. J. Clin. Lab. Invest., *29:* (Suppl. 124) 21, 1972.

Mancini, G., Carbonara, A. O., and Heremans, J. F.: Immunochemical quantitation of antigens by single radial immunodiffusion. Immunochemistry, *2:* 235, 1965.

Patterson, R.: *Allergic Diseases-Diagnosis and Management.* Philadelphia: J. B. Lippincott, Co., 1972.

Rapp, H. J., and Borsos, T.: *Molecular Basis of Complement Action.* New York: Appleton-Century-Crofts, 1970.

Rose, N. R., and Friedman, H.: *Manual of Clinical Immunology.* Washington, D.C.: American Society for Microbiology, 1976.

Samter, M.: *Immunologic Diseases* (2nd ed.). Boston: Little, Brown and Co., 1971.

Theofilopoulous, A. N., Wilson, C. B., and Dixon, F. J.: The Raji cell radioimmune assay for detecting immune complexes in human sera. J. Clin. Invest., *57:* 169, 1976.

Vyas, G. N., Stites, D. P., and Brecher, G.: *Laboratory Diagnosis of Immunologic Disorders.* New York: Grune and Stratton, 1975.

Weir, D. M.: *Handbook of Experimental Immunology,* (2nd ed.). Oxford: Blackwell Scientific Publications, Vol. 1–3, 1973.

Wide L., Bennich, H., and Johansson, S. G. O.: Diagnosis of allergy by an in vitro test for allergen antibodies. Lancet, *2:* 1105, 1967.

Zubler, R. H., Nydegger, U., Perrin, L. H., Fehr, K., McCormick, J., Lambert, P. H., and Miescher, P. A.: Circulating and intra-articular immune complexes in patients with rheumatoid arthritis. J. Clin. Invest., *57:* 1308, 1976.

INDEX